The concept of vascular biology has emerged and expanded rapidly over the past 25 years and with research in this area has come an improved understanding of a wide range of clinical conditions. For both specialists and newcomers to the field in search of a broad overview and also for the non-specialist requiring an up-to-date insight into progress and its implications, this book provides a much needed concise resource. The multidisciplinary team of contributors cover topics ranging from normal and pathological aspects of endothelial function to the role of the vasculature in haemostatis, atherosclerosis and hypertension. This carefully illustrated and highly readable text provides both a valuable source of practical information and clear explanations of the impact of new techniques of cellular and molecular biology on recent and future developments.

AN INTRODUCTION TO VASCULAR BIOLOGY

From physiology to pathophysiology

AN INTRODUCTION TO VASCULAR BIOLOGY

From physiology to pathophysiology

Edited by

ALISON HALLIDAY

*Consultant Vascular Surgeon, Epsom Hospital, Surrey and
St George's Hospital, London*

BEVERLEY J. HUNT

*Consultant and Hon. Senior Lecturer in Haematology,
Department of Haematology and Rheumatology, Guys and
St Thomas's Trust, London*

LUCILLA POSTON

*Professor of Fetal Health, Department of Obstetrics and
Gynaecology, United Medical and Dental Schools, London*

MICHAEL SCHACHTER

*Senior Lecturer, Department of Clinical Pharmacology, Imperial
College School of Medicine at St Mary's, London*

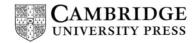

CAMBRIDGE
UNIVERSITY PRESS

PUBLISHED BY THE PRESS SYNDICATE OF THE UNIVERSITY OF CAMBRIDGE
The Pitt Building, Trumpington Street, Cambridge CB2 1RP, United Kingdom

CAMBRIDGE UNIVERSITY PRESS
The Edinburgh Building, Cambridge CB2 2RU, United Kingdom
40 West 20th Street, New York, NY 10011-4211, USA
10 Stamford Road, Oakleigh, Melbourne 3166, Australia

First published 1998

Printed in the United Kingdom at the University Press, Cambridge

Typeset in $9\frac{1}{2}$/12 pt. Times [VN]

A catalogue record for this book is available from the British Library

Library of Congress Cataloguing in Publication data

An Introduction to vascular biology / edited by A. Halliday ... [et al.].
p.   cm.
ISBN 0 521 58998 3 (pbk.)
1. Blood-vessels – Diseases.   2. Blood-vessels – Physiology.
I. Halliday, A. (Alison)
RC691.I595   1998 97-23258 CIP
616.1′3 – dc21

ISBN 0 521 62330 8 hardback
ISBN 0 521 58998 3 paperback

Contents

Contributors

M. D. Brown
School of Sport and Exercise Sciences, University of Birmingham, Birmingham B15 2TT, UK

R. Bucala
Picower Institute for Medical Research, Manhasset, New York 11030-3816, USA

P. Chan
Surgical Sciences, Northern General Hospital, Sheffield S5 7AU, UK

A. P. Cockell
Fetal Health Research Group, Division of Obstetrics and Gynaecology, St. Thomas' Hospital, London SE1 7EH, UK

S. Egginton
Department of Physiology, University of Birmingham, Birmingham B15 2TT, UK

J. R. Gosney
Department of Pathology, University of Liverpool, Liverpool L69 3BX, UK

A. M. Henney
Department of Cardiovascular Medicine, Wellcome Trust Centre for Human Genetics, University of Oxford, Oxford OX3 7BN, UK

S. Hepple
University of Sheffield and Northern General Hospital, Sheffield S5 7AU, UK

O. Hudlická
Department of Physiology, Medical School, University of Birmingham, Birmingham B15 2TT, UK

A. D. Hughes
Department of Clinical Pharmacology, St. Mary's Hospital, London W2 1NY, UK

B. J. Hunt
Departments of Haematology and Rheumatology, Guy's and St Thomas' Trust, St Thomas' Hospital, London SE1 7EH, UK

K. M. Jurd
Department of Haematology, Guy's and St. Thomas' Trust, St Thomas' Hospital, London SE1 7EH, UK

P. T. Khaw
Wound Healing Research Unit, Departments of Pathology and Glaucoma, Institute of Ophthalmology and Moorfield's Eye Hospital, Bath St, London EC1V 9EL, UK

K. M. McCulloch
Clinical Research Initiative in Heart Failure, West Medical Building, University of Glasgow, Glasgow G12 5QQ, UK

J. C. McGrath
Department of Physiology and Pharmacology, University of Strathclyde, Glasgow G1 1XW, UK

N. L. Occleston
Pfizer Central Research, Discovery Biology Tissue Repair Group, Sandwich, Kent CT13 9NJ, UK

J. D. Pearson
Vascular Biology Research Centre, Biomedical Sciences Division, King's College London, London W8 7AH, UK

L. Poston
Division of Obstetrics and Gynaecology, St. Thomas' Hospital, London SE1 7EH, UK

R. Poston
Department of Experimental Pathology, Guy's Hospital, London SE1 9RT, UK

J. T. Powell
Department of Surgery, Charing Cross Hospital, London W6 8RF, UK

M. L. Rose
Heart Science Centre, Harefield Hospital, London UB9 6JH, UK

M. Schachter
Department of Clinical Pharmacology, St. Mary's Hospital, London W2 1NY, UK

A. Stitt
Department of Ophthalmology, The Queen's University of Belfast, UK

H. A. J. Struijker-Boudier
Department of Pharmacology, University of Limbourg, 6200 MD Maastricht, The Netherlands

H. Vlassara
Picower Institute for Medical Research, Manhasset, New York 11030-3816, USA

S. Ye
Wellcome Trust Centre for Human Genetics and Department of Cardiovascular Medicine, University of Oxford, Windmill Road, Oxford OX3 7BN, UK

Introduction

This book is written for physiologists, doctors, PhD students and for those who are curious about how blood vessels and endothelium develop, perform and misbehave.

It is divided into three areas: development and physiology; atherosclerosis, hypertension and diabetes; and other specific pathological problems. The reader is expected to have a general knowledge of university physiology and biochemistry. Some chapters such as angiogenesis, hypertension and aortic aneurysm deal with general principles and are less detailed. The chapters on physiology of blood vessel function repeat and reinforce each other, and can be used as a basis for investigating specific pathological problems in other areas, such as inflammation and sepsis.

Many readers want to learn about atherosclerosis. This major disease process is treated in greater depth and can be related to allied clinical problems like diabetes, re-stenosis and aortic aneurysm. The authors have included up-to-date references with a special emphasis on general reviews and seminal papers. Each year much information is added to vascular biological knowledge. We hope that this introduction will stimulate you to read and enjoy learning about this fascinating subject.

Part 1
Development and control of blood vessel function

1

Angiogenesis: basic concepts and methodology

O. HUDLICKÁ, M. D. BROWN and S. EGGINTON

Introduction

Growth of new blood vessels during development of an organism can occur by two processes. The first, vasoculogenesis, involves differentiation of endothelial cells in situ from more primitive mesenchymal cells. The second process involves sprouting and growth of capillaries from existing vessels into avascular parts of tissues and is called angiogenesis. In adult organisms, the main mode of vessel growth is angiogenesis as vasculogenesis does not seem to occur. Angiogenesis is a very important physiological process, being responsible for vessel growth in most organs during postnatal development and also during endurance training, exposure to cold or high altitude. It is the primary form of vascularization during embryogenesis in the brain and the kidney. It is also responsible for vessel growth in pathological conditions where it may be either beneficial or detrimental. Angiogenesis is essential in wound healing including situations such as gastrointestinal ulcers, stroke, myocardial infarction and heart hypertrophy or regeneration. On the other hand, inhibition of angiogenesis would be important in disease states such as tumours, retinopathies, rheumatoid arthritis and psoriasis where uncontrolled blood vessel growth occurs.

It is generally accepted that the initiation and process of angiogenesis occurs as follows (Fig. 1.1A). The first event is disruption or disturbance of the basement membrane that encompasses endothelial cells of existing capillaries, occurring through the action of various protease enzymes which are activated possibly by growth or mechanical factors (see later). This allows migration of endothelial cells into the extravascular space followed by proliferation and formation of capillary sprouts which eventually connect to neighbouring vessels, permitting flow (Hudlická & Tyler, 1986). An alternate mechanism of angiogenesis called intussusceptive growth was described, originally in the lung, by Burri & Tarek (1990) (Fig. 1.1B). They observed fusion of opposing capillary walls, narrowing a capillary to a complete occlusion, with subsequent ingrowth of surrounding mesenchymal tissue eventually dividing the capillary into two. The factors which promote this mechanism are not clear but as it occurs mainly during development in most organs, it is possible that growth of the surrounding mesenchymal tissue is faster than growth of endothelial cells and pressure exerted by the tissue causes the initial

A.

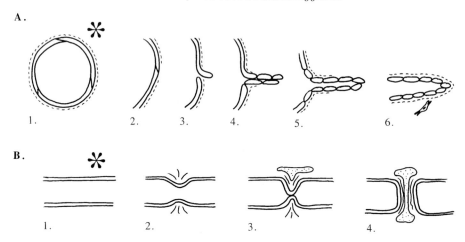

Fig. 1.1(A). Classical view of capillary growth by abluminal sprouting. The angiogenic signal (1) results in focal disruption of the basement membrane (2), allowing endothelial cell migration (3) followed by proliferation (4), inter cellular tube formation (5), re-establishment of the basement membrane and migration of pericytes (6). Lumen formation may also take place by intracellular vacuolization. (B) Scheme of intussusceptive growth by luminal division. The angiogenic signal (1) leads to protrusion of the capillary wall into the vessel lumen, accompanied by interstitial filaments (2). This is followed by migration of interstitial cells (3) and eventual formation of a connective tissue bridge to separate new daughter vessels (4).

capillary collapse. This highlights the importance of interactions between endothelial cells and their extracellular components which is inevitable given that new vessels must have the space in which to grow. Another growth mechanism is longitudinal splitting of existing capillaries, particularly in the heart (van Groningen et al, 1991). The growth of larger vessels such as arteries and arterioles can occur either by a process in which capillaries, either preexisting or new, become invested with contractile elements (Skalak & Price, 1996) or by enlargement of the diameter and/or length of existing large vessels, by proliferation of both endothelial and smooth muscle cells (Hudlická & Brown, 1994).

There are many factors which initiate and regulate angiogenesis depending upon the circumstances under which vessel growth takes place. In vitro and in vivo studies have implicated mechanical, humoral or growth factors and these are discussed in more detail later.

Methods of studying angiogenesis

Tissue cultures

Tissue cultures of endothelial cell (EC) lines from a variety of sources – tumours, skin, retina, glomeruli, placenta, large vessels (aorta) and microvessels (e.g. adrenal capillaries) – and of smooth muscle cells (SMC) have been used widely for testing the angiogenic potential of substances such as growth factors, and for studying the responses of cells to mechanical stimuli. Motility and migration of cells can be directly observed (speed or distance of movement) and quantitative assessment of cell proliferation in culture is routinely made by simple cell counts or by incorporation of [^{3}H]thymidine or its analogue, bromodeoxyuridine (BrdU), into cell nuclei prior to mitotic division and subsequent scintillation counting or derivation of a labelling index from immuno labelling or autoradiography. Such analysis has shown that EC proliferation in vitro is stimulated by fibroblast growth factors (FGFs), transforming growth factor beta (TGF-β1), vascular endothelial growth factor (VEGF) and platelet-derived growth factor (PDGF). Migration, however, is enhanced by insulin-like growth factor (IGF-1).

The source of endothelial cell used for culture is extremely important (Lelkes et al, 1996) because responses from cells of different origin vary considerably. For example, endothelial cells derived from human dermal microvasculature (HMVEC) form capillary-like tubes much faster than human umbilical vein cells (HUVEC); and fibroblast growth factor stimulates increased production of the tissue plasminogen activator (t-PA) in aortic ECs but inhibits production of t-PA in HUVEC. Cells of different origin also deposit different amounts of components such as fibronectin in the subendothelial extracellular matrix and their response to mechanical distortion in terms of expression of angiogenic factors (HMVEC exposed to cyclic strain showed increased expression of tissue factor while HUVEC did not) and growth response (stretch enhanced growth rate of EC derived from aorta and pulmonary artery but not from vena cava, Iba et al, 1991) may well be different. It is thus important when studying the potency of stimulators or inhibitors of angiogenesis that EC are isolated from microvessels from the appropriate organs.

Tissue culture systems enable study of interactions with the extracellular environment notably the substratum upon which cells are grown. Endothelial cells form capillary-like tubes faster when grown on matrigel (a mixture of basement membrane components extracted from Englebreth–Holm–Swarm tumour) than on collagen, fibronectin, gelatin or plastic (Grant et al, 1992). Extracellular matrix molecules also dictate whether the cells will proliferate, migrate, differentiate or undergo involution illustrated by the fact that cells will migrate but not divide when grown on matrigel (Hudlick & Brown, 1993).

The great advantage of using tissue cultures is that the effects of individual factors, be they polypeptides, cytokines, adhesion molecules, components of extracellular matrix or individual mechanical factors (e.g. shear stress – altering the velocity of flow of the medium in contact with the cultured cells, or stretch – growing cells on a deformable substratum), can be studied. Cultures have also been useful for manipulating cellular receptors to elucidate the signalling mechanisms involved in angiogenesis and for studying EC expression of mRNA for different growth factors induced in response to, for example, hypoxia. It is also possible to coculture combinations of smooth muscle cells, pericytes and endothelial cells and thus to study their interactions under simplified conditions.

The disadvantage of tissue cultures is that it is not possible to replicate the real complexity of in vivo interactions. The phenotype of cells changes when they are transferred from tissues to tissue culture and they may then behave in a very different way. Thus evidence for the involvement of various stimulatory or inhibitory factors on angiogenesis which is derived from tissue culture studies should be confirmed by studies in vivo. Various models of angiogenesis and studies on growth of vessels in live animals or humans have been developed (for a review see Hudlická & Tyler, 1986).

In vivo models of angiogenesis

One of the most commonly used assays for angiogenesis is chicken chorioallantoic membrane (CAM), a thin vascular membrane that is easily accessible by making a small window in the shell of a 7–8 day incubated egg. Small quantities of putative angiogenic agents may be applied to the surface of the membrane either directly, on a filter paper, or in disks which ensure slow release. Similar methods of application can be used to assess angiogenesis in a normally avascular rabbit or rat cornea. Chambers implanted in different positions in animals (rabbit ear, hamster dorsal skinfold) or even humans (skin) enable observation of vessel growth either during the process of wound healing or regeneration or under various interventions applied either locally or systemically. In these situations angiogenesis is assessed by the number, length and direction of growing vessels, a process which can be aided by image analysis techniques. Except where the tissue is essentially two dimensional, there is a likelihood of underestimating microvascular volume unless appropriate stereological analyses (see Assessment of microcirculatory growth) are used. Sterile polyester sponges (Andrade et al, 1987) or foam discs have been used to study inflammatory angiogenesis and to assess angiogenesis-promoting or -inhibiting substances. Vessel growth is measured either by histological techniques and direct counts of vessel number, by the total amount of haemoglobin and/or blood flow (^{133}Xenon clearance or microspheres) or by [^{3}H]thymidine incorporation.

Angiogenesis in situ

Intravital observations

Growth of arterioles, venules and capillaries can be investigated by intravital microscopic observations in living organisms. This method was used in the very elegant experiments by Clark (1918) who observed that the progression and regression of vessels in the tadpole tail were dependent on the velocity of blood flow. More recently, Rhodin & Fujita (1989) combined intravital observations of vessels with electron microscopy in the rat mesentery during early postnatal development. Their results are a classical description of growth of the microcirculation. Capillary sprouts originated as endothelial spurs from arteriolar-venular arcades and continued to grow forming solid sprout tips which progressively lengthened by migration of ECs. The extended leading tip displayed pseudopodia devoid of basement membrane, its cytoplasm containing an array of microtubules, filaments and many small vesicles. The sprout lumen arose between endothelial cells of the solid sprout. Mesenteric connective tissue fibroblasts approached and settled down on the sprouts and were converted to pericytes which reinforced the wall of the delicate new capillary. Perivascular cells surrounding the arteriolar feeder of the capillary arcades represented precursors of smooth muscle cells which later became apposed to the newly formed capillaries. Intravital observations have been made of the patterns of capillary growth in tumours (e.g. Reinhold & Berg-Block, 1983) and capillary sprouts were demonstrated even in normal muscles exposed to chronically increased activity (Myrhage & Hudlická, 1978). In addition to providing data on vessel diameters and lengths, intravital observations can allow quantification of changes in vascular branching pattern (internode length, number of branches of a given order, branching angle) particularly in thin tissues such as the mesentery or essentially planar muscles like the spinotrapezius. While measurements of maximal conductance within whole organs can be used to demonstrate growth of large vessels (see below), they say very little about the growth of capillaries. They are important, however, particularly when based on observations of flow velocity and vessel diameters, for estimation of wall shear stress and tension, thereby enabling determination of the involvement of mechanical factors in the initiation of angiogenesis.

Assessment of large vessel growth

Methods for studying vessel growth in the whole organism differ depending on whether the emphasis is to be on growth of large or small vessels. Larger vessel growth has been studied by methods which identify structural features of the vascular bed, e.g. angiography, vascular casts, standard histological techniques to depict arteries/arterioles or veins/venules, and labelling of proliferating components, endothelial or smooth muscle cells, in the vessel walls. All the above methods have also been used to study growth of the vasculature in many angiogenic conditions – tumours, retinopathies, wound healing, brain infarction, placental development and the development of collateral circulation in ischaemic hearts or skeletal muscles. Angiography shows visible filling of existing and newly formed vessels and is used mainly to asses the development of the collateral circulation. The recent development of computerized angiography (Fujita et al, 1993) enables quantitative evaluation but in general it is difficult to identify the categories of vessels according to branching system and size and to determine which are the new vessels.

There is increasing evidence that individual vessel function is dependent not only on the local environment but also on their position within the branching network. The analysis of vascular topology and its alteration during angiogenesis is an important aspect. India ink injection and 'clearing' of tissue with various chemicals was used to visualize vascular beds in different organs in the last century. Currently, vascular casts are used, produced by infusion of curable latex or resin, which hardens and is exposed by digestion of the surrounding tissue at high pH. Providing that filling is complete and that there is no rupture of vessels, which requires tight control over viscosity and perfusion pressure, this method can be used to demonstrate both large and small vessels in casts prepared for scanning electron microscopy; however, three dimensional reconstruction of such casts and quantification remains very difficult. The total cast volume (weight corrected for density) as a proportion of total organ volume gives some indication of changes in vascular supply but it is difficult to partition any evident growth among the various vessel categories and quantitative data of this nature is therefore limited. Vascular casting has been used to study angiogenesis in many organs and tissues – skeletal muscles, heart, ovaries, kidney, cornea – as well as in tumours. Casting with carmine dye in gelatin has also been used to demonstrate inflammatory angiogenesis in mouse granuloma (Colville-Nash et al, 1995).

Standard histological techniques and light microscopy are inadequate on their own for large vessel identification and evaluation of their growth, for it is not always possible to unequivocally discriminate between arterial and venous vessels at this resolution. Although vessels other than capillaries can be stained in several tissues for the presence of enzymes such as adenosine triphosphatase (ATPase) or adenosine diphosphatase (ADPase) (Padykula & Herman, 1955), the reaction is very pH labile and not reliable for identification purposes. Vascular endothelium in larger vessels can also be stained using assorted lectins which bind to characteristic carbohydrate residues on the lumen surface, but staining intensity is variable throughout the vascular tree (Lis & Sharon, 1986). It is therefore important that staining characteristics of a particular lectin in vessels of a particular tissue are well documented before using this method quantitatively to ascribe growth to one or other size class of either arterial or venous vessels. Immunohistological methods staining for alpha-smooth muscle actin distinguish arterial vessels down to small sizes and have been successfully used, for example to show arteriolar growth in skeletal muscles subjected to electrical stimulation (Hansen-Smith et al, 1996) or chronic vasodilatation (Skalak & Price, 1996). Nevertheless, if larger vessels such as arterioles are to be included in a quantitative analysis, their relatively low density compared with that of capillaries needs to be accommodated by ensuring a large enough sample area, this being inversely related to vessel density.

In ischaemic tissue, larger vessels grow predominantly as part of the collateral vascular tree (Schaper et al, 1988; see also Hudlická et al, 1992). This has been studied in detail in the heart in response to either abrupt or gradual occlusion of a major coronary artery. Incorporation of [^{3}H]thymidine followed by autoradiography has been used to locate proliferation in smooth muscle and endothelial cells of both large and small vessels. A significant increase in labelling index of both types of vessels in ischaemic pig hearts was observed at the same time as an increase in density and cross-sectional area of arterioles (White & Bloor, 1992). Studies such as these have shown that in pigs, as in humans, it is primarily small vessels and capillaries which grow in response to ischaemia, but in dog hearts, it is the larger epicardial arteries. It is still difficult to assess whether this proliferation is due to expansion of preexistent vessels or to de novo synthesis.

The capacity of the whole vascular bed can also be assessed in vivo by measuring the maximal vascular conductance (maximal blood flow/blood pressure). As the capillaries exert little resistance to flow, increases in maximal conductance are used as an index of growth of arterioles and conduit arteries. This approach has been used to determine that there is larger vessel growth in the myocardium in response to endurance exercise training and in skeletal muscles where angiogenesis was induced by chronic electrical stimulation (Hudlická et al, 1992). Laughlin & McAllister (1992) pointed out that maximal conductance is only valid as a measure if certain haemodynamic conditions are fulfilled to maintain perfusion pressure. In ischaemic myocardium, there is a correlation between the increase in arteriolar density and cross-sectional area and rise in maximum conductance over time (White & Bloor, 1992).

Assessment of microcirculatory growth

Most angiogenesis in the adult organism occurs by capillary growth, thus methods for evaluation of this are of fundamental importance. The specificity of markers for micro-vessels becomes crucial because most quantitation is based on examination and count-ing vessels under the light microscope. Capillary supply can be evaluated from sections stained by the periodic acid- Schiff/amylase. This method identifies carbohydrate moie-ties of basement membrane and has been used to show the increase in capillary supply of human skeletal muscles after endurance training. Basement membrane of both capilla-ries and other tissue elements can also be depicted by staining with silver methenamine, or with antibodies to laminin, fibronectin or type IV collagen. Enzymatic markers of the capillary endothelium are ideal especially for use on frozen tissue sections although heterogeneity is found among species, between organs and during ontogenetic develop-ment. For example, alkaline phosphatase, a reliable indicator of endothelial cells in both frozen and paraffin-embedded adult skeletal muscle, cannot be demonstrated in rat or rabbit neonatal muscle, or in human tissue, and it is detectable in rat but not rabbit brain capillaries. Variable staining may even be seen within a given microvascular network as alkaline phosphatase activity decreases, and serine protease activity in-creases, towards the venular ends of capillaries in heart and skeletal muscle. With a different substrate, however, and using a different chromogen, alkaline phosphatase staining can be shown to yield the same capillary counts in skeletal muscle as obtained with low power electron microscopy, confirming its suitability as an anatomical marker of microvessels. One further caveat is the fact that in certain pathological situations, e.g. myocardial infarction, in which capillaries are affected, the enzyme and consequently staining properties appear to be lost. Other enzymatic markers are ATPase and car-bonic anhydrase, used with varying success.

Particular markers are used for endothelium in human tissue. Antibodies to von Willebrand factor are widely used to locate ECs in biopsies and tumours of many origins, and combined with labelling by [³H]thymidine or other markers of nuclear division to assess proliferative status and are therefore useful as a prognostic indicator. More recently, other EC surface antigens such as CD34/QBend10 are being exploited as vessel markers. For human tissue, as with animal tissue, lectin staining of the sugar residues of cell surface glycoproteins is extremely useful, with specific lectins being suitable for particular species. Lectin *Ulex europeaus* is widely used to depict capillaries in human tissues while *Griffonia simplicifolia* reacts with vessels in many animal tissues. Colocaliz-ation of these markers with labelling of proliferating cells is increasingly used. In addition to incorporation of [³H]thymidine and BrdU during the S-phase of division, antibodies are available to nuclear components specific to other time points of the cell division cycle, such as proliferating cell nuclear antigen (PCNA) found in G1 + S + G2 phases or Ki-67 antigen, maximally expressed in S-phase. Such methods have been used to demonstrate

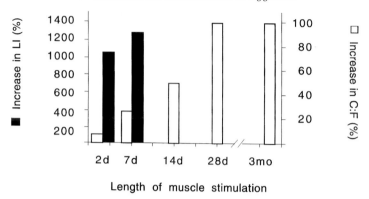

Fig. 1.2. Percentage increase in capillary supply (C:F, open bars) and labelling index (LI, closed bars) of capillary-linked nuclei with varying duration of indirect electrical stimulation. An increase in C:F is apparent after 7 days stimulation, reaching a maximum after approximately 4 weeks, while the increase in labelling index precedes this.

specific EC proliferation in hypo- and hyperthyroid hearts (Heron & Rakusan, 1995) or hearts with irradiation damage or infarction. The ability to detect EC proliferative sites not only enables quantitation of angiogenesis but also the spatiotemporal involvement of other factors such as growth factors in relation to angiogenic locations. For example, in rat brain infarction FGF II immuno expression is elevated earlier than the appearance of cell proliferation, which involves ECs, pericytes, macrophages and glial cells (Liu & Chen, 1994), whereas in chronically stimulated skeletal muscles, BrdU incorporation into capillary-linked nuclei is high (Pearce & Hudlická, 1995) at the same time as levels of endothelial cell stimulating angiogenic factor (ESAF) and anatomical evidence of capillary growth (Fig. 1.2) (Brown et al, 1995).

    After capillaries have been detected by a suitable marker, their growth is assessed by evaluation of the physical extent of the capillary bed. Simple vessel counts in models such as the chambers, sponges, or tissue sections, etc. are used providing the sampling field is constructed so that the counts are not biased due to peripherally located vessels (edge effect). If at the same time as angiogenesis is occurring, there is expansion of the surrounding tissue, as during development, hypertrophy or tumour growth, this will influence straightforward vessel counts by increasing vessel separation. It may be more useful to express capillary supply in terms of a ratio of numbers of vessels to units of tissue area, for example capillary/fibre ratio in skeletal or cardiac muscle. Even this approach may not take account of three-dimensional aspects of growth and vessel tortuousity unless stereological analyses are employed. Stereology is the application of geometrical probability theory that permits extrapolation of structural information from n to n + 1 dimensions (e.g. length to surface, area to volume), providing random sampling criteria are applied. This type of analysis takes into account the fact that in many tissues, capillaries form a complex three-dimensional network with numerous interconnections such that both the effective capillary length and surface area are greater than those estimated from simple counts in transverse sections. An index such as length density, Jv, which evaluates the length of capillaries per unit volume of tissue, can be multiplied by true tissue volume to arrive at an absolute value for the length of the capillary bed in km. Length density is derived on the basis of a constant of proportionality estimated from capillary density counts made in sections taken at mutual right angles (for ease of sectioning these are usually transverse and longitudinal sections). The impact of vessel tortuousity on quantitative assessment varies considerably in importance in different organs, being highly significant in the brain where capillaries have a very randomly oriented three-dimensional architecture and even accounting for 1.6 – 42% of length density in skeletal muscle where capillaries lie alongside muscle fibres. If mean capillary dimensions are known then capillary volume and surface densities can be calculated from the product of Jv and capillary cross-sectional area and perimeter, respectively. Such structural indices will give estimates of the maximal capacity of a microvascular network and permit more accurate evaluation of angiogenic growth (Egginton, 1990) (Fig. 1.3).

Electron microscopy has demonstrated not only the presence of capillary sprouts but also the initial stages of capillary angiogenesis, identified from signs of EC activation. These include increased organelle content (mitochondria, cytoplasmic vacuoles, endoplasmic reticulum and occasionally Golgi apparatus) or altered structure (greater electron translucency of the cytoplasm, increased luminal or abluminal surface roughness). EC proliferation can be detected as increased numbers of cell profiles per capillary, usually requiring high magnification (around $\times$ 29 000) and enhanced contrast (osmium ferricyanide postfixation or tannic acid mordanting) to help in identification of cell boundaries. Other changes in fine structure, such as breakage of the basal lamina, may best be studied by labelling specific constituents such as laminin or collagen type IV. Mitotic nuclei may be rare by virtue of the low probability of fixing cells during the short time spent in this phase of the cell cycle but labelling after BrdU incorporation or for PCNA is possible by linking antibodies to these to an electron opaque stain (usually colloidal gold). While this is a time-consuming process, especially if silver enhancement of the minute particles (usually 5–10 nm diameter) is required to assist evaluation, the great advantage is the spatial resolution afforded which enables unequivocal identification of cell types undergoing proliferation.

Also at high magnifications, the nature of interaction between ECs and perivascular cell types such as pericytes may be observed. For example, the extent of capillary abluminal perimeter surface covered by pericytes is reduced during angiogenesis in skeletal muscle and heart (Egginton et al, 1996). Capillary morphology (area, perimeter, thickness), can be quantified from electron micrographs at lower magnification in terms of cell dimensions by manual planimetry or from stereological principles using a transparent overlay of a counting frame (Fig. 1.3). Digitizing for subsequent image analysis is useful if enhancement is required, although fully automated analysis is difficult to set up. The smaller size of newly formed vessels and the extent of EC swelling quickly become apparent from such data especially if frequency distributions of size are studied rather than mean values. Examining fine structure or gross morphology of individual capillaries can provide a lot of detail about a very small fraction of the total

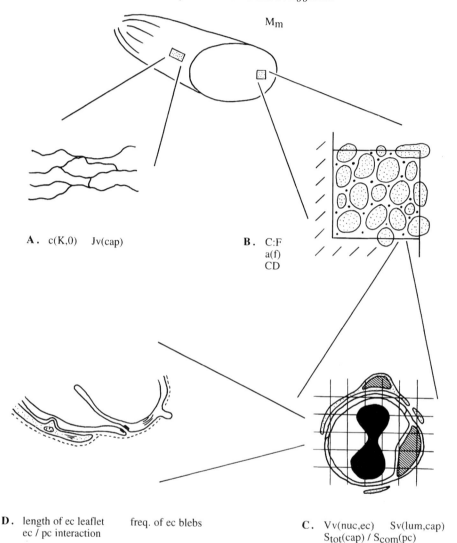

Fig. 1.3. Sampling of skeletal muscle to quantify angiogenesis. In order to quantify absolute values, a reference such as muscle mass Mm or cross-sectional area is required. (A) Longitudinal sections can be used to estimate the degree of capillary tortuousity by calculating the proportionality constant [c(K,O)] which is used to convert numerical capillary density obtained from transverse sections to capillary length density, Jv(cap). (B) Transverse sections can provide unbiased estimates of capillary to fibre ratio [C:F], mean fibre cross-sectional area and capillary density mm^{-2} [CD], provided an appropriate sampling regimen is adopted. (C) Sterological analysis of capillary fine structure evaluates morphology by means of ratios of endothelial cell nuclear volume density [Vv(nuc,ec)] which might be an indication of cell proliferation, surface density of lumen [Sv(lum,cap)] or relative coverage of capillary surface by pericytes. Stot (cap): capillary perimeter surface; S_{com}(pc): surface of capillary covered by pericyte. (D) Capillary ultrastructure can also be used as an index of endothelial cell activation, e.g. length of endothelial cell [ec] leaflets, frequency of ec blebs at the abluminal surface and degree of ec-pericyte [pc] interdigitation.

capillary bed, but such studies should be combined with analysis of larger sample areas under the light microscope to confirm angiogenesis.

The advantages of studying angiogenesis in situ are obvious. It is possible to observe the whole process and its different stages from capillary sprouting to the formation of new vascular networks using intravital microscopy and to assess quantitatively and qualitatively the appearance of vessel growth under varying circumstances unaffected by the introduction of foreign bodies as is the case with implantation of chambers or sponges. The use of immunohistochemistry or in situ hybridization techniques permits study of the involvement of growth factors and systemic administration of growth factors or inhibitors also helps to identify agents involved in angiogenesis. The greatest disadvantage is the difficulty encountered in attempting to elucidate signal transduction on a molecular basis and to quantify precisely either mechanical or humoral/growth factors involved.

Factors involved in angiogenesis

Numerous mechanical, hormonal, humoral or growth factors, are implicated in the initiation and/or process of angiogenesis. Their involvement varies according to the physiological or pathological conditions under which angiogenesis takes place. A summary of these factors is given in Tables 1.1 and 1.2. By reviewing the basic mechanism of cell proliferation, it becomes obvious that angiogenesis is very complex and requires a finely regulated interplay of the various components (Fig. 1.4) (Hudlická & Brown, 1993).

Physiological angiogenesis during development has recently been reviewed by Rhodin & Fujita (1989) in the mesentery and Stingl & Rhodin (1994) in skeletal muscle, in endurance training by Hudlická et al (1992) and in female reproductive organs by Reynolds et al (1996). Under these conditions as well as on exposure to cold or high altitude, angiogenesis is always linked with increased blood flow and thus increased velocity of red blood cells (Vrbc) and possibly increased vessel diameter and increased capillary pressure (P). This results in elevated wall shear stress (τ = viscosity $[4Vrbc/r]$) and increased wall tension (T = Pr) where r is vessel radius. Both factors may initiate angiogenesis by disturbing the layer of glycocalyx on the luminal side of capillaries or basement membrane thus fulfilling the first condition for angiogenesis – the disturbance of basement membrane (Fig. 1.1A) (Hudlická et al, 1992; Hudlická & Brown, 1993). They can also modify the endothelial cell cytoskeleton and disturb the extracellular matrix (Davies, 1995) thus making space for endothelial cell migration. The extracellular matrix itself can be modified by growth of the surrounding tissue during development or with hypertrophy, e.g. in endurance training. Increased shear stress causes the release of various cytokines, including prostaglandins and nitric oxide, from endothelial cells. Recently, inhibitors of release of both these substances have been shown to attenuate capillary growth in muscles with chronically increased activity, and nitric oxide donors to increase endothelial cell migration and proliferation in vitro. In addition, physiological angiogenesis is stimulated by increased levels of thyroid hormones in training or

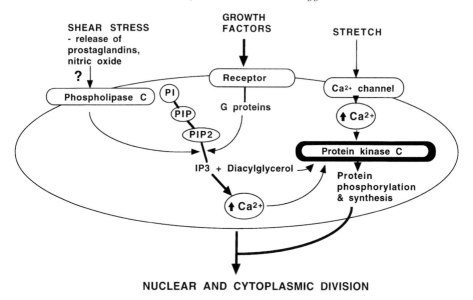

Fig. 1.4. Suggestion of factors possibly involved in endothelial cell proliferation. PI: phosphatidyl inositol; PIP: phosphatidyl inositol phosphate; PIP2: phosphatidyl inositol diphosphate; IP3: phosphatidyl triphosphate.

exposure to cold, and by oestrogens in female reproductive organs. The role of different growth factors in physiological vessel growth is far from clear, although the possibility that VEGF is directly involved in capillary growth during hypoxia and during increased muscle activity is very likely while the involvement of fibroblast growth factors I and II seems to be inconclusive.

Growth factors are of primary importance in angiogenesis occurring under pathological conditions. Folkman (1974) pointed out the importance of growth of vessels in tumours which cannot enlarge beyond a certain size without ingrowth of capillaries from the host. This ingrowth is stimulated by what was first called tumour angiogenic factor. Later, Folkman & Shing (1992) reviewed a variety of peptides as well as other substances with angiogenic potential. The main peptides which have been cloned include FGF I and II (acidic and basic fibroblast growth factor), VEGF (vascular endothelial cell growth factor), ECGF (endothelial cell derived growth factor), TGF-α (transforming growth factor), TNF-α (tumour necrosis factor), PDGF (platelet derived growth factor) and angiogenin. Other factors include prostaglandins, adenosine, heparin, hyaluronic acid and possibly nitric oxide which, however, has also been described as inhibitor of angiogenesis. Inhibitors of angiogenesis in vivo are TGF-β (transforming growth factor beta) and angiostatin. Several new stimulators, as well as inhibitors of angiogenesis are reported in literature every year. Some of these factors are also involved in wound healing which is dealt with in Chapter 13.

Table 1.1. *Mechanical factors involved in endothelial or smooth muscle cell proliferation*

Force	Cell type and response time	Effect	Significance
LSS 0.2–4.0	BAEC 15–40 s	↑ in $[Ca^{2+}]_i$	Role of Ca^{2+} in mitosis
LSS 0–51	BAEC > 1 h HUVEC	↑ in PDGF-A mRNA	Enhanced mitogen secretion; VSM growth
LSS > 10	HUVEC 2 H	Stimulation of IL6	Cytokine secretion
LSS > 10	BAEC < 3 h	Induction of protein kinase C	Regulation of protein phosphorylase
LSS 10	BAEC 30 min	↑ c-myc, c-jun	Induction of early growth genes
LSS 4–25	BAEC 1–2 h	↑ c-fos	Induction of early growth genes
LSS 20	BAEC 2 h	↑ TGFbeta mRNA	Inhibition of VSM growth
LSS 15–36	BAEC 0.5–9 h, peak at 6 h	↑ FGF I mRNA	Regulation of peptide growth factor
LSS 30:60 cyclic stretch	BAEC, HUVEC, > 15–30 s	↑ IP3 (in BAEC)	Second messenger
Cyclic strain at 1 Hz, 24%	HSVC	↑ transient IP3	Second messenger
Turbulent flow, shear stress 1.5–15	BAEC > 3 h	Cell proliferation	Loss of contact inhibition
Disturbed laminar flow	BAEC 12 h	Cell cycle stimulation	Stimulated cell turnover
Change in cell tension, via ECM	Capillary EC 1 h	Changed matrix-integrin binding	Integrins regulate cell growth

Note: LSS: laminar shear stress in dyne/cm²; BAEC: bovine aortic endothelial cells; HUVEC: human umbilical vein endothelial cells; HSVC: human saphenous vein cells; VSM: vascular smooth muscle; ECM: extracellar matrix.
Source: Davies (1995).

Myocardial infarction may be considered as it is a specific example of wound healing. Although some capillary proliferation has been found within the infarcted region, hardly any growth exists in the border zone of infarction and the remaining myocardium, which undergoes hypertrophy, actually has a lower capillary supply (see Hudlická & Brown, 1994). Arterioles as well as larger vessels grow to some extent and it has been postulated that their growth is stimulated by factors identified in infarcted hearts such as a low molecular weight angiogenic factor (Kumar et al, 1983), FGF I (Schaper, 1993) or VEGF (Sharma & Zimmermann, 1993). Indeed, there is evidence that chronic administration of FGF I and VEGF promotes coronary collateral growth in ischaemic hearts and in ischaemic skeletal muscles as well. In contrast to infarction, in pressure overload hypertrophic hearts growth of vessels is not adequate to ensure sufficient supply of

Table 1.2. *Examples of growth, hormonal and humoral factors involved in angiogenesis*

Factor	Stimulatory action on	Inhibitory action on	Identified in
FGF I	EC, VSM		Developing heart, blood vessels, adult heart
FGF II	EC, VSM, growth of collaterals in ischaemic heart and limbs		Tumours, retina, brain
VEGF	EC, growth of collaterals		Tumours, macrophages, brain, hypoxic tissue, endometrium
PDGF	EC, VSM, rabbit cornea		Platelets
ESAF	EC		Tumours, synovial fluid in rheumatoid arthritis, stimulated muscles
Prostaglandins	CAM, cornea		Healing wounds
Nitric oxide	MVEC, CAM	CAM	Everywhere, endothelium
Thrombin	CAM		Blood
TGF-α	EC, cheek pouch		Tumours
TGF-β	EC (tube formation) 1 ng/ml	5–10 ng/ml	Myocardium (normal adult, hypertrophy, adjacent to infarct)
Angiogenin	CAM, rabbit cornea		Liver
PA	Tube fomation		Tip of capillary sprouts
Metalloproteinases	Degradation of BM		Everywhere
Heparin	Binds growth factors		Developing heart (protamine inhibits capillary growth)
Thyroxine	Capillaries in heart, skeletal muscle		
Angiotensin II	VSM	EC	
Steroids	Tumours		
Thrombospondin		EC	
Angiostatin		EC, tumours	Some tumours, cartilage

Note: BM: basement membrane; EC: endothelial cells; ESAF: endothelial cell stimulating angiogenic factor; FGF: fibroblast growth factor; PA: plasminogen activators; PDGF: platelet derived growth factor; TGF: transforming growth factor; VEGF: vascular endothelial growth factor; VSM: vascular smooth muscle cells.
Source: Klagsbrun & D'Amore, 1991; Hudlická et al, 1992; Lelkes et al, 1996; Hudlická & Brown, 1996.

oxygen, eventually leading to heart failure. Coronary vessel growth can occur in young animals' hearts in pressure overload hypertrophy and to some extent even in adult hearts with volume overload hypertrophy (Tomanek & Torry, 1994; Hudlická & Brown, 1996) and in these situations, mechanical rather than growth factors are probably more important as initiators of angiogenesis.

Retinopathies represent a specific case of pathological growth of vessels. Although Stefanson et al (1982) described increased blood flow in retinopathies of varying origin and it may thus be assumed that mechanical factors connected with increased blood flow could be of some importance, a recent review of mechanisms of retinal neovascularization by D'Amore (1994) highlights the importance of assorted growth factors. These include VEGF, FGF I and II, IGF-1, Scatter factor and some interleukins. Inhibitory factors such as thrombospondin and TGF-β maintain the balance between absence and presence of growth. While hypoxia activates predominantly VEGF, other insults may disturb the basement membrane of retinal capillary endothelial cells and result in the release of FGF II. Growth of retinal capillaries, which does not occur in normally healthy eyes, is also inhibited by the physical contact of the endothelium with pericytes, a process mediated by TGF-β.

Conclusions

Angiogenesis is quite clearly a very complex process involving an array of mechanical and chemical stimulators and inhibitors. Under normal circumstances, these keep tight control on the growth of vasculature which can be modified according to physiological or pathological circumstances. Although many factors can induce or inhibit vessel growth when introduced into a system, these are not necessarily responsible for or even connected with the natural occurrence of angiogenesis. There is, for instance, no doubt that FGF II (basic FGF) is an important angiogenic factor which is released by tumours and stimulates growth of collateral circulation; however, it does not seem to play a role in capillary growth in either skeletal muscle or the heart under physiological circumstances (Hudlická et al, 1992). It is equally important to realize that although experiments with tissue cultures are crucial to elucidate signal transduction, angiogenic stimulators or inhibitors can act in a completely different way depending on the type of cells and conditions in vitro and in vivo.

References

Andrade, S. P., Fan, T. P. D. & Lewis, G. P. (1987). Quantitative in-vivo studies on angiogenesis in a rat sponge model. *British Journal of Experimental Pathology*, **68**, 755–66.

Brown, M. D., Hudlická, O., Makki, R. F. & Weiss, J. B. (1995). Low-molecular-mass endothelial cell-stimulating angiogenic factor in relation to capillary growth induced in rat skeletal muscle by low-frequency electrical stimulation. *International Journal of Microcirculation*, **15**, 111–16.

Burri, P. H. & Tarek, M. R. (1990). A novel mechanism of capillary growth in the rat pulmonary circulation. *Anatomical Record*, **228**, 35–45.

Clark, E. R. (1918). Studies on the growth of blood vessels in the tail of the frog. *American Journal of Anatomy*, **23**, 37–88.

Colville-Nash, P. R., Alam, C. A., Appleton, I., Brown, J. R., Seed, M. P. & Willoughby, D. A. (1995). The pharmacological modulation of angiogenesis in chronic granulomatous inflammation. *Journal of Pharmacology and Experimental Therapeutics*, **274**, 1463–72.

D'Amore, P. (1994). Mechanism of retinal and choroidal neovascularization. *Investigations in Ophthalmology and Visual Sciences*, **35**, 3974–9.

Davies, P. F. (1995). Flow-mediated endothelial mechanotransduction. *Physiological Reviews*, **75**, 519–60.

Egginton, S. (1990). Morphometric analysis of tissue capillary supply. In *Advances in Comparative and Environmental Physiology*, vol. 6, ed. R. G. Boutilier, pp. 73–141. Berlin: Springer.

Egginton, S., Hudlická, O., Brown M. D., Graciotti, L. & Granata, A. L. (1996). In vivo pericyte-endothelial cell interaction during angiogenesis in adult cardiac and skeletal muscle. *Microvascular Research*, **51**, 213–28.

Folkman, J. (1974). Tumor angiogenic factor. *Cancer Research*, **34**, 2109–23.

Folkman, J. & Shing, Y. (1992). Angiogenesis. *Journal of Biological Chemistry*, **267**, 10931–4.

Fujita, M., Ohno, A., Miwa, K., Moriuchi, I., Mifune, J. & Sasayama, S. (1993). A new method for assessment of collateral development after acute myocardial infarction. *Journal of the American College of Cardiology*, **21**, 68–72.

Grant, D. S., Kinsella, J., Cid, M. C. & Kleinman, H. K. (1992). Specific laminin domains mediate endothelial cell adhesion. In *Angiogenesis in Health and Disease*, ed. M. E. Maragoudakis, P. Gullino & P. I. Lelkes, pp. 99–110. New York: Plenum Press.

Hansen-Smith, F. M., Hudlická, O. & Egginton, S. (1996). In vivo angiogenesis in adult rat skeletal muscle: early changes in capillary network architecture and ultrastructure. *Cell and Tissue Research*, **286**, 123–36.

Heron, M. I. & Rakusan, K. (1995). Proliferating cell nuclear antigen (PCNA) detection of cellular proliferation in hypothyroid and hyperthyroid rat hearts. *Journal of Molecular and Cellular Cardiology*, **27**, 1393–1403.

Hudlická, O. & Brown, M. D. (1993). Physical forces and angiogenesis. In *Mechanoreception by the Vascular Wall*, ed. G. M. Rubanyi, pp. 197–241. New York: Futura Publishing Co.

Hudlická, O. & Brown, M. D. (1994). Growth of blood vessels in normal and diseased hearts. *Therapeutic Research*, **15**, 93–145.

Hudlická, O. & Brown, M. D. (1996). Postnatal growth of the heart and its blood vessels. *Journal of Vascular Research*, **33**, 266–87.

Hudlická, O. & Tyler, K. R. (1986). *Angiogenesis. The Growth of the Vascular System.* London: Academic Press.

Hudlická, O., Brown, M. D. & Egginton, S. (1992). Angiogenesis in skeletal and cardiac muscle. *Physiological Reviews*, **72**, 369–417.

Iba, T., Sain, T., Sonoda, T., Rosales, O. & Sumpio, B. E. (1991). Stimulation of endothelial secretion of tissue-type plasminogen activator by repetitive stretch. *Journal of Surgical Research*, **50**, 457–60.

Klagsbrun, M. & D'Amore, P. A. (1991). Regulation of angiogenesis. *Annual Reviews of Physiology*, **53**, 217–39.

Kumar, S., Shahabuddin, S., Haboudi, N., West, D., Arnold, F., Reid, H. & Carr, T. (1983). Angiogenesis factor from human myocardial infarcts. *Lancet*, **II**, 364–68.

Laughlin, M. H. & McAllister, R. M. (1992). Exercise training- induced coronary vascular adaptation. *Journal of Applied Physiology*, **73**, 2209–25.

Lelkes, P. I., Manolopoulos, V., Silverman, M., Zhang, S., Karmiol, S. & Unsworth, B. R. (1996). On the possible role of endothelial cell heterogeneity in angiogenesis. In *Molecular, Cellular and Clinical Aspects of Angiogenesis*, ed. M. Maragoudakis, pp. 1–17. New York: Plenum Press.

Lis, L. & Sharon, N. (1986). Biological properties of lectins. In *The Lectins: Properties Functions and Applications in Biology and Medicine*, eds. I. E. Liener, N. Sharon & I. J. Goldstein, pp. 266–93. Orlando: Academic Press.

Liu, H. M. & Chen, H. H. (1994). Correlation between fibroblast growth factor expression

2

Flow-mediated responses in the circulation

A. P. COCKELL and L. POSTON

Introduction

ynamic forces are now established as important modulators of vascular tone
lar wall remodelling, and have also been implicated in atherogenesis. Blood
perience two primary haemodynamic forces. First, the circumferential force
he wall tension resulting from the blood pressure and, second, the frictional
hear stress which results from blood flow along the vessel wall. Although the
ential force has important influences on vascular tone, it is the intention of this
ew to concentrate upon flow associated events in the vasculature.

cently little was known of the mechanisms whereby the physical force of flow
ransduced into a wide range of associated intracellular biochemical events. It
ognized that the endothelial cell, uniquely situated at the interface between the
the vascular wall, is the key player in this haemodynamic signal transduction
The shear stress experienced by the endothelium is a function of the 'axial'
radient (Fig. 2.1) which occurs as blood flows through the vessel (Malek &
94) and, physiologically, is of the order of 0–50 dyne/cm^2 (Fig. 2.2).

Flow and vascular tone

first reported to be important in the control of vascular tone in 1933
mayr, 1933) when it was observed that the femoral artery in the dog hind limb
response to hyperaemia. It is now evident that responses to flow may be
temporal groupings, ranging from extremely rapid to relatively slow and that
ct a wide range of intracellular events (Davies, 1995). Experimentally, the
hear stress have most frequently been investigated by determining the reflow *in vitro* in isolated conduit arteries (Rubanyi et al, 1986; Cooke et al,
there are fewer reports in isolated resistance sized arteries (Koller et al, 1994;
Poston, 1996a), or in isolated vascular beds (Smiesko et al, 1989; Griffith &
1990). There is increasing evidence to suggest that flow-induced dilatation
y dependent on experimental conditions, e.g. initial wall tension, and that it
nicked by changes in pH or pO$_2$. Indeed, in carefully controlled studies we

and cell proliferation in experimental brain infarct: studied v
nuclear antigen immunohistochemistry. *Journal of Neuropa*
Neurology, **53**, 118–26.

Myrhage, R. & Hudlická, O. (1978). Capillary growth in chronica
muscle as studied by intravital microscopy and histological r
Microvascular Research, **16**, 73–90.

Padykula, H. A. & Herman, E. (1955). The specificity of the histc
ATPase. *Journal of Histochemistry and Cytochemistry*, **3**, 17

Pearce, S. C. & Hudlická, O. (1995). Possible involvement of prc
growth in chronically stimulated skeletal muscles. *Microcir*

Reinhold, H. S. & van den Berg-Blok, A. (1983). Vascularization
Development of the Vascular System. CIBA Foundation Syr

Reynolds, L. P., Redmer, D. A., Grazul-Bilska, A. T., Killilea, S.
Angiogenesis in female reproductive organs. In *Molecular,*
of Angiogenesis, ed. M. Maragoudakis, pp. 125–39. New Yc

Rhodin, J. A. G. & Fujita, H. (1989). Capillary growth in the mes
Journal of Submicroscopic Cytology and Pathology, **21**, 1–3

Schaper, W. (1993). New paradigms for collateral vessel growth
Cardiology, **88**, 193–8.

Schaper, W., Gorge, G., Winkler, B. & Schaper, J. (1988). The c
heart. *Progress in Cardiovascular Disease*, **31**, 57–77.

Sharma, H. S. & Zimmermann, R. (1993). Growth factors and
collaterals. In *Growth Factors and the Cardiovascular Syst*
pp. 119–48. Boston: Kluwer Academic Publishers.

Skalak, T. C. & Price, R. J. (1996). The role of mechanical stres
remodeling. *Microcirculation*, **3**, 143–65.

Stefanson, E., Landers, M. B. & Wolbarsht, M. L. (1982). The
vasodilatation in diabetic retinopathy. In *Diabetic Neura*
Friedman & F. A. L'Esperance, pp. 117–51. New York: G

Stingl, J. & Rhodin, J. A. G. (1994). Early postnatal growth of s
the rat. *Cell and Tissue Research*, **275**, 419–34.

Tomanek, R. J. & Torry, R. J. (1994). Growth of the coronary
Cell and Molecular Biology Research, **40**, 129–36.

Van Groningen, J. P., Weninck, A. C. & Testers, L. H. (1991).
in number by splitting of existing vessels. *Acta Embryolo*

White, F. C. & Bloor, C. M. (1992). Coronary vascular remoc
during chronic ischemia. *American Journal of Cardiovas*

Haemoc
and vasc
vessels e
which is
force or
circumfe
short rev
Until
could be
is now re
blood an
pathway.
pressure
Izumo, 1

Flow wa
(Schretze
dilates in
defined b
these refl
effects of
sponse to
1991), bu
Cockell &
Edwards,
may be ve
may be m

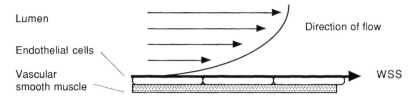

Fig. 2.1. Wall shear stress (WSS) is the force per unit area acting in the direction of blood flow (*Q*) at the endothelial surface dependent on the blood's viscosity, μ. In laminar flow, the magnitude of the shear stress is proportional to the third power of the internal radius of the vessel (*r*): WSS $= \dfrac{4 \times \mu \times Q}{\pi \times r^3}$.

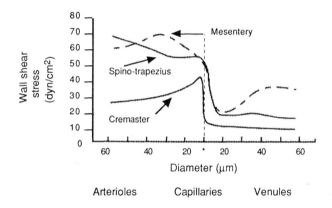

Fig. 2.2. Physiological values for wall shear stress. Representative arteriovenous distributions of wall shear stress from measurements of red cell velocity in the microcirculation of mesentery, spinotrapezius muscle and cremaster muscle from studies in cat, rat and rabbit. Reproduced with permission from 'Shear stress in the circulation', H. L. Lipowsky, 1995. In *Flow-Dependent Regulation of Vascular Function*, ed. J Bevan, G Kaley, G. M. Rubanyi. Oxford University Press, New York, USA.

have observed minimal flow-induced dilatation in resistance sized arteries from different vascular beds of the rat (Cockell & Poston, 1996b; Tribe et al, 1996). More recently flow-induced relaxation in humans has been observed *in vivo* by the imaging of conduit arteries using high resolution Doppler ultrasound (Meredith et al, 1996).

The endothelium dependence of flow-induced dilatation has been proven in conduit arteries from experimental animals (Pohl et al, 1986; Rubanyi et al, 1986) and in resistance sized arterioles (Koller & Kaley, 1991; Koller et al, 1993). There is evidence for some species and/or vascular bed variability as flow-induced relaxation persists after endothelium removal in some circulations, e.g. rabbit ear resistance artery (Bevan et al, 1988).

Nitric oxide and prostacyclin mediated responses

Relaxation to flow involves the release of nitric oxide (NO) and, to a lesser extent, prostacyclin (PGI_2). PGI_2 involvement has been proven by showing flow-induced synthesis of 6-ketoprostaglandin $F_{1\alpha}$, a stable metabolite of PGI_2 (Rubanyi et al, 1986; Hecker et al, 1993), whereas the contribution of NO is usually evaluated by determining responses to flow in the presence and absence of specific inhibitors of endothelial NO synthase (NOS-III). Using this approach, NO has been implicated in flow-induced dilatation in rabbit thoracic aorta (Cooke et al, 1990), rat gracilis arterioles (Koller et al, 1994) and, from our laboratory, in human placental arteries (Learmont & Poston, 1996) and small mesenteric arteries from pregnant rats (Cockell & Poston, 1996b). Others have implicated NO by showing that the effluent emerging from perfused arteries stimulates soluble guanylyl cyclase (Hecker et al, 1993), the enzyme activated by NO to form cGMP, which relaxes the vascular smooth muscle. In addition to activation of vascular smooth muscle, NO acts in an autocrine fashion to stimulate guanylyl cyclase in endothelial cells and measurement of endothelial cell cGMP provides an alternative endpoint for the estimation of NO synthesis. Using this assay as an indirect estimate of NO release, cGMP has been shown to be increased in a graded fashion with laminar flow in cultured endothelial cells (Ohno et al, 1993). Laminar and pulsatile flow have also been found to increase the expression of NOS-III mRNA in endothelial cells (Noris et al, 1995; Ranjan et al, 1995), but turbulent flow had no effect when NOS-III was assessed by a biochemical assay (Noris et al, 1995).

Flow-induced vasoconstriction

Whereas most investigators associate flow with dilatation, flow-induced vasoconstriction may also occur, although it has been suggested that this is only evident if the pre-existing wall tension is above a certain value. Experimentally, this has been demonstrated in pial arteries from the rabbit brain in which the normal vasodilatation to flow occurs when vessels are pressurized to 30 mmHg, but constriction is evident only when the pressure is raised to 90 mmHg (Garcia-Roldan & Bevan, 1990). This dual response could represent an effective autoregulatory mechanism, where flow is maintained if the blood pressure is low but if the blood pressure rises, the end organ will be protected by the flow-induced constriction.

It is likely that flow-induced constriction results from increased synthesis of an endothelium derived constrictor and endothelin (ET-1) is an obvious candidate. Early observations suggested that flow led to both an increase in synthesis and release of ET-1 (Yoshizumi et al, 1989), but more recently a biphasic response has been described with stimulation being followed by inhibition (Kuchan & Frangos, 1993). Another report suggests that ET-1 plays no role at all, as ET-1 mRNA expression in cultured endothelial cells was not significantly affected by changes in shear stress (Noris et al, 1995).

In addition to vasodilator and vasoconstrictor responses, flow is also a potent stimulus to the synthesis of a number of other factors involved in different aspects of vascular function, particularly smooth muscle growth (which is considered in more detail below).

Shear may also affect haemostasis. PGI_2 and NO produced in response to flow, are not only potent vasodilators but also have powerful anti-aggregatory properties and are thought to contribute tonically to thrombus prevention. Flow also increases the expression of other factors which play an important role in haemostasis, including tissue plasminogen activator (tPA) and tPA inhibitor (tPAI). In addition, the expression of some cellular adhesion molecules is affected by elevation of shear, particularly the intercellular adhesion molecule-1 (ICAM-1), which is increased and the vascular endothelial cell adhesion molecule (VCAM-1) which is decreased (Davies & Tripathi, 1993; Davies, 1995). The physiological relevance of these apparently opposing effects is unknown.

How is the flow stimulus detected by the endothelial cells?

The complexity of the mechanotransduction pathways by which the frictional force is detected by endothelial cells is gradually being unravelled. The frictional force is obviously initially experienced at the luminal surface of the cell, but this is probably not the site of flow detection. Evidence now points to an important role for transduction of the frictional force through the cytoskeleton to focal adhesion sites on the basal side of the cell (Fig. 2.3). The dramatic realignment of filamentous actin (F-actin) stress fibres which occurs 12–15 h after the onset of increased shear implicates cytoskeletal proteins as the principal force transmission structure of endothelial cells. In the presence of physiological shear, F-actin is predominantly located in the periphery of the cell particularly at cell–cell junctions where it is thought to play a role in cell permeability. In the presence of high shear long, thicker strands of F-actin are observed centrally in association with elongation of the cell.

The role of focal adhesion sites is implied by their rapid remodelling which occurs in response to flow. This has been observed in elegant experiments in which these sites have been 'visualised' using tandem scanning confocal image analysis (Davies et al, 1994). Focal adhesion sites are rich in integrins, the β-containing integrins predominantly. The integrin family are transmembrane proteins that span the plasma membrane and bind to extracellular adhesion proteins, connecting to the cytoskeleton via linker proteins on the inside of the cell (Fig. 2.3). The method by which flow, integrins and cellular responses are interrelated has yet to be fully elucidated, although certain elements of the pathway have been identified (Davies, 1995). Flow-mediated activation of integrins leads to phosphorylation of a tyrosine kinase (125 kDa tyrosine kinase, known as FAK). Tyrosine kinases are a group of enzymes recently identified as playing an important role in signal transduction pathways leading to a variety of responses, including cell growth. Activation of the tyrosine kinase leads to recruitment and activation of other protein kinases which in turn phosphorylate a further focal adhesion molecule protein, paxillin. Paxillin has also been shown to change its alignment in response to flow, suggesting a probable role in mechanotransduction.

A second mechanotransduction pathway, implicating G proteins, has also been proposed, but whether this involves the basal focal adhesion sites or activation of luminal membrane receptors is unknown. Until recently, the supportive evidence was

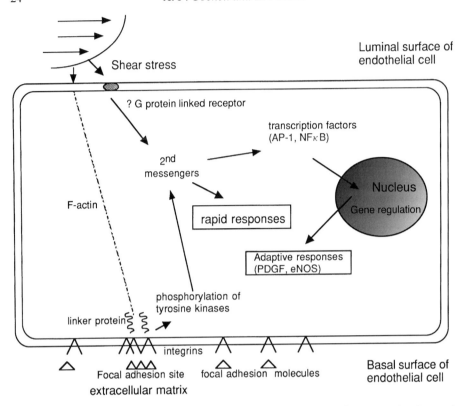

Fig. 2.3. Signal transduction mechanisms. Mechanisms for the mechanotransduction pathways in the endothelial cell. The cytoskeleton plays an important role in the transmission of the force stimulus.

largely indirect, relying upon the observation that a number of intracellular messengers, stimulated by a G protein dependent mechanism, were also generated in response to flow. These included inositol triphosphate (IP_3), diacylglycerol (DAG), protein kinase C (PKC) and increased intracellular calcium. Involvement of the G_i subtype of G proteins was suggested by the observation in some, but not all experiments, of the pertussis toxin sensitivity of NO release (Ohno et al, 1993) and PGI_2 release (Berthiaume & Frangos, 1992). These early, but indirect suggestions of G protein involvement have been strengthened by a recently published study using endothelial cells, in which G proteins were assayed by immunoprecipitation. This has now shown activation of G protein sub-units $G_{\alpha q/\alpha 11}$ and $G_{\alpha i3/\alpha o}$ in responses to flow (Gudi et al, 1996). Activation of G protein linked receptors stimulates mitogen activated protein (MAP) kinases which are intimately involved in growth responses and flow has also been found to increase MAP kinase activity in cultured endothelial cells (Tseng et al, 1995). Whilst implicating G proteins, this does not suggest their exclusive involvement, as flow-mediated MAP kinase activation also occurs in response to activation of β1 integrins (associated with focal adhesion sites) or through tyrosine kinases (Ishida et al, 1996).

The shear stimulus therefore is known to activate intracellular second messenger pathways, either through integrin activation or focal adhesion sites, or through stimulation of G proteins. Second messenger pathways may include protein kinase C, the MAP kinases and the tyrosine kinases. In turn these lead to the characteristic immediate and delayed responses to shear stress.

Immediate response to flow

Acute responses to flow include an immediate rise in intracellular calcium in most cells studied (Schwarz et al, 1992; Shen et al, 1992) and this is likely to be the result of flow-induced opening of endothelial cell potassium channels with subsequent hyperpolarization (Nakache & Gaub, 1988; Cooke et al, 1991). Hyperpolarization increases endothelial cell calcium, which in turn is a potent stimulus to the activation of NOS-III (Luckhoff & Busse, 1990). The stimulus to opening of potassium channels is unknown but could result from direct displacement of the luminal channel protein by shear stress or from the activation of a mechanoreceptor (either cytoskeletal or G protein). The necessity of a rise in intracellular calcium for flow-induced relaxation would, however, not appear universal as a recent study has shown a component of flow-induced NO mediated relaxation to be calcium-independent (Ayajiki et al, 1996). This calcium-independent NO release showed strong dependence on tyrosine kinase-induced phosphorylation of cellular proteins (including MAP kinases) and on intracellular pH.

Other immediate responses to shear stress include the release of vasoactive agonists such as adenosine triphosphate (ATP) and substance P and these in turn may stimulate NO release. Synthesis of these vasoactive agents may also be related to increases in IP_3, DAG and PKC activity, all of which have been documented in the rapid response to elevated shear stress (Davies, 1995).

Longer term responses to flow

In addition to the immediate responses to flow, the continued presence of shear stress can regulate endothelial cell gene expression. Endothelial cell protein synthesis can be altered by haemodynamic forces and this can occur through genomic mechanisms. The first protein thus implicated was tPA, as tPA mRNA expression was upregulated in cultured endothelial cells exposed to laminar shear stress (Diamond et al, 1990). Others have since found evidence for *in vitro* shear stress regulation of a number of genes involved in cell growth including the 'early growth response genes' c-*myc*, c-*fos* and c-*jun*, platelet-derived growth factors A and B (PDGF-A, PDGF-B) and transforming growth factor -β1 (TGF-β1). The expression of these growth factors might be expected, directly or indirectly through synthesis of other growth factors, to act in a paracrine fashion to alter vascular smooth muscle cell growth. In view of the important role of NO in flow-induced dilatation, it is not surprising that among the genes upregulated by flow is that which encodes for NOSIII (for a review see Resnick & Gimbrone, 1995). Expression of some molecules show biphasic responses (e.g. ET-1 and thrombomodulin) and some are down regulated by shear (e.g. VCAM-1).

The identification of de novo protein synthesis in response to flow implies that the genes responsible are sensitive to shear stress. The mechanism by which this occurs has been the subject of intense interest and it is now known that one of the fundamental prerequisites for the response to flow is the presence on the gene of a common base sequence known as the 'shear stress response element' (SSRE). The SSRE was first identified in the PDGF-B gene as a 6 base pair stretch now identified as the sequence GAGACC (Resnick & Gimbrone, 1995). This sequence is common to other endothelial genes unrelated to PDGF-B, such as NOSIII, tPA, TGF-β1, c-fos, ICAM-1 and monocyte chemotactic protein-1 (MCP-1).

The activation of the SSRE (or other shear sensitive elements) probably results from synthesis of a number of cellular transcription factors. Shear stress has been found to influence a number of recognized transcription and transactivation factors including nuclear factor kappa beta (NFκB) and the c-fos/c-jun complex (AP1) (Lan et al, 1994). An increase in NFκB factor expression in endothelial cells may be seen within 10 min of exposure to shear stress (Resnick & Gimbrone, 1995) and it is suggested that NFκB may bind to the SSRE sequence and so play a functional role in the response to flow (Khachigian et al, 1995).

Although involved in the increase in mRNA for many proteins, the SSRE does not explain all flow-mediated de novo protein synthesis. Therefore some genes have an apparently functionless SSRE sequence, e.g. that encoding for MCP-1, and others are responsive to shear in the absence of the SSRE sequence, e.g. PDGF-A (Resnick & Gimbrone, 1995).

Flow, vascular remodelling and atherosclerosis

Arteries develop structural reorganization in response to flow. The most obvious example is the alignment and elongation of the endothelial cells in the direction of flow (Flaherty et al, 1972). The alignment of the cells confers a degree of rigidity on the endothelial cell and may reduce the shear stress gradients, so providing an adaptive mechanism to reduce the force stimulus. The reorganization of the endothelial cells is associated with the redistribution of cytoskeletal proteins including microtubules, vimentin rich intermediate filaments, paxillin and F-actin (as discussed earlier in relation to signal transduction). The rearrangement may not only be involved in mechano-signal transduction but also in the associated adhesion to components of the extracellular matrix, so conferring stability upon the cell (Davies, 1995).

If increased flow is maintained for a considerable period of time, the arteries become permanently dilated. This is a result of structural modification associated with an increase in lumen diameter and a greater medial cross-sectional area (Zarins et al, 1987). Structural changes may result from hyperplasia and/or redistribution of vascular smooth muscle cells within their matrix, i.e. remodelling. The mechanisms associated with flow-induced hyperplasia presumably involves increased expression of the genes for a number of growth factors, as previously described, and also upregulation of other growth factors associated with increased activity of the tyrosine kinases and MAP kinases. Remodelling involves degradation or rearrangement of matrix proteins but remodelling in response to flow has not been extensively investigated. In other experimental situations involving remodelling without changes in flow, various agents have been implicated including plasminogen activators (Clowes et al, 1990) and the matrix metalloproteinases (Dollery et al, 1995), both leading to degradation of matrix proteins.

Flow-induced structural changes may occur in several physiological and pathophysiological situations (for a review see Langille, 1995). Shear stress may play an important role in the remodelling which occurs in the uterine vascular bed during the menstrual cycle and in many different vascular beds during pregnancy, although the relative contribution of haemodynamic and hormonal influences are not known. Elegant experiments in chick embryos (Rychter, 1962) have shown the importance of flow in the normal development of the aortic arch. Furthermore, the abrupt changes in blood flow, which occur in some vascular beds at the time of birth, may have profound influences on vessel development. This is suggested by the strong correlation with blood flow and vessel growth which has been observed in the weeks following birth (Langille et al, 1991).

The relation between shear stress, vascular restructuring and/or growth has led to speculation of an association between shear and the formation of atherosclerotic lesions. The distribution of shear in the aorta, carotid and femoral arteries which are all particularly prone to atheroma formation is, however, complex. The shear at any given point is influenced by many factors such as the vessel size, wall elasticity, curvature, local geometry and branching. An association, nonetheless, has been made between low levels of shear stress and focal areas of disease. In support of this 'low shear' theory of atherosclerosis, intimal thickening in human arteries is greater in areas of low shear (Friedman et al, 1986) and in a pig model of atherosclerosis (Gerrity et al, 1985), focal areas of disease are associated with non-aligned endothelial cells (indicative of low shear).

The failure of therapeutic angioplasty procedures is frequently due to subsequent intimal proliferation and some authors attribute this to changes in shear stress. In a rat model of carotid artery angioplasty, in which vascular damage was induced by balloon-catheter injury, increasing the blood flow (and therefore the shear stress) was found to reduce early neointimal proliferation (Kohler & Jaiwien, 1992).

Vasodilatation to flow in vascular disease

The recognition of the important role of flow in the maintenance of vascular dilatation and hence in the control of peripheral resistance, has stimulated interest in responses to shear stress in vascular disease. As there is limited availability of arteries from human subjects studies of isolated arteries have been few, although in our laboratory we have recently shown flow-induced dilatation to be reduced in small arteries from pregnant women with preeclampsia (Cockell & Poston, 1996c). These arteries were dissected from biopsies of subcutaneous fat obtained during caesarean section and were compared with those from normotensive pregnant or non-pregnant women. Interestingly the NO-mediated response to flow in the normotensive women was greatly increased compared with that observed in arteries from non-pregnant women, which suggests that an increased response to shear stress may underlie peripheral vasodilatation in normal pregnancy; however, absence of this response may contribute to the elevation of the blood pressure in pre-eclampsia. In similar experiments, poor dilatation to flow has also been documented in isolated arterioles from spontaneously hypertensive rats (Koller & Huang, 1994) and in the coronary circulation of the atherosclerotic pig (Kuo et al, 1992).

The estimation of flow-induced responses *in vivo* has recently been facilitated by the use of high resolution Doppler ultrasound. Flow-induced dilatation may be assessed in the human by imaging the brachial or radial artery. Enhanced flow is induced by reactive hyperaemia in the hand, distal to the site of measurement, and changes in the artery diameter recorded. This hyperaemic flow-induced dilatation in the forearm, has been proven to be partly mediated by NO (Meredith et al, 1996) and abnormal responses have been identified in children and adults at risk of atherosclerosis (Celermajer et al, 1992), in subjects with non-insulin dependent diabetes (Goodfellow et al, 1996) and, most recently, in cigarette smokers and passive smokers (Celermajer et al, 1996).

Conclusion

Despite the recognition more than 60 years ago that flow was an important modulator of vascular tone, it has only been in the last decade that the extent and physiological importance of flow-mediated responses have been appreciated. The flow-mediated release of potent vasodilators in response to shear stress suggests that flow tonically reduces the blood pressure. Furthermore, we are now beginning to appreciate the complexity of the underlying pathways involved in the transduction of the flow signal to cellular responses. The demonstration that flow affects vascular growth and remodelling offers an exciting challenge to unravel the complex interaction between flow, growth factors and the biochemical pathways contributing to the rearrangement of matrix proteins. In the clinical setting, it is becoming increasingly apparent that abnormal responses to flow or abnormal flow patterns within arteries may contribute to cardiovascular dysfunction. A more detailed understanding of the physical and biochemical events underlying flow mediated responses is likely to have an important role to play in the prevention and treatment of cardiovascular disease.

References

Ayajiki, K., Kindermann, M., Hecker, M., Fleming, I. & Busse, R. (1996). Intracellular pH and tyrosine phosphorylation but not calcium determine shear stress-induced nitric oxide production in native endothelial cells. *Circulation Research*, **78**, 750–8.

Berthiaume, F. & Frangos, J. A. (1992). Flow-induced prostacyclin production is mediated by a pertussis toxin-sensitive G protein. *FEBS Letters*, **308**, 277–9.

Bevan, J. A., Joyce, E. H. & Wellman, G. C. (1988). Flow-dependent dilation in a resistance artery still occurs after endothelium removal. *Circulation Research*, **63**, 980–5.

Celermajer, D. S., Adams, M. R., Clarkson, P., Robinson, J., McCredie, R., Donald, A. & Deanfield, J. E. (1996). Passive smoking and impaired endothelium-dependent arterial dilatation in healthy young adults. *New England Journal of Medicine*, **334**, 150–4.

Celermajer, D. S., Sorenson, K. E., Gooch, V. M., Spiegelhalter, D. J., Miller, O. I., Sullivan, I. D., Lloyd, J. K. & Deanfield, J. K. (1992). Non-invasive detection of endothelial dysfunction in children and adults at risk of atherosclerosis. *Lancet*, **340**, 1111–15.

Clowes, A. W., Clowes, M. M., Au, Y. P. T., Reidy, M. A. & Belin, D. (1990). Smooth muscle cells express urokinase during mitogenesis and tissue-type plasminogen activator during migration in injured rat carotid artery. *Circulation Research*, **67**, 61–7.

Cockell, A. P. & Poston, L. (1996a). Pregnancy is associated with enhanced flow-induced dilatation in isolated human subcutaneous arteries. Abs. *Proceedings of International Society for the Study of Hypertension in Pregnancy*. Seattle USA (abstract).

Cockell, A. P. & Poston, L. (1996b). Isolated mesenteric arteries from pregnant rats show enhanced flow-mediated relaxation but normal myogenic tone. *Journal of Physiology*, **495**, 545–51.

Cockell, A. P. & Poston, L. (1996c). Flow-induced vasodilatation is reduced in isolated human subcutaneous arteries from pregnant women with pre-eclampsia and diabetes. *Journal of Vascular Research*, **33,** 27 (abstract).

Cooke, J. P., Rossitch, E., Andon, N. A., Loscalzo, J. & Dzau, V. J. (1991). Flow activates an endothelial potassium channel to release an endogenous nitrovasodilator. *Journal of Clinical Investigation*, **88**, 1663–71.

Cooke, J. P., Stamler, J., Andon, N. A., Davies, P. F., McCinley, G. & Loscalzo, J. (1990). Flow stimulates endothelial cells to release a nitrovasodilator that is potentiated by reduced thiol. *American Journal of Physiology*, **259**, H804–H812.

Davies, P. F. (1995). Flow-mediated endothelial mechanotransduction. *Physiological Reviews*, **75**, 519–60.

Davies, P. F. & Tripathi, S. C. (1993). Mechanical stress mechanisms and the cell: an endothelial paradigm. *Circulation Research*, **72**, 239–45.

Davies, P. F., Robotewskyj, A. & Griem, M. L. (1994). Quantitative studies of endothelial cell adhesion: directional remodelling of focal adhesion sites in response to flow forces. *Journal of Clinical Investigation*, **93**, 2031–8.

Diamond, S.L., Sharefkin, J. B., Dieffenbach, C., Frasier-Scott, J., McIntire, L. V. & Eskin, S. G. (1990). Tissue plasminogen activator messenger RNA levels increase in cultured human endothelial cells exposed to laminar shear stress. *Journal of Cell Physiology*, **143**, 364–71.

Dollery, C. M., McEwan, J. R. & Henney, A. M. (1995). Matrix metalloproteins and cardiovascular disease. *Circulation Research*, **77**, 863–8.

Flaherty, J. J., Pierce, J. E., Ferrans, V. J., Patel, D. J., Tucker, W. K. & Fry, D. L. (1972). Endothelial nuclear patterns in the canine arterial tree with particular reference to hemodynamic events. *Circulation Research*, **30**, 23–33.

Friedman, M. H., Peters, O. J., Bargeron, C. J., Hutchins, G. M. & Mark, F. F. (1986). Shear-dependent thickening of the human arterial intima. *Atherosclerosis*, **60**, 161–71.

Garcia-Roldan, J.-L. & Bevan, J. A. (1990). Flow-induced constriction and dilation of cerebral resistance arteries. *Circulation Research*, **66**, 1445–8.

Gerrity, R. V., Goss, J. A. & Soby, L. (1985). Control of monocyte recruitment by chemotactic factors in lesion prone areas of swine aorta. *Atherosclerosis*, **5**, 55–66.

Goodfellow, J., Ramsey, M. W., Luddington, L. A., Jones, C. J. H., Coates, P. A., Dunstan, F., Lewis, M. J., Owens, D. R. & Henderson, A. A. (1996). Endothelium and inelastic arteries: an early marker of vascular dysfunction in non-insulin dependent diabetes. *British Medical Journal*, **312**, 744–5.

Griffith, T. M. & Edwards, D. H. (1990). Myogenic autoregulation of flow may be inversely related to endothelium-derived relaxing factor activity. *American Journal of Physiology*, **258**, H1171–H1180.

Gudi, S. R. P., Clark., C. B. & Frangos, J. A. (1996). Fluid flow rapidly activates G proteins in human endothelial cells: involvement of G proteins in mechanotransduction. *Circulation Research*, **79**, 834–9.

Hecker, M., Mülsch, A., Bassenge, E. & Busse, R. (1993). Vasoconstriction and increased flow: two principal mechanisms of shear stress-dependent endothelial autocoid release. *American Journal of Physiology*, **265**, H828–H833.

Ishida, T., Peterson, T. E., Kovach, N. L. & Berk, B. C. (1996). MAP kinase activation by flow in endothelial cells. *Circulation Research*, **79**, 310–16.

Khachigian, L. M., Resnick, N., Gimbrone, M. A. & Collins, T. (1995). Nuclear factor -$_K$B interacts functionally with the PDGF-B chain shear-stress-response-element in vascular endothelial cells exposed to shear stress. *Journal of Clinical Investigation*, **96**, 1169–75.

Kohler, T. R. & Jaiwien, A. (1992). Flow affects development of intimal hyperplasia after arterial injury in rats. *Arteriosclerosis and Thrombosis*, **12**, 963–71.

Koller, A. & Huang, A. (1994). Impaired nitric oxide-mediated flow-induced dilation in arterioles of spontaneously hypertensive rats. *Circulation Research*, **74**, 416–21.

Koller, A. & Kaley, G. (1991). Endothelial regulation of wall shear stress and blood flow in skeletal muscle microcirculation. *American Journal of Physiology*, **260**, H862–H868.

Koller, A., Sun, D. & Kaley, G. (1993). Role of shear stress and endothelial prostaglandins in flow- and viscosity- induced dilatation of arterioles in vitro. *Circulation Research*, **72**, 1276–84.

Koller, A., Sun, D., Huang, A. & Kaley, G. (1994). Corelease of nitric oxide and prostaglandins mediates flow-dependent dilation of rat gracilis muscle arterioles. *American Journal of Physiology*, **267**, H326–H332.

Kuchan, M. J. & Frangos, J. A. (1993). Shear stress regulates endothelin-1 release via protein kinase C and cGMP in cultured endothelial cells. *American Journal of Physiology*, **264**, H150–H156.

Kuo, L., Davis, M. J., Cannon, M. S. & Chilian, W. M. (1992). Pathophysiological consequences of atherosclerosis extend into the coronary microcirculation. Restoration of endothelium-dependent responses by L-arginine. *Circulation Research*, **70**, 465–76.

Lan, Q., Mercurius, K. O. & Davies, P. F. (1994). Stimulation of transcription factors NF$_K$ B and AP-1 in endothelial cells subjected to shear stress. *Biochemical and Physical Research Communications*, **201**, 950–6.

Langille, B. L. (1995). Blood flow-induced remodelling of the artery wall. In *Flow-Dependent Regulation of Vascular Function*, ed. J. Bevan, G. Kaley & G. Rubanyi, 277–99. New York: Oxford University Press.

Langille, B. L., Brownlee, R. D. & Adamson, S. L. (1991). Perinatal aortic growth in lambs: relation to blood flow changes at birth. *American Journal of Physiology*, **259**, H1247–H1253.

Learmont, J. G. & Poston, L. (1996). Nitric oxide is involved in flow-induced dilation of isolated human small fetoplacental arteries. *American Journal of Obstetrics and Gynecology*, **174**, 583–8.

Luckhoff, A. & Busse, R. (1990). Calcium influx into endothelial cells and formation of endothelium-derived relaxing factor is controlled by the membrane potential. *Pflugers Archives European Journal of Physiology*, **416**, 305–11.

Malek, A. M. & Izumo, S. (1994). Molecular aspects of signal transduction of shear stress in the endothelial cell. *Journal of Hypertension*, **12**, 989–99.

Meredith, I. T., Currie, K. E. & Anderson, T. J., Roddy, M. A., Ganz, P. & Creager, M. A. (1996). Post-ischaemic vasodilation in human forearm is dependent on endothelium-derived nitric oxide. *American Journal of Physiology*, **270**, H1435–H1440.

Nakache, M. & Gaub, H. E. (1988). Hydrodynamic hyperpolarisation of endothelial cells. *Proceedings of the National Academy of Sciences USA*, **85**, 1841–3.

Noris, M., Morigi, M., Dondelli, R., Aiello, S., Foppolo, M., Todeschini, M., Orisio, S., Remuzzi, G. & Remuzzi, A. (1995). Nitric oxide synthesis by cultured endothelial cells is modulated by flow conditions. *Circulation Research*, **76**, 536–43.

Ohno, M., Gibbons, G. H., Dzau, V. J. & Cooke, J. P. (1993). Shear stress elevates endothelial cGMP. Role of a potassium channel and G protein coupling. *Circulation*, **88**, 193–7.

Pohl, U., Holtz, J., Busse, R. & Bassenge, E. (1986). Crucial role of endothelium in the vasodilator response to increased flow in vivo. *Hypertension*, **8**, 37–44.

Ranjan, V., Xiao, Z. & Diamond, S. L. (1995). Constitutive NOS expression in cultured endothelial cells is elevated by fluid shear stress. *American Journal of Physiology*, **269**, H550–H555.

Resnick, N. & Gimbrone, J. R. (1995). Hemodynamic forces are complex regulators of endothelial gene expression. *FASEB Journal*, **9**, 874–82.

Rubanyi, G. M., Romero, J. C. & Vanhoutte, P. M. (1986). Flow-induced release of endothelium-derived relaxing factor. *American Journal of Physiology*, **250**, H1145–H1149.

Rychter, Z. (1962). Experimental morphology of the aortic arches and heart loop in chick embryos. *Advances in Morphology*, **2**, 333.

Schretzenmayr, A. (1933). Uber kreislaufregulatorische vorgange an den großen arterien bei der muskelarbeit. *Pflugers Archiv. fur Gesamte die Physiolie*, **232**, 743–8.

Schwarz, G., Callewaert, G., Droogmans, G. & Nilius, B. (1992). Shear stress-induced calcium transients in endothelial cells from human umbilical cord veins. *Journal of Physiology*, **458**, 527–38.

Shen, J., Luscinskas, F. W., Connolly, A., Forbes Dewey, C. & Gimbrone, M. A. (1992). Fluid shear stress modulates cytosolic free calcium in vascular endothelial cells. *American Journal of Physiology*, **262**, C384–C390.

Smiesko, V., Lang, D. J. & Johnson, P. C. (1989). Dilator response of rat mesenteric arcading arterioles to increased blood flow velocity. *American Journal of Physiology*, **257**, H1958–H1965.

Tribe, R. M., Thomas, C.R. & Poston, L. (1996). Flow-induced responses in isolated small arteries using a pressure myograph. *Journal Vascular Research*, **33**, 48 (abstract).

Tseng, H., Peterson, T. E. & Berk, B.C. (1995). Fluid shear stress stimulates mitogen-activated protein kinase in endothelial cells. *Circulation Research*, **77**, 869–78.

Yoshizumi, M., Kurihara, H., Sugiyama, T., Takaku, F., Yanagisawa, M., Masaki, T. & Yasaki, Y. (1989). Haemodynamic shear stress stimulates endothelin production by cultured endothelial cells. *Biochemical and Physical Research Communications*, **161**, 859–64.

Zarins, C. K., Zatina, M. A., Giddens, D. P., Ku, D. N. & Glagov, S. (1987). Shear stress regulation of artery lumen diameter in experimental atherogenesis. *Journal of Vascular Surgery*, **5**, 413–20.

3

Endothelial cell control of vascular tone and permeability

J. D. PEARSON

Introduction

Knowledge of endothelial cell biology, and an appreciation of its importance for the maintenance of many aspects of vascular homeostasis, are still increasing rapidly. Much of the advance stems from the introduction, just over 20 years ago, of routine methods for the successful isolation and culture of large vessel endothelial cells, which led rapidly to the realization that endothelium is a metabolically active partner in the processes of thrombus formation, coagulation and fibrinolysis, control of vessel tone, and leukocyte traffic across blood vessels. More recently, the advent of new techniques to isolate and culture microvascular endothelial cells, still not routinely available for all vascular beds, has allowed a greater understanding of the functional diversity of endothelial cells from large and small vessels and in different organs. Current growth points in endothelial biology include attempts to understand the mechanisms underlying the complex phenotypic changes induced when the cells are exposed to inflammatory cytokines (involving altered adhesivity for leukocytes, and potentially prothrombotic modulation of function, discussed in more detail in Chapter 14); recognition that interactions with the immune system are likely to be critical for the success of organ and vessel grafts or transplants (Chapter 15); novel insights into the molecular control of angiogenesis, particularly as anti-angiogenic strategies hold considerable promise for the prevention of tumour growth and metastasis; and intense interest in devising sensitive, selective and accurate ways to monitor human endothelial cell function relatively non-invasively in vivo, as abnormalities of endothelial cell function are increasingly implicated in a wide range of diseases.

The classically recognized role of endothelium, albeit originally regarded as rather passive, is the control of blood vessel permeability to solutes and macromolecules. An interacting role, preeminently recognized in the seminal paper by Furchgott & Zawadzki (1980), is the control of vessel tone and hence blood pressure. These two roles of the endothelium are of fundamental importance to vascular physiology and pathophysiology. This chapter summarises our current understanding of the most important biochemical mediators and pathways involved in the endothelial control of vascular tone and permeability, with reference to the main methods used to study them, particularly using cultured endothelial cells.

Endothelial cell control of vascular tone

Prostacyclin

The first endothelium-derived vasodilator to be identified was the labile prostaglandin I_2 (PGI_2; prostacyclin) (Moncada et al, 1976). PGI_2 was also recognised to be a potent inhibitor of platelet aggregation, and it was not long before it became clear that release of PGI_2 from intact endothelial cells was rapidly and transiently stimulated by a variety of mediators (including thrombin, ATP, ADP and serotonin) generated extracellularly during thrombus formation. Subsequently it was shown that these agonists each activate specific receptors of the seven transmembrane spanning family on the endothelial surface, and that consequent mobilization of intracellular Ca^{2+} stores to raise cytoplasmic Ca^{2+} concentrations, $[Ca^{2+}]_i$, was critical for PGI_2 synthesis and release (for a review see Carter & Pearson, 1992).

PGI_2 was originally detected by bioassay of the inhibition of platelet aggregation (MacIntyre et al, 1978), and while this remains a relatively cheap and sensitive technique, which is also specific if set up carefully (e.g. to eliminate the contribution of other endothelium-derived platelet-active mediators, notably nitric oxide – see pp. 35–38) it has generally been supplanted by radio or enzyme immunoassay of the hydrolytic breakdown product from PGI_2, 6-keto-$PGF_{1\alpha}$. Commercial kits are convenient and will detect PGI_2 released over a period of a few minutes from monolayers of endothelial cells grown in 24-well plates.

The main sources of difficulty in establishing reproducible assays from PGI_2 release are twofold. (Similar considerations apply to assays for nitric oxide (NO) release.) First, individual endothelial cell cultures usually respond similarly in terms of sensitivity to a given agonist only if studied at the same (early) passage number, and even then may have different absolute levels of basal or stimulated PGI_2 release. Second, it is now well recognized that PGI_2 synthesis can be stimulated by applying physical forces, particularly shear stress, to the cells (Frangos et al, 1985; Grabowski et al, 1985). The signal transduction pathways involved are not fully understood, although elevation of $[Ca^{2+}]_i$ may be less important for shear stress induced PGI_2 production than activation of protein kinases. We have shown recently that agonist-induced PGI_2 synthesis requires activation of p42 MAP kinase in addition to elevation of $[Ca^{2+}]_i$ (Wheeler-Jones et al, 1996.)

Assays involving pipetting of solutions on and off cell monolayers inevitably introduce shear forces and hence cause PGI_2 release independently of the particular agonist being tested, so the experimental protocols must be designed to minimize and standardize this effect. An example of such a protocol is shown in Fig. 3.1 (Carter et al, 1988). An alternative approach is to eliminate changes in shear forces from the assay system, e.g. by using constant flow superfusion of endothelial cells grown on microcarrier beads and packed into small columns (Pearson et al, 1983). This system, while possessing several advantages (notably for detailed time course studies or repeated additions of different stimuli), is more expensive to set up as it requires specialized stirrer flasks for cell culture and has other disadvantages: the large cell surface area relative to volume of perfusion

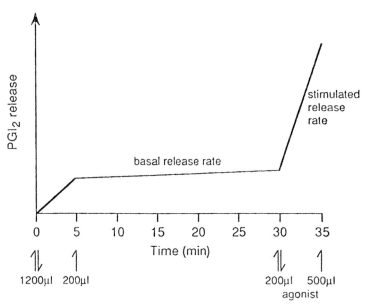

Fig. 3.1. Determination of basal and stimulated PGI_2 release from endothelial cells cultured in 24-well trays. All operations are carried out at $37\,^{\circ}C$. Growth medium is replaced with 1.0 ml of serum-free Hepes-buffered medium for 30 min. Then (at 0 min in this graph) the medium is carefully removed and replaced with 1.2 ml of the same medium. Five min later a 0.2 ml aliquot is removed. Twenty-five min later a further 0.2 ml is carefully removed, to allow the determination of basal PGI_2 release in isolation from the transient release due to physical forces at 0 min, and immediately carefully replaced with 0.2 ml containing an agonist. Five min later a sample (e.g. 0.5 ml) of the medium is removed to determine agonist-stimulated release.

medium makes the system ideal for investigating uptake and/or metabolism of added stimuli (Gordon et al, 1986), but these two factors complicate the interpretation of dose–response experiments.

The relation between PGI_2 synthesis and elevation of $[Ca^{2+}]_i$ has been determined by parallel spectrometric measurements of $[Ca^{2+}]_i$ using suspensions, or better, mono-layers on coverslips of endothelial cells preloaded with a $[Ca^{2+}]$-sensitive ratiometric fluorescent dye such as fura-2 (Hallam et al, 1988). The advent of fluorescent imaging systems capable of resolving spatial and temporal changes in $[Ca^{2+}]_i$ in single cells with high resolution led to the recognition that $[Ca^{2+}]_i$ within individual endothelial cells in culture can oscillate and/or exhibit waves across cells in response to exposure to an agonist such as thrombin or histamine (Jacob, 1991). How this complex behaviour relates to PGI_2 synthesis is not understood, as there is no straightforward method to measure single cell PGI_2 production in real time. An approach that may be successful, although I am not aware that it has been tested for PGI_2, involves quantitation of lysis of neighbouring added red blood cells by antigen antibody complexes, when the medium contains complement and antibody to the secreted mediator. This method has been used, for example, to detect cytokine secreting cells within mixed populations (Lewis et al, 1991). From spectrometric studies of endothelial monolayers it is apparent that under normal conditions mean $[Ca^{2+}]_i$ must be substantially elevated, between five and ten fold above resting levels, to induce PGI_2 synthesis (Fig. 3.2). Thus release occurs predominantly rapidly (within seconds) and transiently (complete within a few minutes) as internal stores of Ca^{2+} are initially translocated to the cytosol; thereafter mean $[Ca^{2+}]_i$ are insufficient to sustain PGI_2 synthesis.

Nitric oxide

The importance of PGI_2 as a vasodilator has been overshadowed (although it should not be ignored) by the explosion of knowledge and interest in NO as a potent endothelium-derived vasodilator and novel biological signalling molecule in several other contexts. PGI_2 and NO act additively as vasodilators and synergistically to block platelet activation (Radomski et al, 1987). First recognized as endothelium-derived

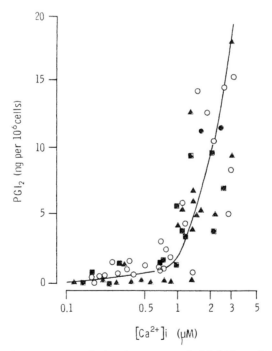

Fig. 3.2. Concentration–response relation between peak $[Ca^{2+}]_i$ and PGI_2 synthesis in human umbilical vein endothelial cells. Experiments were carried out in the absence of added extracellular Ca^{2+}. Identical curves were found when $[Ca^{2+}]_i$ was raised by varying doses of ionomycin (○), ATP (■) or the more potent analogue 2-chloro-ATP (▲). Reproduced with permission from Carter et al (1988) in *British Journal of Pharmacology*, 95, 1181–90.

relaxing factor (EDRF) by Furchgott & Zawadzki (1980), EDRF was subsequently identified as NO, synthesized from arginine, by Palmer et al (1988). The rapid discovery of arginine analogues that selectively inhibit NO synthase not only led to the demonstration that NO is an important endothelium-derived vasodilator contributing to the minute by minute regulation of vascular tone in most vascular beds, and hence of systemic blood pressure, but also provided helpful tools for quantifying NO release in ex vivo or in vitro assay systems (Rees et al, 1990).

NO release from isolated vessels with intact endothelium, or from cultured endothelial cells, can thus be measured by bioassay of the relaxation of a preconstricted, endothelium-denuded vessel, which is exposed to the perfusate from the first vessel or from endothelial cells (Palmer et al, 1988). Relaxation can be estimated when the effects of eicosanoids such as PGI_2 are inhibited with for example indomethacin, and when the production of NO is abolished by arginine analogues such as L-NMMA or L-NAME, and compared with dilatation induced by exogenous NO.

Like PGI_2 release, NO synthesis by endothelial cells is rapid, relatively short-lived, normally requires elevation of $[Ca^{2+}]_i$ (although rises of only two to threefold above resting are probably sufficient) and takes place in response to many of the same agonists that cause PGI_2 production (for a review see Busse & Fleming, 1995). In vivo or in isolated vessels, acetylcholine is an effective agonist for NO synthesis, but endothelial cells in culture do not respond, apparently because of rapid loss of muscarinic receptors. Shear stress is also an important physiological inducer of NO synthesis : in this case changes in $[Ca^{2+}]_i$ are less important than as yet not fully defined protein kinase signalling cascades, which may have common elements with those activated for PGI_2 synthesis, and mechanotransduction via the cell cytoskeleton (Ayajiki et al, 1996; Corson et al, 1996; Hutcheson & Griffith, 1996).

There are several chemical assay techniques to measure NO, or more usually its breakdown products nitrite and nitrate. The simplest colorimetric assay for nitrite, using the Griess reagent, while suitable for detecting the production of NO over several hours from cells such as macrophages containing the inducible isoform of NO synthase, is insufficiently sensitive to detect transient NO release from endothelial cells in response to vasoactive agonists. A fluorimetric variant of this assay, introduced by Misko et al (1993), is, however, straightforward and sufficiently sensitive (detection limit $\cong 10\,nM$) to measure release of NO from endothelial cells in multiwell trays. The chemiluminescent assay originally used by Palmer et al (1988) requires expensive specialised equipment and is less sensitive. NO is efficiently trapped by oxyhaemoglobin, leading to the formation of methaemoglobin, and this reaction forms the basis of an alternative sensitive assay method, in principle capable of monitoring rates of NO release in real time from superfused cells (Kelm et al, 1991). The need for a dual wavelength spectrometer (to measure the difference spectrum between absorption at 401 and 411 nm) and to prepare freshly pure solutions of oxidized haemoglobin have limited its use. More recently, there has been significant progress in the production of sensitive porphyrin-based NO-selective electrodes. While not yet routinely available and still undergoing development it seems likely that this technology will become a preferred method to measure NO release directly from cultured cells: it has already been used successfully by several groups (Guo et al, 1996; Wiemer et al, 1996; Zeng & Quon, 1996; for a review, see Wink et al, 1995).

Perhaps the most widely adopted method at present, however, for detecting NO production by endothelial cells relies on the knowledge that a major target for the action of NO in many cell types (including both smooth muscle cells and endothelial cells themselves) is the soluble guanylyl cyclase enzyme. Hence NO production can be monitored by quantifying changes in cGMP, either within the endothelial cells generating NO, or in a target cell type to which the endothelial cell medium is rapidly transferred (Bogle et al, 1996). Increases in cGMP are usually stabilized by the presence of a phosphodiesterase inhibitor such as IBMX or zaprinast, and levels are measured in lysed cells by specific radio or enzyme immunoassay using commercially available reagents. An example of this, in an experiment is which alterations in arginine transport and NO production in response to bradykinin were measured concomitantly (Bogle et al, 1991), is shown in Fig. 3.3.

There is still increasing interest in the measurement of endothelium-derived NO, because of the accumulating evidence that NO production or its action is impaired at an early stage of atherogenesis (Zeiher et al, 1991), by mechanisms that have yet to be fully understood. These may include dysregulation of agonist-stimulated signal transduction, and/or inactivation of NO by excess production of oxygen-derived free radicals such as superoxide or radicals present on oxidized lipoproteins (for a review see Lüscher & Noll,

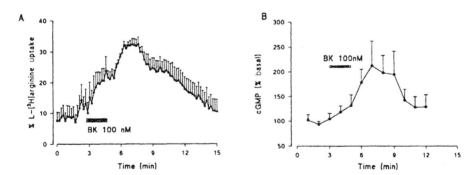

Fig. 3.3. Parallel stimulation of L-arginine influx and NO release from superfused cultures of porcine aortic endothelial cells grown on microcarrier beads, in response to 100 nM bradykinin (BK). (A) shows fractional [^{3}H]arginine uptake from the superfusion medium. (B) Secretion of NO was measured by taking samples of the effluent superfusate each minute and determining their ability to stimulate elevation of cyclic GMP concentrations after 30 s exposure in 2 cm^{2} wells of the kidney epithelial cell line LLC-PK$_1$. The LLC-PK$_1$ cells were pretreated with the phosphodiesterase inhibitor isobutylmethylxanthine (0.5 M for 10 min) and in control experiments it was shown that rises in cGMP induced by the endothelial cell perfusate were blocked by the addition of the NO synthase inhibitor nitro-L-arginine, (100 μM). Reproduced with permission from Bogle et al (1991), in *Biochemical Biophysical Research Communications*, **180**, 926–32.

1995). A further possibility is that arginine transport into endothelial cells is impaired. It was recognized when the biosynthetic pathway for NO was discovered that supply of extracellular arginine could be rate limiting for endothelial NO release (Palmer et al, 1988), and subsequently shown that arginine transport is transiently upregulated by NO-producing agonists (Bogle et al, 1991). The mechanism for enhanced arginine influx is likely to be related to agonist-induced membrane hyperpolarization, although this is not apparently involved in regulating NO biosynthesis.

Hence methods to monitor rapid arginine influx into endothelial cells, which primarily occurs via the cationic y^+ amino acid transporter, are also useful. This can be done routinely by short-term incubation of cells in monolayers with [^{3}H]arginine, or, as in Fig. 3.3, by measuring uptake of arginine by superfused cultures. A variation of this assay can also be used as an indicator of NO production: while NO is being formed, the conversion of added [^{3}H]arginine to [^{3}H]citrulline is significantly enhanced, and measurement of [^{3}H]citrulline, which can be simply separated from [^{3}H]arginine by charge on small disposable Dowex columns, provides an estimate of the fold increase in NO generation when an agonist is added (Bredt & Snyder, 1989).

Endothelium-derived hyperpolarising factor (EDHF)

In several vascular beds in different species, it has been shown that endothelium-dependent vasodilatation can take place, in response to agonists such as acetylcholine, even though eicosanoid and NO production or action are fully inhibited. This phenomenon can be reproduced in bioassay systems where mediators are transferred to an endothelium-denuded vessel, indicating that a further distinct endothelium-derived vasodilator is produced (for a review see Cohen & Vanhoutte, 1995). This factor acts by hyperpolarizing smooth muscle cells, and thus in the absence of its identification it is named EDHF. The factor acts to open K^+ channels in smooth muscle cells, and opinions are divided as to whether EDHF may be a cytochrome P450-dependent metabolite of arachidonic acid. Until EDHF is fully characterized chemically, direct assays will not be possible, and its overall contribution to endothelium-dependent vasodilatation remains uncertain.

Endothelin-1 (ET-1)

ET-1, originally isolated and identified from supernatants of endothelial cell cultures by Yanagisawa et al (1988), is the most potent vasoconstrictor agent yet described. In the few years since its discovery, details of the biosynthetic pathway for the mature bioactive peptide ET-1, via sequential cleavage of preproendothelin and big endothelin, have been elucidated; at least two classes of ET receptors have been identified; and potent and selective synthetic agonists have been designed (for a review see Levin, 1995). There is also increasing evidence that overproduction of ET-1 occurs in a variety of diseases, including coronary heart disease and chronic heart failure (Love et al, 1996; Salomone et al, 1996), and in at least some forms of hypertension (Ergul et al, 1996). Hence there is a need to understand the regulation of ET-1 synthesis and secretion by endothelial cells, which is still not well characterized. As a result of the long duration (many minutes or hours) of pressor action of ET-1 in vivo, and its very low circulating levels in healthy subjects, it seems likely that the main control of ET-1 production is at the level of transcription of preproendothelin mRNA, although control of its formation from big endothelin by endothelin coverting enzyme may also be relevant.

Assay of ET-1 in cell culture supernatants is now relatively straightforward, and commercial radioimmunoasssay kits are available, although several groups had developed their own versions earlier. This required careful choice of immunogen and screening to obtain antibodies that do not cross-react between ET-1 and big endothelin (Corder et al, 1993). A limited range of stimuli has been shown to enhance ET-1 secretion over a period of hours from endothelial cell cultures; these include thrombin, insulin, hypoxia, calcium ionophores within a limited concentration range (high levels inhibit), endotoxin and several inflammatory cytokines (e.g. interleukin 1 (IL-1) or tumour necrosis factor (TNF)) (Yanagisawa et al, 1988; Brunner et al 1994; Bodi et al, 1995; Corder et al, 1995). In most cases these stimuli act predominantly to increase the steady state level of preproendothelin mRNA. There is also apparent cross talk between ET-1 production and NO and PGI_2 production. Inhibition of endogenous NO or PGI_2 synthesis enhances ET-1 release while added exogenous NO or PGI_2 reduces it (Boulanger & Lüscher, 1990; Razandi et al, 1996). Both NO and PGI_2 have been shown to inhibit ET-1 production by cGMP-dependent pathways. Conversely, at low concentrations, ET-1 acting on ETB receptors on endothelial cells stimulates PGI_2 and NO synthesis.

Like NO and PGI_2 synthesis, the level of ET-1 release from endothelial cells is enhanced by physical forces including shear and distension (Macarthur et al, 1994; Wang et al, 1995). Interestingly, Macarthur et al (1994) found that ET-1 release was increased almost immediately (as well as over a longer period) by shear forces and they detected a significant intracellular pool of mature ET-1 (Fig. 3.4), suggesting that there is also a regulated acute release mechanism for ET-1. This is consistent with the finding that infusion of a selective ET receptor antagonist into the human brachial artery in vivo causes rapid vasodilatation (Haynes et al, 1995), and indicates that more work is required to understand the acute ET-1 release process. Recently a modified enzyme immunoassay using chemiluminescent detection, with markedly enhanced sensitivity, has been reported (Iwata et al, 1996), which may facilitate studies of this type.

Control of endothelial monolayer permeability

Increased microvascular (predominantly venular) permeability to macromolecules is a hallmark of the acute inflammatory response. Although a part of the efflux of macromolecules may be due to transcytosis via endothelial vesicles, the mechanisms and regulation of which are poorly understood, there is no doubt that during inflammation the flux is predominantly paracellular and involves the regulated opening of junctional complexes between adjacent endothelial cells (for a review see Michel, 1996). Technically

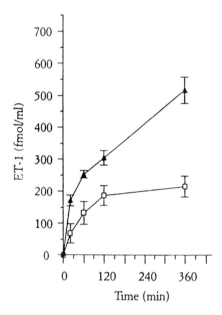

Fig. 3.4. Stretch-induced secretion of ET-1 from bovine aortic endothelial cells. Cells were grown on the flexible surface of 'Petriperm' dishes and either left unstretched (□) or stretched at 0.2 HZ (▲). Reproduced with permission from Macarthur et al (1994), in *Biochemical, Biophysical Research Communications*, **200**, 395–400.

demanding methods have been developed to try to examine in intact vessels in vivo the intracellular signalling pathways involved in increasing permeability (Easton & Fraser, 1994; He & Curry, 1994), but despite acknowledging that the absolute values for permeability of macromolecules across in vitro monolayers of endothelial cells are often considerably higher than in vivo estimates, in vitro experiments have proved invaluable in probing the mechanisms and cellular components involved. Interestingly, considering that most of the earlier in vitro studies used macrovascular endothelial cells rather than the pathophysiologically more relevant microvascular cells, the pathways elucidated (with a few exceptions) are generally applicable.

The basic technique was introduced by Taylor et al (1981) and Shasby et al (1982), and requires the growth of confluent endothelial monolayer on a porous filter surface so that molecular flux across the monolayer can be detected by sampling medium beneath the filter. Various substrates, often precoated with matrix proteins to assist cell adhesion and spreading, have been used but commercially available 'transwell' filter systems are now reproducible and relatively inexpensive. These consist of presterilized polycarbonate membranes with good cell attachment and adequate light transmission properties, set in inserts that drop into standard tissue culture wells. Levels of fluid in the compartment above the monolayer and beneath are equalized to eliminate convective flow, and tracer molecules can be added to and sampled from either compartment. Trans-monolayer electrical resistance (a correlate of hydraulic conductivity) can also be measured. Flux determinations often use radiolabelled or fluorescently tagged macro-molecules such as albumin, or an enzyme (e.g. horseradish peroxide) that can be conveniently quantified by subsequent assay (Fig. 3.5). More complex systems have been designed in which fluid flow over the endothelial monolayer can be introduced : these are usually custom built, but as there is evidence that shear and/or pressure modulates basal permeability values, they may be of value to study the mechanisms involved. Permeability can also be determined rapidly by single pass simultaneous superfusion of several tracers of different size through columns containing endothelial cells cultured on porous microcarrier beads, by an adaptation of the indicator dilution technique (Eaton et al, 1991). While this technique is potentially powerful, in practice it is not straightfor-ward to set up and requires carefully designed protocols, and has not yet been used by many groups.

Numerous transwell studies have provided a general picture of the initial signalling pathways and some of their counter regulators (for reviews see Lum & Malik , 1994; Pearson, 1994). Elevation of $[Ca^{2+}]_i$, in response to classical inflammatory mediators such as histamine, bradykinin or thrombin provides one input signal leading to in-creased permeability. Activation of certain protein kinase C isoforms provides a second. Elevated permeability is reduced by agents that elevate cAMP (including β adrenocep-tor agonists and PGI_2) or cGMP (e.g. NO) (Fig. 3.6; Draijer et al , 1995; Suttorp et al,

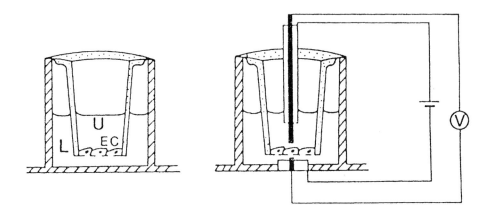

Fig. 3.5. Schematic view of the transwell system for measuring molecular permeability of cultured endothelial cell monolayers. Endothelial cells (EC) are seeded at high density on polycarbonate filters and left for several days to form a tightly confluent monolayer before experiments. L: lower compartment; U: upper compartment. The right hand panel shows the electrodes required to measure transendothelial resistance. Alternating current (50 μA, 1 pulse/min) is passed across the monolayer by two source electrodes 2 cm apart, and two further electrodes 3 mm apart detect the potential difference across the monolayer. Repro-duced with permission from *Thrombosis Research*, **60**, 240–6 by Langeler and van Hinsbergh (1988).

1996), although one distinct exception has been found using rat coronary microvascular endothelial cells, where adenosine or other agents that elevate cAMP *increase* permeability (Hempel et al, 1996). It would also not be surprising to find additional or different mechanisms in the brain microvascular endothelium, where the exceptionally low permeability in vivo forms the blood–brain barrier, and is known to be at least in part maintained by a factor or factors derived from neighbouring glial cells (Rubin et al, 1991).

Reorganization of the cytoskeleton and cellular contraction are involved, as reagents that block actin depolymerization can inhibit agonist-induced increases in permeability (Lum & Malik, 1994). This is almost certainly due to direct links between actin and one or more of the components making up the junctional complexes, notably vinculin, catenins and the homophilic transcellular linking protein, VE-cadherin (for a review see Dejana, 1996). Recent work has implicated tyrosine phosphorylation of one or more of these components as a necessary distal signal to cause increased permeability (Staddon et al, 1995 a, b). Protein phosphatase inhibitors enhance permeability, acting to increase

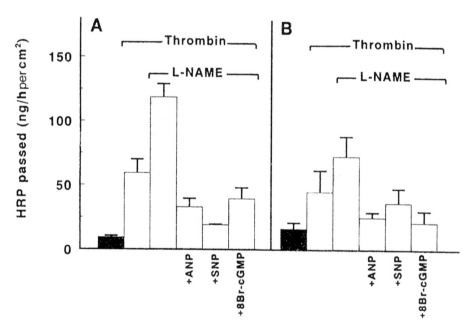

Fig. 3.6. NO acting via cGMP opposes enhanced endothelial monolayer permeability. Passage of horse radish peroxidase (HRP) across transwell filters with monolayers of human aortic (A) or pulmonary artery (B) endothelial cells was increased by thrombin (1 U/ml), and further increased on addition of the NO synthase inhibitor L-NAME (100 μM). These increases were inhibited by agents that elevate cGMP; either atrial natriuretic peptide (ANP; 0.1 μM), sodium nitroprusside (SNP; 100 μM) or 8-Br-cGMP (1 mM). Reproduced with permission from Draijer et al (1995), in *Circulation Research*, **76**, 199–208.

phosphorylation of junctional components or of myosin light chain kinase (required for actin-myosin mediated contraction) (Verin et al, 1995).

Enhanced permeability has also long been recognized to accompany neutrophil adhesion and emigration across the endothelium in vivo (Wedmore & Williams, 1981). How this is achieved is still not fully understood, but in vitro systems provide useful models to dissect the mechanisms involved. H_2O_2 is an effective inducer of increased endothelial permeability; however, although secretion of H_2O_2 by activated neutrophils may facilitate their emigration it is not believed to be necessary for induction of the process. Recent in vitro evidence indicates that β_2 integrin-mediated adhesion of neutrophils to endothelial cells provides a further specific signalling pathway leading to disorganization of the junctional complexes between endothelial cells, and hence enhanced permeability (Del Maschio et al, 1996), although previous studies have shown that under appropriate conditions neutrophil emigration, despite causing increased endothelial $[Ca^{2+}]_i$, need not cause detectable increases in macromolecular permeability (Huang et al, 1993, 1998).

There is a final, more complicated, link between endothelial NO production and permeability in the presence of leukocytes. In both in vivo and in vitro studies NO inhibits neutrophil adhesion to endothelial cells, in addition to reducing enhanced permeability. It is not clear that this involves any direct effect of NO on the neutrophil, and ongoing experiments, particularly by Kubes' group, have implicated the anti-oxidant properties of NO. Leukocyte rolling and adhesion observed by intravital microscopy is enhanced by local mast cell activation and involves local production of superoxide or related free radicals. Endothelium-derived NO, or exogenous NO donors, reduce mast cell activation and local oxidant levels, thus reducing leukocyte adhesion (Gaboury et al, 1996). H_2O_2 sensitive fluorescent dyes (e.g. dihydrorhodamine 123 or dichlorofluorescein) can be used to monitor directly the level of H_2O_2 either extracellularly or, in in vitro studies, intracellularly by preloading cells with lipophilic esterified fluorochrome (Suematsu et al, 1993; Kurose et al, 1995). Fluorescence can then be measured in real time, either by spectrometry or by imaging, as for $[Ca^{2+}]_i$ measurements (Fig. 3.7). Experiments of this type indicate that endothelial cells themselves can produce oxidants, particularly when NO synthesis is inhibited (Niu et al, 1996), although it is likely that the main source is the neutrophils during an inflammatory response. Superoxide anion production by endothelial cells can be measured in vitro by a chemiluminescence assay based on lucigenin (Ohara et al, 1993), a fluorescence assay after loading cells with dihydroethidine (Carter et al, 1994), or less sensitively by spectrometric assay of the superoxide dismutase-inhibitable oxidation of cytochrome C (Holland et al, 1990).

Conclusions

Endothelial cells regulate vascular tone and permeability. Both these processes are vital for the control of healthy vascular homeostasis, and their disturbance contributes to a wide variety of vascular pathologies : therefore knowledge of the molecular pathways

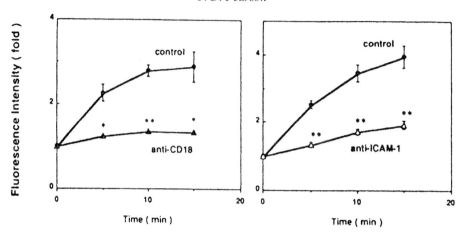

Fig. 3.7. Use of peroxide-sensitive fluorophore to demonstrate stimulation of peroxide levels in cultured bovine carotid artery endothelial cells when exposed to phorbol ester-activated human neutrophil granulocytes. Endothelial cells were preincubated with dichlorofluorescein diacetate ($5\,\mu M$, 30 min) and washed. Fluorescence emission was monitored after addition of neutrophils in the absence (control) or presence (anti-CD18, anti-ICAM-1) of antibodies that block neutrophil adhesion to endothelial cells. These records were obtained from images of 20 individual endothelial cells at each time point. Reproduced with permission from Fujita et al (1994), in *Archives of Biochemistry and Biophysics*, **309**, 62–9.

involved is required for rational approaches to therapy designed, for example, to restore impaired endothelium-dependent vasodilatation or to reduce excessive increases in vascular permeability. The ability to isolate and culture endothelial cells has led directly to significant advances in identifying powerful endothelial mediators of vascular tone, the regulation of their synthesis, the sequential molecular interactions involved in leukocyte adhesion and emigration (not discussed here, but described in Chapter 14), and the signalling pathways modulating paracellular junctional integrity and hence macromolecular permeability across the endothelium. The work described in this chapter provides an introduction and summary to the in vitro methods currently in use to study the secretion of vasoactive mediators by endothelial cells and the measurement of permeability, together with indications of the current questions being asked using these methods, in the hope that it will suggest practical ways for the reader to investigate new questions relating to endothelial cell pathophysiology. This chapter has not reviewed methods to isolate and culture endothelial cells, which can be found elsewhere (Warren, 1990; Hewett & Murray, 1993), but it is relevant to conclude by urging the use, in future, of microvascular cells from specific vascular beds where feasible and appropriate. Despite the functional similarities of cultured endothelial cells from large and small vessels, phenotypic differences related to organ of origin or vessel type exist in vivo and are likely to be at least in part retained in culture.

Acknowledgements

I thank the British Heart Foundation, the Wellcome Trust and the Medical Research Council for their support of the research from our group described in this chapter.

References

Ayajiki, K., Kindermann, M., Hecker, M., Fleming, I. & Busse, R. (1996). Intracellular pH and tyrosine phosphorylation but not calcium determine shear stress-induced nitric oxide production in native endothelial cells. *Circulation Research*, **78**, 750–8.

Bodi, I., Bishopric, N. H., Discher, D. J., Wu, X. & Webster, K. A. (1995). Cell-specificity and signalling pathways of endothelin-1 gene regulation by hypoxia. *Cardiovascular Research*, **30**, 975–84.

Bogle, R. G., Baydoun, A. R., Pearson, J. D. & Mann, G. E. (1996). Regulation of L-arginine transport and nitric oxide release in superfused porcine aortic endothelial cells. *Journal of Physiology*, **490**, 229–41.

Bogle, R. G., Coade, S. B., Moncada, S., Pearson, J. D. & Mann, G. E. (1991). Bradykinin and ATP stimulate L-arginine uptake and nitric oxide release in vascular endothelial cells. *Biochemical and Biophysical Research Communications*, **180**, 926–32.

Boulanger, C. & Lüscher, T. F. (1990). Release of endothelin from the porcine aorta. Inhibition of endothelium-derived nitric oxide. *Journal of Clinical Investigation*, **85**, 587–90.

Bredt, D. S. & Snyder, S. H. (1989). Nitric oxide mediates glutamate-linked enhancement of cGMP levels in the cerebellum. *Proceedings of the National Academy of Sciences of the United States of America*, **86**, 9030–3.

Brunner, F., Stessel, H., Simecek, S., Graier, W. & Kukovetz, W. R. (1994). Effect of intracellular Ca^{2+} concentration on endothelin-1 secretion. *FEBS Letters*, **350**, 33–6.

Busse, R. & Fleming, I. (1995). Regulation and functional consequences of endothelial nitric oxide formation. *Annals of Medicine*, **27**, 331–40.

Carter, T. D. & Pearson, J. D. (1992). Regulation of prostacyclin release in endothelial cells. *News in Physiological Sciences* **7**, 64–9.

Carter, T. D., Hallam, T. J. & Pearson, J. D. (1988). Regulation of P_{2y}-purinoceptor mediated prostacyclin release from human endothelial cells by cytoplasmic calcium concentration. *British Journal of Pharmacology*, **95**, 1181–90.

Carter, W. O., Narayanan, P. K. & Robinson, J. P. (1994). Intracellular hydrogen peroxide and superoxide anion detection in endothelial cells. *Journal of Leukocyte Biology*, **55**, 153–58.

Cohen, R. A. & Vanhoutte, P. M. (1995). Endothelium-dependent hyperpolarization. Beyond nitric oxide and cyclic GMP. *Circulation*, **92**, 3337–49.

Corder, R., Carrier, M., Khan, N., Klemm, P. & Vane J. R. (1995). Cytokine regulation of endothelin-1 release from bovine aortic endothelial cells. *Journal of Cardiovascular Pharmacology*, **26**, S56–S58.

Corder, R., Harrison, V. J., Khan, N., Anggard, E. E. & Vane, J. R. (1993). Effects of phosphoramidon in endothelial cell cultures on the endogenous synthesis of endothelin-1 and on conversion of exogenous big endothelin-1 to endothelin-1. *Journal of Cardiovascular Pharmacology*, **22**, S73–S76.

Corson, M. A., James, N. L., Latta, S. E., Nerem, R. M., Berk, B. C. & Harrison, D. G. (1996). Phosphorylation of endothelial nitric oxide synthase in response to fluid shear stress. *Circulation Research*, **79**, 975–82.

Dejana, E. (1996). Endothelial adherens junctions. Implications in the control of vascular permeability and angiogenesis. *Journal of Clinical Investigation*, **98**, 1949–53.

Del Maschio, A., Zanetti, A., Corada, M., Rival, Y., Ruco, L., Lampugnani, M. G. & Dejana, E. (1996). Polymorphonuclear leukocyte adhesion triggers the disorganisation of endothelial cell-to-cell adherens junctions. *Journal of Cell Biology*, **135**, 479–510.

Draijer, R., Atsma, D. E., van der Laarse, A. & van Hinsbergh, V. W. M. (1995). cGMP and nitric oxide modulate thrombin-induced endothelial permeability: Regulation via different pathways in human aortic and umbilical vein endothelial cells. *Circulation Research*, **76**, 199–208.

Easton, A. S. & Fraser, P. A. (1994). Variable restriction of albumin diffusion across inflamed cerebral microvessels of the anaesthetised rat. *Journal of Physiology*, **475**, 147–57.

Eaton, B. M., Toothhill, V. J., Davies, H. A., Pearson, J. D. & Mann G. E. (1991). Permeability of human venous endothelial cell monolayers perfused in microcarrier cultures: effects of flow rate, thrombin, and cytochalasin D. *Journal of Cellular Physiology*, **149**, 88–99.

Ergul, S., Parish, D. C., Puett, D. & Ergul, A. (1996). Racial differences in plasma endothelin-1 concentrations in individuals with essential hypertension. *Hypertension*, **28**, 652–5.

Frangos, J. A., Eskin, S. G., McIntire, L. V. & Ives, C. L. (1985). Flow effects on prostacyclin production by cultured human endothelial cells. *Science*, **227**, 1477–9.

Fujita, H., Morita, I. & Murota, S. (1994). A possible mechanism for vascular endothelial cell injury elicited by activated leukocytes. A significant involvement of adhesion molecules, CD11/CD18, and ICAM-1. *Archives of Biochemistry and Biophysics*, **309**, 62–9.

Furchgott, R. F. & Zawadski, J. V. (1980). The obligatory role of endothelial cells in the relaxation of arterial smooth muscle by acetylcholine. *Nature*, **288**, 373–6.

Gaboury, J. P., Niu, X. F. & Kubes, P. (1996). Nitric oxide inhibits numerous features of cell-induced inflammation. *Circulation*, **93**, 318–26.

Gordon, E. L., Pearson, J. D. & Slakey, L. L. (1986). The hydrolysis of extracellular adenine nucleotides in cultured endothelial cells from pig aorta: feed-forward inhibition of adenosine production at the cell surface. *Journal of Biological Chemistry* **261**, 15496–504.

Grabowski, E. F., Jaffe, E. A. & Weksler, B. B. (1985). Prostacyclin production by cultured endothelial cell monolayers exposed to step increases in shear stress. *Journal of Laboratory and Clinical Medicine*, **105**, 36–43.

Guo, J. P., Murohara, T., Buerke, M., Scalia, R. & Lefer, A. M. (1996). Direct measurement of nitric oxide release from vascular endothelial cells. *Journal of Applied Physiology*, **81**, 774–9.

Hallam, T. J., Pearson, J. D. & Needham, L. A. (1988). Thrombin-stimulated elevation of human endothelial cell cytoplasmic free calcium concentration causes prostacyclin production. *Biochemical Journal*, **251**, 243–9.

Haynes, W. G., Strachan, F. E. & Webb D. J. (1995). Endothelin ET_A and ET_B receptors cause vasoconstriction of human resistance and capacitance vessels in vivo. *Circulation*, **92**, 357–63.

He, P. & Curry, F. E. (1994). Endothelial cell hyperpolarization increases $[Ca^{2+}]_i$ and venular microvessel permeability. *Journal of Applied Physiology*, **76**, 2288–97.

Hempel, A., Noll, T., Muhs, A. & Piper, H. M. (1996). Functional antagonism between cAMP and cGMP on permeability of coronary endothelial monolayers. *American Journal of Physiology – Heart and Circulatory Physiology*, **270**, H1264–H1271.

Hewett, P. W. & Murray, J. C. (1993). Human microvessel endothelial cells: isolation, culture and characterisation. *In Vitro Cellular and Developmental Biology*, **29A**, 823–30.

Holland, J. A., Pritchard, K. A., Pappolla, M. A., Wolin, M. S., Rogers, N. J. & Stemerman, M. B. (1990). Bradykinin induces superoxide anion release from human endothelial cells. *Journal of Cellular Physiology*, **143**, 21–5.

Huang, A. J., Furie, M. B., Nicolson, S. C., Fischbarg, J., Liebovitch, L. S. & Silverstein, S. C. (1988). Effects of human neutrophil chemotaxis across human endothelial cell monolayers on the permeability of these monolayers to ions and macromolecules. *Journal of Cellular Physiology*, **135**, 355–66.

Huang, A. J., Manning, J. E., Bandak, T. M., Ratau, M. C., Hauser, K. R. & Silverstein, S. C. (1993). Endothelial cell cytosolic free calcium regulates neutrophil migration across monolayers of endothelial cells. *Journal of Cell Biology*, **120**, 1371–80.

Hutcheson, I. R. & Griffith, T. M. (1996). Mechanotransduction through the endothelial cytoskeleton: mediation of flow- but not agonist-induced EDRF release. *British Journal of Pharmacology*, **118**, 720–6.

Iwata, R., Hayashi, T., Nakao, Y., Yamaki, M., Yoshimasa, T., Ito, H. & Saito, Y. (1996). Direct determination of plasma endothelin-1 by chemiluminescence enzyme immunoassay. *Clinical Chemistry*, **42**, 1155–8.

Jacob, R. (1991). Calcium oscillations in endothelial cells. *Cell Calcium*, **12**, 127–34.

Kelm, M., Feelisch, M., Deussen, A., Strauer, B. E. & Schrader, J. (1991). Release of endothelium derived nitric oxide in relation to pressure and flow. *Cardiovascular Research*, **25**, 831–6.

Kurose, I., Wolf, R., Grisham, M. B., Tak Yee, A. W., Specian, R. D. & Granger, D. N. (1995). Microvascular responses to inhibition of nitric oxide production: role of active oxidants. *Circulation Research*, **76** 30–9.

Langeler, E. G. & van Hinsbergh, V. W. M. (1988). Characterisation of an in vitro model to study the permeability of human arterial endothelial cell monolayers. *Thrombosis and Haemostasis*, **60**, 240–6.

Levin, E. R. (1995). Endothelins. *New England Journal of Medicine*, **333**, 356–63.

Lewis, C. E., McCracken, D., Ling, R., Richards, P. S., McCarthy, S. P. & McGee, J. O. D. (1991). Cytokine release by single, immunophenotyped human cells : use of the reverse haemolytic plaque assay. *Immunological Reviews*, **119**, 23–39.

Love, M. P., Haynes, W. G., Gray, G. A., Webb, D. J. & McMurray, J. J. V. (1996). Vasodilator effects of endothelin-converting enzyme inhibition and endothelin ET(A) receptor blockade in chronic heart failure patients treated with ACE inhibitors. *Circulation*, **94**, 2131–7.

Lum, H. & Malik, A. B. (1994). Regulation of vascular endothelial barrier function. *American Journal of Physiology – Lung Cellular and Molecular Physiology*, **267**, L223–L241.

Lüscher, T. F. & Noll, G. (1995). The endothelium as a regulator of vascular tone and growth. In *The Endothelium in Cardiovascular Disease*, ed. T. F. Lüscher, pp. 1–24. Berlin: Springer.

Macarthur, H., Warner, T. D., Wood, E. G., Corder, R. & Vane, J. R. (1994). Endothelin-1 release from endothelial cells in culture is elevated both acutely and chronically by short periods of mechanical stretch. *Biochemical and Biophysical Research Communications*, **200**, 395–400.

MacIntyre, D. E., Pearson, J. D. & Gordon, J. L. (1978). Localisation and stimulation of prostacyclin production in vascular cells. *Nature*, **271**, 549–51.

Michel, C. C. (1996). Transport of macromolecules through microvascular walls. *Cardiovascular Research*, **32**, 644–53.

Misko, T. P., Schilling, R. J., Salvemini, D., Moore, W. M. & Currie, M. G. (1993). A fluorometric assay for the measurement of nitrite in biological samples. *Analytical Biochemistry*, **214**, 11–16.

Moncada, S., Gryglewski, R., Bunting, S. & Vane, J. R. (1976). An enzyme isolated from arteries transforms prostaglandin endoperoxides to an unstable substance that inhibits platelet aggregation. *Nature*, **263**, 663–5.

Niu, X. F., Ibbotson, G. & Kubes, P. (1996). A balance between nitric oxide and oxidants regulates mast cell dependent neutrophil-endothelial cell interactions. *Circulation Research*, **79**, 992–9.

Ohara, Y., Peterson, T. E. & Harrison, D. G. (1993). Hypercholesterolemia increases endothelial superoxide anion production. *Journal of Clinical Investigation*, **91**, 2546–51.

Palmer, R. M. J., Ashton, D. S. & Moncada, S. (1988). Vascular endothelial cells synthesize nitric oxide from L-arginine. *Nature*, **333**, 664–6.

Pearson, J. D. (1994). Endothelial cells: biology and immunopathology. *In: Handbook of Immunopharmacology: The Microcirculation*, ed. S. D. Brain, pp. 9–23. Academic Press.

Pearson, J. D., Slakey, L. L. & Gordon, J. L. (1983). Stimulation of prostaglandin production through purinoceptors on cultured porcine endothelial cells. *Biochemical Journal*, **214**, 273–6.

Radomski, M. W., Palmer, R. M. J. & Moncada, S. (1987). Comparative pharmacology of endothelium-dependent relaxing factor, nitric oxide and prostacyclin in platelets. *British Journal of Pharmacology*, **92**, 181–7.

Razandi, M., Pedram, A., Rubin, T. & Levin, E. R. (1996). PGE_2 and PGI_2 inhibit ET-1 secretion from endothelial cells by stimulating particulate guanylate cyclase. *American Journal of Physiology – Heart and Circulatory Physiology*, **270**, H1342–H1349.

Rees, D. D., Palmer, R. M. J., Schulz, R., Hodson, H. F. & Moncada, S. (1990). Characterisation of three inhibitors of endothelial nitric oxide synthase in vitro and in vivo. *British Journal of Pharmacology*, **101**, 746–52.

Rubin, L. L., Hall, D. E., Porter, S., Barbu, K., Cannon, C., Horner, H. C., Janatpour, M., Liaw, C. W., Manning, K., Morales, J., Tanner, L. I., Tomaselli, K. J. & Bard, F. (1991). A cell culture model of the blood-brain barrier. *Journal of Cell Biology*, **115**, 1725–35.

Salomone, O. A., Elliott, P. M., Calvino, R., Holt, D. & Kaski, J. C. (1996). Plasma immunoreactive endothelin concentration correlates with severity of coronary artery disease in patients with stable angina pectoris and normal ventricular function. *Journal of the American College of Cardiology*, **28**, 14–19.

Shasby, D. M., Shasby S. S., Sulllivan, J.M. & Peach, M. J. (1982). Role of endothelial cell cytoskeleton in control of endothelial permeability. *Circulation Research*, **51**, 657–61.

Staddon, J. M., Herrenknecht, K., Smales, C. & Rubin L. L. (1995a). Evidence that tyrosine phosphorylation may increase tight junction permeability. *Journal of Cell Science*, **108**, 609–19.

Staddon, J. M., Smales, C., Schulze, C., Esch, F. S. & Rubin L. L. (1995b). A p120-related protein (p100), and the cadherin/catenin complex. *Journal of Cell Biology*, **130**, 369–81.

Suematsu, M., Scmid-Schonbein, G. W., Chavez-Chavez, R. H., Yee, T. T., Tamatani, T., Miyasaka, M., Delano, F. A. & Zweifach, B. W. (1993). In vivo visualisation of oxidative changes in microvessels during neutrophil activation. *American Journal of Physiology*, **264**, H881–H891.

Suttorp, N., Hippenstiel, S., Fuhrmann, M., Krull, M. & Podzuweit, T. (1996). Role of nitric oxide and phosphodiesterase isoenzyme II for reduction of endothelial hyperpermeability. *American Journal of Physiology – Cell Physiology*, **270**, C778–C785.

Taylor, R. F., Price, T. H., Schwartz, S. M. & Dale, D. C. (1981). Neutrophil-endothelial cell interactions on endothelial monolayers grown on micropore filters. *Journal of Clinical Investigation*, **67**, 584–7.

Verin, A. D., Patterson, C. E., Day, M. A. & Garcia J. G. N. (1995). Regulation of endothelial cell gap formation and barrier function by myosin-associated phosphatase activities. *American Journal of Physiology – Lung Cellular and Molecular Physiology*, **269**, L99–L108.

Wang, D. L., Wung, B. S., Peng, Y. C. & Wang, J. J. (1995). Mechanical strain increases endothelin-1 gene expression via protein kinase C pathway in human endothelial cells. *Journal of Cellular Physiology*, **163**, 400–6.

Warren, J. B. (ed) (1990). *The Endothelium: An Introduction to Current Research*. New York: Wiley-Liss.

Wedmore, C. V. & Williams, T. J. (1981). Control of vascular permeability by polymorphonuclear leukocyes in inflammation. *Nature*, **289**, 646–50.

Wheeler-Jones ,C. P. D., Houliston, R., May, M. J. & Pearson, J. D. (1996). Inhibition of MAP kinase kinase (MEK) blocks endothelial PGI_2 release but has no effect on von Willebrand factor secretion or E-selectin expression. *FEBS Letters*, **388**, 180–4.

Wiemer, G., Pierchala, B., Mesaros, S., Scholkens, B. A. & Malinski, T. (1996). Direct measurement of nitric oxide release from culutured endothelial cells stimulated by bradykinin or ramiprilat. *Endothelium*, **4**, 119–25.

Wink, D. A., Christodoulou, D., Ho, M., Krishna, M. C., Cook, J. A., Haut, H., Randolph, J. K., Sullivan, M., Coia, G., Murray, R. & Meyer, T. (1995). A discussion of electrochemical techniques for the detection of nitric oxide. *Methods: A Companion to Methods in Enzymology*, **7**, 71–7.

Yanagisawa, M., Kurinara, H., Kimura, S., Tomobe, Y., Kobayashi, M., Miksui, Y., Yazaki, Y., Goto, K. & Masaki, T. (1988). A novel potent vasoconstrictor peptide produced by endothelial cells. *Nature*, **332**, 411–15.

Zeiher, A. M., Drexler, H., Wollschlager, H. & Just, J. N. (1991). Endothelial dysfunction of the coronary microvasculature is associated with impaired coronary blood flow regulation in patients with early atherosclerosis. *Circulation*, **84**, 1984–992.

Zeng, G. & Quon, M. J. (1996). Insulin-stimulated production of nitric oxide is inhibited by Wortmannin: direct measurement in vascular endothelial cells. *Journal of Clinical Investigation*, **98**, 894–8.

4

Contractile mechanisms of vascular smooth muscle

A. D. HUGHES

Introduction

Under physiological circumstances the primary role of differentiated smooth muscle is to generate force to undue contraction. In blood vessels the degree of contraction governs the arterial resistance and venous distensibility. The amount of force produced by a smooth muscle cell therefore needs to be finely regulated by a variety of extracellular factors: both physical and chemical (Somlyo & Somlyo, 1994). Despite the diversity of extracellular contractile stimuli, extensive evidence indicates that a rise in the concentration of free Ca^{2+} ($[Ca^{2+}]_i$) is the predominant *intracellular* signal responsible for activation of the contractile machinery of the cell. This chapter gives an overview of the process of contraction in differentiated vascular smooth muscle: how intracellular $[Ca^{2+}]_i$ is regulated, the role of ion channels in this process and how force is generated and translated through the intracellular structures of the vascular smooth muscle cell into contraction. In some cases events in vascular smooth muscle have been inferred from findings in other smooth muscles, but wherever possible the specific circumstances obtaining in vascular smooth muscle have been described. More comprehensive reviews of specific areas covered are cited at the end of the chapter.

Types of stimulus for contraction and relaxation

Stimuli that act directly on vascular smooth muscle can broadly be grouped into three categories.

Agents acting at G protein-linked receptors

The majority of classical vasoconstrictors such as α-adrenoceptor agonists, angiotensin II, serotonin and vasopressin and vasodilators such as β-adrenoceptor agonists, vasoactive intestinal peptide and calcitonin gene-related peptide act at G protein-linked receptors. This superfamily of receptors possess seven transmembrane domains and as a result of their snake-like appearance are also sometimes known as serpentine receptors. In the interior of the cell these receptors couple to heterotrimeric G proteins which act as transducers linking the ligand receptor complex to a variety of intracellular signals (e.g.

$[Ca^{2+}]_i$ in the case of contractile stimuli, cyclic nucleotides or K channels in the case of relaxant agents). Heterotrimeric G proteins are membrane associated proteins composed of α, β and γ subunits with the α subunit possessing GTP-ase activity (Bourne, 1995). In the absence of receptor activation they exist in an inactive heterotrimeric complex with GDP. The ligand receptor complex acts as a GDP/GTP exchange factor for the α subunit of the heterotrimeric complex promoting formation of a dissociated α subunit•GTP complex and a free $\beta\gamma$ dimer (Fig. 4.1). The α subunit•GTP complex and the $\beta\gamma$ dimer probably remain associated with the cell membrane and there is evidence that both may play signalling roles. Specificity in signalling (i.e. why one agonist increases $[Ca^{2+}]_i$, while another increases cyclic adenosine monophosphate for instance) is probably accomplished by the existence of multiple isoforms of heterotrimeric G proteins (particularly the α subunit) which interact preferentially with particular receptors and effector systems. After signalling activation of the intrinsic GTPase of the α subunit catalyses hydrolysis of GTP to GDP which completes the cycle and results in reformation of the inactive $\alpha\beta\gamma$ heterotrimer•GDP complex.

Growth factors

It is now recognized that vascular growth factors such as platelet-derived growth factor (PDGF) and epidermal growth factor (EGF) can affect tone as well as acting as mitogens

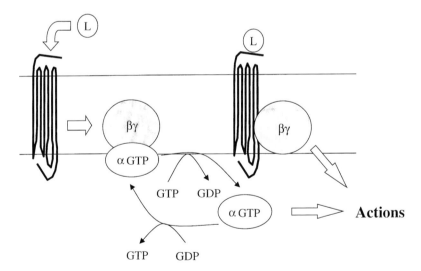

Fig. 4.1. Regulation of heterotrimeric G proteins. Under resting conditions heterotrimeric G proteins exist in the cell membrane in a GDP-bound state. Following stimulation of the receptor by a ligand (L), GDP on the α-subunit is exchanged for GTP and the α-subunit•GTP complex dissociates from the $\beta\gamma$ subunits and both α and $\beta\gamma$ subunits are free to interact with effectors. GTP is then hydrolysed allowing reformation of the GDP-bound inactive heterotrimer.

for vascular smooth muscle cells (Berk & Alexander, 1989). The majority of growth factors act by binding to and inducing dimerization of transmembranous receptors which are intrinsic tyrosine kinases. Dimerization results in trans-autophosphorylation of tyrosine residues in the intracellular domain of the receptor and leads to recruitment and activation of a range of signalling molecules (Schlessinger & Ullrich, 1992). There is increasing evidence that both growth factor-activated, and non-receptor tyrosine kineases (e.g. pp60[src]) play extensive roles in cell physiology not merely restricted to growth. It should be noted that although heterotrimeric G protein-linked receptors and growth factor receptors posses unique signalling characteristics increasing evidence suggests substantial cross-talk between these systems (Daub et al, 1996). It seems likely that boundaries between classical vasoconstrictors and growth factors will become increasingly blurred in the future.

Pressure/tension

The ability of vascular smooth muscle to respond to increased transmural pressure by increased tone was first recognized by Bayliss in 1902. The current view is that wall tension or stress, rather than pressure per se is the stimulus for contraction and that myogenic vasoconstriction and flow- (or endothelial shear stress) dependent vasodilatation may provide the homeostatic background on which other vasoactive agents act. While the myogenic response is a very important determinant of tone, perhaps particularly in the microvasculature, the biochemical mechanisms underlying its transduction are still poorly understood; stretch-induced production of vasoconstrictors or growth factors, stretch sensitivity of ion channels, stretch-dependent activation of signalling enzymes and the sensitivity of cell–cell or cell–matrix interactions to tensile stress are all possible candidates for this role (Osol, 1955).

In addition to those agents that have a direct action on vascular smooth muscle cells many substances influence vascular tone indirectly by having an action via another cell type such as the endothelium, mast cells or nerves supplying the blood vessel.

Regulation of $[Ca^{2+}]_i$

The pivotal role of Ca^{2+} in muscle contraction has been recognized for many years. In smooth muscle increases in $[Ca^{2+}]_i$ may arise from two sources: a net influx of extracellular Ca^{2+} or release of Ca^{2+} from storage sites within the cell (Van Breemen & Saida, 1989). The relative importance of influx or release of stores varies between blood vessels of differing calibre and site of origin as well as depending on the applied stimulus. In the resistance vasculature (i.e. vessels with internal diameters less than 0.5 mm; Mulvany & Aalkjaer, 1990) and microvasculature (arterioles and precapillary vessels) Ca^{2+} entry through voltage-operated calcium channels appears to predominate.

How Ca²⁺ is regulated

Ion channels and membrane potential

Like all cells, the vascular smooth muscle cell maintains a low $[Ca^{2+}]_i$ (approximately 100 nM) in the face of an immense electrochemical gradient (extracellular Ca^{2+} approximately 1.6 mM, membrane potential approximately -60 mV) (Himpens et al, 1992). Despite the powerful Ca^{2+} buffering capacity of the cell, opening of channels permeable to Ca^{2+} ions can cause $[Ca^{2+}]_i$ to rise to near micromolar levels which are sufficient to activate the contractile (and other) processes. There is evidence that $[Ca^{2+}]_i$ is compartmentalized within the cell and that localized increases in $[Ca^{2+}]_i$ may play important roles (Nelson et al, 1995), especially in modulating ion channel activity. The most important channel admitting Ca^{2+} into vascular smooth muscle cells is the voltage-operated calcium channel. As its name implies this channel is primarily regulated by the cell's membrane potential and the likelihood of the channel opening (open probability) increases with depolarization. Consequently the regulation of membrane potential is an important determinant of Ca^{2+} influx in vascular smooth muscle cells.

Ions are not distributed uniformly inside and outside the cell (Fig. 4.2) and their uneven distribution allied to variable permeability to each ion generates an electrical potential (membrane potential) across the cell membrane. Essentially membrane potential in vascular smooth muscle is governed by the distributions and permeabilities to four ions, K^+, Cl^-, Na^+ and Ca^{2+}, with K^+ and Cl^- being the most important under resting conditions.

Measurements of membrane potential, ionic concentrations and ionic permeabilities by radiotracer flux techniques in isolated blood vessels indicate that resting membrane potential is fairly close to that predicted by theory, although some ion pumps such as the Na-K-ATPase also generate electric potentials and may contribute up to 10 mV hyperpolarization under certain circumstances (Hermsmeyer, 1982). Most studies of isolated vascular smooth muscle suggest that the resting membrane potential is approximately

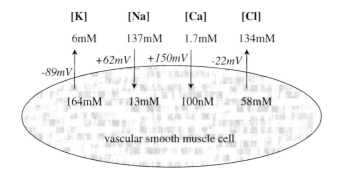

Fig. 4.2. Determinants of membrane potential (E_m). The diagram shows the approximate extracellular and intracellular concentrations and reversal potential (in italics) of the major ionic species governing E_m in vascular smooth muscle cells.

$-60\,\text{mV}$, although *in vivo* vascular smooth muscle cells are likely to be more de-polarized than this (approximately $-40\,\text{mV}$) as a result of 'myogenic' pressure-induced depolarization and prevailing tonic contractile influences such as the sympathetic nervous system and circulating factors. In general vascular smooth muscle cells act as an electrically coupled unit and unlike most excitable cells vascular smooth muscle cells rarely display action potentials, but show graded depolarization to stimuli.

Ion channel types present in vascular smooth muscle

Potassium channels

Changes in the permeability of the cell membrane to K^+ ions (accomplished by opening or closing K channels) are a major mechanism regulating membrane potential and tone in vascular smooth muscle. Four types of K channel are present in vascular smooth muscle: voltage-dependent (K_V) channels, Ca^{2+}-activated (K_{Ca}) channels, inward recti-fier (K_{IR}) channels and ATP-sensitive (K_{ATP}) channels, although their relative import-ance depends on the vascular bed studied. Opening of these channels increases K^+ permeability and induces membrane hyperpolarization. K channel opening probably accounts for the rarity of action potentials recorded from vascular smooth muscle cells. K channels are a major target for physiological regulators of membrane potential in vascular smooth muscle (Brayden & Nelson, 1992; Nelson & Quayle, 1995). Many vasodilators (e.g. β-adrenoceptor agonists, calcitonin-gene related peptide, nitric oxide), either directly or by elevating cyclic nucleotides, increase the open probability of K channels such as the K_{Ca} or K_{ATP} channel. Recent evidence also implicates the K_{Ca} channel in modulating myogenic tone at least in some blood vessels. Additionally a number of therapeutically important vasoactive drugs act at K channels, such as minoxidil, nicorandil or cromakalim which open K_{ATP} channels, and thiazide diuretics which open K_{Ca} channels (Table 4.1).

Chloride channels

In contrast to many cell types Cl^- permeability is an important influence on membrane potential in vascular smooth muscle cells (Amedee et al, 1990). The non-passive distribu-tion of Cl^- (i.e. not in accordance with electrochemical equilibrium) allied to the relatively high conductance to Cl^- of the vascular smooth muscle cell membrane accounts in part for membrane potential being significantly different from the reversal potential for K^+ ions (E_K). Unlike skeletal muscle, Cl^- is actively concentrated inside the vascular smooth muscle cell probably as a result of the activity of the Na–K–Cl cotransporter and HCO_3^-/Cl^- exchange and the distribution of Cl^- across the cell membrane establishes a Cl^- equilibrium potential of approximately $-25\,\text{mV}$. The major Cl channel in vascular smooth muscle appears to be the Ca^{2+}-activated Cl channel (Pacaud et al, 1992; Klockner, 1993). This small conductance channel is opening by increases in $[Ca^{2+}]_i$ and appears to play a large role in the responses of some blood

Table 4.1. *Ion channels in vascular smooth muscle*

Channel	Physiological role	Opener	Inhibitor/blocker
Potassium channels			
K_V	Regulation of membrane potential Hypoxic pulmonary vasoconstriction	Depolarization	4-aminopyridine, quinidine, phenylcyclidine, tedisamil, tetraethylammonium
K_{IR}	Resting membrane potential K^+-induced dilatation	Depolarization	Ba^{2+}
K_{Ca}	Myogenic tone 'Brake' on agonist-induced depolarization	$[Ca^{2+}]_i$ Depolarization Thiazides NS004	Charybdotoxin, iberiotoxin
K_{ATP}	Metabolic regulation of tone Reactive hypertaemia Autoregulation Endotoxic shock	$[ATP]_I$ Cromakalim, diazoxide, minoxidil, nicorandil, pinacidil, RP-49356	Sulphonylureas, U-37883A, Ba^{2+}
Chloride channels			
Cl	Agonist-induced depolarization	$[Ca^{2+}]_i$	Niflumic acid, stilbenes (e.g. DIDS, SITS), frusemide
Cation channels			
ROC	Agonist-induced depolarization	G protein-linked receptors	Inorganic cations (e.g. Ni^{2+}, Gd^{3+})
Ca^{2+}-activated	?	$[Ca^{2+}]_i$	
Calcium channels			
L-type	Myogenic tone Agonist-induced calcium entry.	Depolarization, Dihydropyridine agonists (e.g. Bay K8644a).	Dihydropyridine antagonists, phenylalkylamines, benzothiazepines.
T-type	?	Depolarization	Mibefradil

vessels to contractile stimuli. A number of relatively non-selective blockers of this channel have been described but in general much remains to be learned about the biophysics, physiological role and regulation of this channel.

Sodium channels

There is little evidence that tetrodotoxin-sensitive Na^+ selective ion channels such as those found in neurons or cardiac myocytes contribute to membrane potential in vascular smooth muscle cells; however relatively non-selective channels permeable to mono- and divalent cations (see below) may contribute to increased Na^+ permeability following activation of vascular smooth muscle cells by contractile stimuli.

Calcium channels and cation channels

The voltage-operated L-type calcium channel is a major route of Ca^{2+} entry in vascular smooth muscle and the ability of drugs such as amlodipine and verapamil to block this channel account for their vasodilator actions. At resting membrane potentials (approximately $-60\,mV$) few L-type channels are open, nevertheless even this low level of opening allows some Ca^{2+} entry (Gollasch et al, 1992). At more depolarized potentials (less than $-50\,mV$) more channels open and Ca^{2+} enters the cell along its electrochemical gradient. Another sort of voltage-operated calcium channel which is opened a less depolarized potentials, the T-type channel, has also been demonstrated in isolated vascular smooth muscle cells though the physiological significance of this channel is uncertain. Recently a selective blocker of T-type channels, mibefradil has been described. This agent lowers blood pressure and the role of T channels in vascular smooth muscle is likely to be an important topic of future studies. The smooth muscle L-type channel is closely related to the cardiac L-type channel and shows a lesser degree of homology with the skeletal muscle channel. It is sensitive to dihydropyridines (e.g. nifedipine), phenylalkylamines (e.g. verapamil) and benzothiazepines (e.g. diltiazem) and although most of the differences in the actions of calcium channels antagonists on the vasculature as opposed to the heart reflect the different membrane potential of the cells there is evidence that some L-type channel blockers act selectively on the vasculature. The L-type channel is also a major target for physiological modulation and many vasoactive agents affect the opening of this channel directly, as well as influencing opening indirectly through effects on membrane potential (Hughes, 1995). In contrast to cardiac L-type channels, cAMP or agents that elevate cAMP generally inhibit the opening of smooth muscle L-type calcium channels. In contrast vasoconstrictors such as noradrenaline, serotonin, angiotensin II or platelet-derived growth factors increase L-type channel opening. The biochemical mechanism of this effect is uncertain but protein kinase C (PKC) or pp60[src] have been proposed as possible mediators.

Voltage-operated calcium channels are not the only route by which Ca^{2+} can enter the vascular smooth muscle cell. Ca^{2+} can also enter the vascular smooth muscle through non-selective cation channels. Unlike voltage-operated calcium channels which are highly selective for Ca^{2+} over monovalent cations such as Na^+ or K^+, cation channels show limited selectivity for divalent over monovalent cations. Two types of cation channel have been described in vascular smooth muscle: those linked to vasoconstrictor agonists, termed receptor-operated channels (ROC) and those opened as a result of a rise in $[Ca^{2+}]_i$: Ca^{2+}-activated cation channels. The physiological role of the latter is uncertain, however the opening of ROCs following vasoconstrictor activation is an important mechanism of Ca^{2+} entry and depolarization in some vascular smooth muscle.

Intracellular calcium stores

Although release of Ca^{2+} from intracellular stores appears to play a diminished role in smaller blood vessels the intracellular store is not unimportant. There is evidence that even in small arteries release of Ca^{2+} from the stores is crucial for some responses, for example those evoked by brief neural activation. In addition the intracellular store may modulate the consequences of Ca^{2+} entry by influencing the Ca^{2+} buffering properties of the cell. According to this model, termed the superficial buffer barrier by Van Breemen et al. (1995), the intracellular store acts as a Ca^{2+} uptake site in the vicinity of the cell membrane so limiting access of incoming Ca^{2+} to the contractile machinery located nearer the cell interior. The permeability of the store will therefore modulate the extent to which Ca^{2+} entering the cell will cause contraction and also influence the level of Ca^{2+} in the region of the plasma membrane which in turn may affect ion channel opening (Moore et al, 1993; Etter et al, 1994). The effective permeability of the intracellular store is determined by uptake into and efflux from sites in the endoplasmic (sarcoplasmic) reticulum. Uptake into the store is via a Ca^{2+} ATPase probably of the SERCA 2 subtype. Activity of this pump is regulated by phospholamban which inhibits the pump in its dephosphorylated state. Phosphorylation of phospholamban by cyclic adenosine 3,5-monophosphate (cAMP)-dependent protein kinase, cyclic guanosine 3,5-monophosphate (cGMP)-dependent protein kinase, Ca^{2+}-calmodulin-dependent protein kinase II or protein kinase C (PKC) results in activation of the pump and is one mechanism accounting for the relaxant actions of cyclic nucleotides. The endoplasmic reticulum Ca^{2+} ATPase can also be blocked irreversibly by thapsigargin and reversibly by cyclopiazonic acid. Efflux from the store into the cytoplasm is through Ca^{2+}-selective ion channels located in the sarcoplasmic reticulum. Two types of channel have been described in smooth muscle: inositol 1,4,5-trisphosphate (IP_3)-sensitive channels (IP_3R) and ryanodine-sensitive channels (RyR) and there is evidence that these may be localized to particular regions within the cell. IP_3R has been isolated from aortic smooth muscle and is a glycoprotein consisting of a single polypeptide chain resembling a four armed pinwheel. The channel is believed to be formed from these four subunits and opens following binding of IP_3 (K_d approximately 2 nM). The IP_3R has been reported to be phosphorylated by cGMP-dependent protein kinase. IP_3 itself is produced as a result of agonist activation of phospholipase C (PLC) which hydrolyses the minor membrane lipid phosphatidylinositol 4,5 bisphosphate (PIP_2) to IP_3 and diacylglycerol (DAG). A number of isoforms of phospholipase C have been described, but at present the identity of the PLC mediating agonist-induced effects in vascular smooth muscle is uncertain. PLC-β has generally been assumed to be responsible on the basis of findings in non-vascular cells: however some recent studies have failed to demonstrate PLC-β isoforms in vascular smooth muscle. Possibly novel β isoforms or other isotypes such as PLC-γ or PLC-δ are involved. IP_3 is probably the major signal for store release in vascular smooth muscle and in contrast to intestinal smooth muscle or cardiac muscle the physiological role of the RyR is uncertain. The channel is sensitive to Ca^{2+}, adenine nucleotides, Mg^{2+} and pH and in cardiac or intestinal smooth muscle it is involved in Ca^{2+}-induced Ca^{2+} release from the intracellular store, hence contributing to the establishment of Ca^{2+} waves within the cell. As yet, evidence for Ca^{2+}-induced Ca^{2+} release in vascular smooth muscle is inconclusive; however, opening of this channel also accounts for the ability of caffeine to release Ca^{2+} from the intracellular store and transiently contract vascular smooth muscle.

Calcium efflux: Ca-ATPase, Na–Ca exchange

Vascular smooth muscle also extrudes Ca^{2+} into the extracellular medium through the action of Ca^{2+} pumps in the cell membrane (Himpens et al, 1995). Both the plasma membrane Ca-ATPase (PMCA) and the Na^+/Ca^{2+} exchanger (McCarron *et al*, 1994) contribute to this process. The affinity of PMCA for Ca^{2+} is increased by calmodulin (CaM) and by cAMP or cGMP-dependent kinases. In general this is the major efflux pathway for Ca^{2+} in vascular smooth muscle cells. The importance of the Na^+/Ca^{2+} exchanger to overall Ca^{2+} homeostasis in vascular smooth muscle cells is disputed but it may make a major contribution in some tissues (e.g. swine carotid artery). Moreover it appears to be distributed in particular membrane regions in the smooth muscle cell along with the Na^+/K^+ ATPase and to exert an important influence on local $[Ca^{2+}]_i$ in the vicinity of the cell membrane and hence Ca^{2+}-sensitive ion channel activity, Ca^{2+} release from the endoplasmic reticulum, and membrane potential.

Force generation in smooth muscle

Before going on to discuss how a rise in $[Ca^{2+}]_i$ causes force generation the structural elements of the differentiated smooth muscle cell need to be considered as these provide the structural framework on which the contractile elements exert force.

Ultrastructure of the contractile apparatus in smooth muscle

Unlike cardiac and skeletal muscle the organization of the contractile apparatus in smooth muscle is not well defined (Bagby, 1986; Small, 1995). Ultrastructural studies show filamentous structures in the cytoplasm of smooth muscle cells but these lack the regular geometric arrangement seen in striated muscle, hence the smooth appearance of the cell. This should not be taken to mean that the contractile machinery is disorganized but that the 3-diminensional pattern is probably more complex than in striated muscle (Fig. 4.3). The contractile machinery in vascular smooth muscle cells is largely made up of actin (thin filaments) and myosin (thick filaments) (Fig. 4.4). Thin filament (actin-associated) proteins (e.g. caldesmon, calponin) are also present and may play a modulatory role in the contractile process.

It is thought that thin filaments occupy distinct domains within the smooth muscle cell, some being directly involved in the contractile process (contractile domains) and others serving a cytoskeletal function (structural domains). Differences in actin-associated proteins are consistent with this proposal (Table 4.2). In addition to thick and thin filaments, when actin and myosin are removed from the cell a cytoskeletal network of

Table 4.2. *Domains in smooth muscle*

DOMAIN	Antibody positive to
Contractile	Actin
	Myosin
	Tropomyosin
	Caldesmon
Structural	Actin
	Desmin
	Filamin
	Tropomyosin

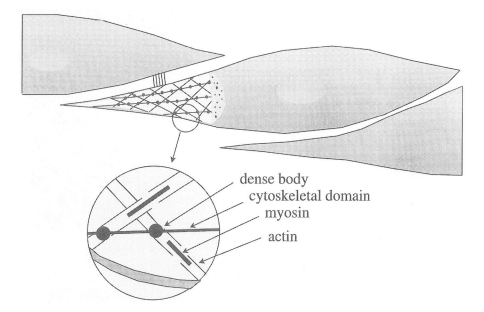

Fig. 4.3. The structural organization of the smooth muscle cell. A schematic depiction of the organization of filaments in a vascular smooth muscle cell. Filaments are organized into distinct structural (cytoskeletal) and contractile domains which interconnect via dense bodies. Modified from Small (1995).

intermediate filaments remains. The major component of these intermediate filament is desmin, though they also contain many other proteins. The cytoskeleton probably couples the contractile machinery to the cell membrane (and hence to other cells and the extracellular matrix), but is not believed to be otherwise involved in contraction, except to limit overextension or excessive shortening of the cell. The connection between the contractile machinery and the cytoskeleton occurs at cytoplasmic dense bodies, α-actinin-rich ovoid structures which are distributed in the cytoplasm in a regular 3-dimensional pattern. It has been speculated that filamin, an actin-associated protein involved in actin polymerization may be an important regulator of the linkage between the cytoskeleton and the contractile machinery. The cytoskeleton also attaches to the cell membrane and makes connection with the extracellular matrix or other cells via specialized junctional regions known as adherens junctions or membrane dense plaques. In chicken gizzard smooth muscle these attachment regions appear as submembraneous dense plaques around separated by similar sized caveolae running along the cell's long axis giving the appearance of longitudinal ribs. Adherens junctions contain a number of specialized proteins including vinculin, paxillin and tensin, which are also present in focal adhesions seen in cultured cells. These proteins are involved in attaching the cytoskeleton to other transmembraneous proteins which couple the cells to other cells (cadherins) or to extracellular matrix proteins (integrins) and may also play signalling roles.

Force generation: actin myosin interaction

The process of contraction is essentially similar in smooth, cardiac and skeletal muscle (Cross, 1989; Stull et al, 1991; Allen & Walsh, 1994). Actin and myosin are motor elements powering contraction (Fig. 4.3) and contraction occurs by a sliding filament action (Fig. 4.5). The contractile process, however, in smooth muscle differs in a number of important ways from that in cardiac and skeletal muscle (Table 4.3).

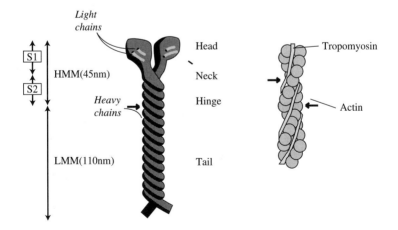

Fig. 4.4. Actin and myosin. Myosin consists of two heavy chain subunits (approximately 230 kDa) and two pairs of light chains (LC_{20} and LC_{17}). Actin exists in monomeric (G) or polymerized (F) forms: an actin filament consisting of a 'double string of beads' in combination with tropomyosin is shown. Each actin molecule usually contains one molecule of ATP and one Ca^{2+} ion. Multiple isoforms of actin exist the α isoform is predominantly found in vascular smooth muscle.

Table 4.3. *Comparison of smooth and skeletal muscle*

Smooth	Skeletal (striated)
Coordinate activity	Individual recruitment of cells
Inefficient	Highly efficient
Direct activation by Ca^{2+} plays no physiological role	Direct activation by Ca^{2+}
Regulator/graded mechanism	On-off mechanism
Low energy (1% skeletal muscle) requirement for sustained force	High energy requirement for sustained force

How increased $[Ca^{2+}]_i$ initiates contraction

The rise in $[Ca^{2+}]_i$ brings about contraction not by directly activating the actin–myosin interaction but through activation of a signal cascade. The first step in this pathway is activation of calmodulin. Calmodulin (CaM) is a widely distributed intracellular protein (17 kDa) that possesses high affinity for Ca^{2+} ions. One molecule of calmodulin binds four molecules of Ca^{2+} via a domain known as the EF hand domain, a domain common in a number of Ca^{2+}-binding proteins. This results in a conformational change in CaM exposing hydrophobic sites which interact with target molecules (Fig. 4.6).

In this way $(Ca^{2+})_4$CaM activates a number of cellular enzymes notably myosin light chain kinase (MLCK). MLCK is a serine/threonine kinase which shows a number of

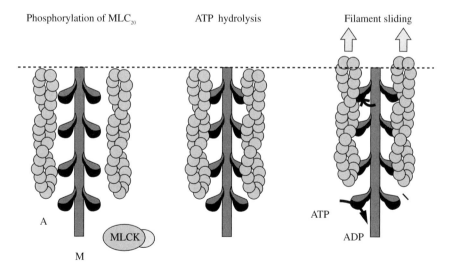

Fig. 4.5. The sliding filament hypothesis. Schematic representation of the process by which force generation occurs as a result in a change in conformation of the myosin head (power stroke) bringing about relative movement between myosin and actin.

structural similarities to other serine/threonine kinases, e.g. 3'5'-cyclic AMP-dependent kinase, calmodulin-dependent kinase II. There are multiple isoforms of MLCK which can be broadly classified into two groups: skeletal muscle and smooth muscle isoforms, the latter group being more substrate specific. Unlike in cardiac and skeletal muscle where Ca^{2+} directly activates the actin–myosin interaction, MLCK is necessary for Ca^{2+} to activate contraction in smooth muscle. Consequently the response to activation in smooth muscle is slow (almost equal to 500 ms) and graded. In the absence of $(Ca^{2+})_4CaM$, MLCK is inactive. This may be because part of MLCK has considerable homology with myosin and effectively acts as pseudosubstrate inhibitor. $(Ca^{2+})_4CaM$ releases this inhibition and allows MLCK to interact with myosin (Figs 4.6 and 4.7).

The $(Ca^{2+})_4CaM\bullet MLCK$ ternary complex catalyses the phosphorylation of myosin at serine 19 on each of the two 20 kDa myosin light chains (MLC_{20}). Phosphorylation at both sites on MLC_{20} is necessary before Mg^{2+}-ATPase activity can increase and actin–myosin crossbridge cycling occur (Fig. 4.7).

Sensitization of the contractile machinery to $[Ca^{2+}]_i$

While there is little doubt that a rise in $[Ca^{2+}]_i$ is the primary signal for contraction in smooth muscle the amount of force generated by the contractile machinery can also be modulated by altering the sensitivity of the contractile machinery to the change in $[Ca^{2+}]_i$ (Katsuyama & Morgan, 1993). Such sensitization is likely to play a significant part in regulating tonic vascular smooth muscle activity and may account for agonist-induced modulation of myogenic tone. Early studies showing that stimulants such as noradrenaline increased tone following depolarization with potassium were originally

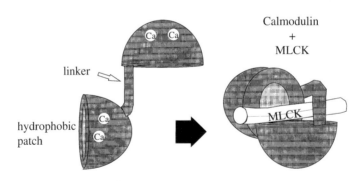

After Kretsinger 1993

Fig. 4.6. Activation of calmodulin (CaM) and its interaction with myosin light chain kinase (MLCK). CaM binds four molecules of Ca^{2+} which results in exposure of hydrophobic regions of the CaM molecule allowing it to bind to MLCK. The image of CaM was obtained from the Protein Data Bank at Brookhaven National Laboratories, USA and visualized using RasMol V2.6 (Roger Sayle, Glaxo Wellcome Research and Development, Stevenage, Hertfordshire, UK). After Kretsinger (1993).

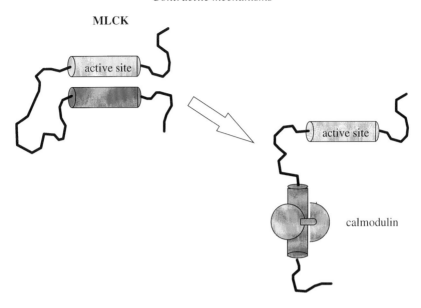

Fig. 4.7. Activation of myosin light chain kinase (MLCK). In the absence of active cal-modulin $((Ca^{2+})_4CaM)$ MLCK is inactive due to an inhibitory interaction between a myosin-like pseudosubstrate region of MLCK and the active site. $(Ca^{2+})_4CaM$ releases this autoinhibition, probably by binding to the pseudosubstrate inhibitory region.

interpreted as indicating receptor-linked influx of Ca^{2+}, over and above that induced by depolarization. With the advent of photometric and fluorescent techniques for the measurement of intracellular Ca^{2+}, however, it has become evident that increases in tone following addition of a contractile agonist to depolarized vessels can occur without any detectable increase in $[Ca^{2+}]_i$. More detailed studies of intact arteries have shown that in general the ratio of force $[Ca^{2+}]_i$ is higher during contractions induced by receptor agonists than in those induced by depolarization by high potassium. Other work has also shown that such agonists induce a greater degree of myosin light chain phosphorylation for a given Ca^{2+} level than potassium depolarization, indicating that this effect of agonists involves an increase in effective Ca^{2+} sensitivity of MLC_{20} phosphorylation.

In contrast, agents which relax vascular smooth muscle may reduce sensitivity of the contractile machinery to Ca^{2+} possibly due to the action of cyclic nucleotides, cAMP and cGMP. cAMP has been reported to increase MLCK phosphorylation, and there-fore it was proposed that this would inhibit MLCK activity, accounting for its relaxant action. While such an effect can be observed following using pharmacological levels of cAMP, with more physiological levels such as those achieved following β-adrenoceptor-induced relaxation there is no change in the $(Ca^{2+})_4CaM$ activation properties of MLCK and the current view is that β- adrenoceptor-induced relaxation of smooth muscle does not involve a change in the K_{CaM} for MLCK. At present how cyclic nucleotides influence Ca^{2+} sensitivity is unclear.

In addition to agonist-induced modulation of Ca^{2+} sensitivity, there is evidence that differences in phasic (e.g. guinea pig ileum) and tonic smooth muscles (e.g. pulmonary artery) may arise through intrinsic differences in sensitivity to Ca^{2+}. Recent work by our group has suggested that constitutive differences in Ca^{2+} sensitivity may also contribute to the differing propensity of blood vessels from different sites to display myogenic activity.

Biochemical mechanisms of sensitization

The biochemical basis of both intrinsic and agonist-activated differences in Ca^{2+} sensitivity is unclear. Work in skinned smooth muscle, using techniques which irreversibly permeabilize the smooth muscle cell but preserve receptor coupling, has replicated the increases in Ca^{2+} sensitivity seen with contractile agonists. Moreover, a number of studies have shown that this effect can be mimicked by application of AlF_4^- or GTP-γ-S, or and blocked by GDP-β-S, non-hydrolysable analogues of GTP and GDP, respectively. In general such findings have been interpreted as indicating that agonist-induced sensitization of vascular smooth muscle occurs by a mechanism involving heterotrimeric G proteins. While the effects of non-hydrolysable analogues of guanine nucleotides are consistent with a role for heterotrimeric G proteins in mediating vasoconstrictor-induced increases in Ca^{2+} sensitivity, it should be noted that there are other members of the GTPase superfamily which may also be affected by nonhydrolysable GTP/GDP analogues in vascular smooth muscle, and as will be discussed below it is possible that other members of the GTPase superfamily participate in the contractile process.

At present there are several hypotheses regarding which second messenger(s) are responsible for agonist-induced sensitization of contraction.

Phospholipase C and protein kinase C

As discussed above many vasoconstrictor receptors induce activation of phospholipase C. In addition to generating IP_3 the DAG which is released by the action of PLC acts as an activator of protein kinase C (PKC), causing its translocation from the cytoplasm to the cell membrane. A number of studies have demonstrated that phorbol esters, tumour-promoting agents which activate PKC, cause an increase in the Ca^{2+}-sensitivity of the contractile machinery (Walsh et al, 1994. Until recently this was widely considered to be the mechanism by which agonists linked to phospholipase C caused the increase in Ca^{2+}-sensitivity; however this view has come into question. Phorbol esters are relatively unphysiological activators of protein kinase C (Wilkinson & Hallam, 1994) and there is increasing doubt about the relevance of their action to physiological activation of the enzyme. Although phorbol esters do increase Ca^{2+} sensitivity their effects are slow (of the order of 30 min), whereas the effects of agonists are rapid (within minutes). Similarly, measurements of PKC translocation have not shown close relations between the degree of translocation and force production for some agonists. Other studies also indicate that the temporal relation between agonist-induced rises in tension and the physiologically produced diacylglycerols is poor in vascular smooth muscle and some agonist cause sensitization despite failing to induce detectable rises in DAG. Furthermore, although myosin is a target for PKC-catalysed phosphorylation it appears that, unlike the action of MLCK, phosphorylation at PKC-susceptible sites is inhibitory. PKC can also induce phosphorylation of MLCK in vitro, but there is little evidence that this process is of physiological significance, and studies comparing MLCK phosphorylation by agonists and K^+ show similar levels of phosphorylation at the key site A. Furthermore, the effects of agonists and GTP-γ-S on Ca^{2+} release and increased Ca^{2+} sensitivity can be dissociated, suggesting that phospholipase C activation is not necessary for sensitization to occur. Other problems centre on putative antagonists of PKC. Many of these agents such as the isoquinolines and staurosporine are now known to be non-selective and to exert inhibitory effects on a range of important signal transduction systems. The results of many early studies which interpreted findings with these agents relatively uncritically therefore require reappraisal. More recently studies with putatively more selective PKC inhibitors (calphostin C and K-252b) or downregulation experiments using prolonged exposures to phorbol esters have failed to inhibit agonist-induced sensitization or had only small effects on agonist-induced tone in smooth muscle. This is not to exclude PKC from playing a role in agonist-induced sensitization, and the ever increasing number of isoforms of PKC being discovered opens new possibilities within this field; nevertheless, the role of PKC in agonist-induced sensitization is still an unresolved question.

Protein phosphatases

Protein phosphatases oppose the influence of kinases as they catalyse the dephosphorylation of cellular proteins. Despite the evidence that the phosphatase activity generally exceeds kinase activity until recently most work has focused on the modulation of MLCK or some other kinase in the contractile process. Control of dephosphorylation of myosin by phosphatases is now attracting increasing attention as a potential regulatory site of action for drugs influencing smooth muscle tone.

There are four classes of serine/threonine phosphatases (PP) in eukaryotic cells: type 1, 2A, 2B and 2C. In cardiac muscle type PP-2A probably represents the major soluble myosin phosphatase activity and in bovine aortic smooth muscle it has been proposed that myosin dephosphorylation is catalysed by multiple PP belonging to the type 2A class. Consistent with this proposal, it has been reported that the addition of exogenous PP-2A causes relaxation of skinned fibres from porcine carotid artery; however PP-1 also binds to contractile proteins in skeletal and cardiac muscles and dephosphorylates myosin light chain *in vitro* and a PP-1 termed smooth muscle myosin phosphatase has recently been isolated and is reported to be relatively specific for myosin. Myosin phosphatase is a trimeric protein consisting of a 37 kDa catalytic subunit in combination with a 20 kDa subunit and a 130 kDa myosin binding subunit which may be regulated by a monomeric small G protein (rho) via rho-dependent kinase. Results of studies with selective inhiabitors, calyculin A and okadaic acid, are consistent with a role for PP-1 in the physiological regulation of tone as calyculin A (non-selective) is more effective than okadaic acid (type 2A selective) in eliciting a contraction in smooth muscle fibres.

Somlyo and colleagues have suggested that heterotrimeric G proteins linked to receptors for contractile stimulants increase tone in part by influencing the activity of myosin light chain phosphatase. They have reported that norepinephrine and GTP-γ-S increase MLC_{20} phosphorylation in skinned smooth muscle in the presence of ML-9, a putative inhibitor of MLCK. G protein-dependent production of arachidonic acid has been proposed to mediate this effect.

Ras proteins: rho regulation of Ca^{2+}-sensitivity

As mentioned above G proteins are not the only GTPases present in smooth muscle which have signalling roles. Smooth muscle also contains abundant monomeric small G proteins approximately 21 kDa proteins belonging to the ras superfamily. Of these smg p21/rap and rho appear to be the dominant forms in vascular smooth muscle. Like heterotrimeric G proteins these GTPases may exist in GDP-bound (inactive) or GTP-bound (active) states. Interconversion of these states is controlled by three types of regulatory proteins: guanine-nucleotide-exchange factors (GEF) such as Sos1, guanine-nucleotide-dissociation inhibitors (GDI) and GTPase-activating proteins (GAPs) (Fig. 4.8).

GEF promote replacement of GDP with GTP, while GDI inhibit this process and probably also inhibit the interaction of ras proteins with GAP for ras (Fig. 4.8). Under resting conditions the majority of small G proteins are believed to be present in the cytosol in inactive form complexed to GDI. GAPs accelerate hydrolysis of GTP to GDP by small G proteins and may therefore inhibit their activity. It is also possible that GAPs also act as effectors for small G proteins, though recently a number of other effectors for ras proteins such as enzymes in the phosphoinositide pathway (e.g. phosphatidylinositol 3-kinase) and a novel group of serine/threonine kinases have been described, including one which modulates myosin phosphatase activity. Overall this regulatory system bears a number of schematic similarities to heterotrimeric G proteins (e.g. Fig. 4.1; where receptors act as GDP-GTP exchange factors). The precise details of the regulation of the ras family is only beginning to be understood and as yet the roles of these and related GTPases in smooth muscle is ill defined. Work in non-muscle cells has suggested that rho is an important regulator of the cytoskeleton and actin polymerization (Symons, 1995). Growth factors which activate membrane associated tyrosine kinases are known to activate ras, and also cause contraction of vascular smooth muscle. Recent work in smooth muscle has indicated that botulinum ADP-ribosyltransferase C3 (C3) and EDIN exoenzyme of *Staphylococcus aureus* (both of which ADP-ribosylate Asn41 in the effector domain of rho) inhibits GTP-γ-S sensitization of saponin skinned smooth muscle. Recently a rho-associated kinase has been reported to phosphorylate the 130 kDa

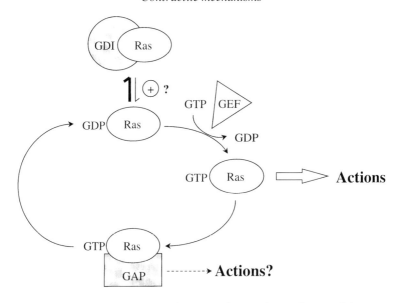

Fig. 4.8. Regulation of ras-like monomeric G proteins. Under resting conditions ras-related GTPases largely exist as a cytoplasmic complex with a GDP-dissociation inhibitor (GDI). Following stimulation ras is released from the GDI by an unknown process and probably translocates to a lipid membrane. The action of a GDP-GTP exchange factor (GEF) promotes release of GDP and GDP is replaced by GTP. GTP-ras is the active signalling molecule. GTPase-activating proteins (GAP) stimulate ras-induced hydrolysis of GTP resulting in formation of inactive GDP-ras which then is complexed with GDI completing the cycle.

myosin binding subunit of myosin phosphatase resulting in inhibition of activity. This provides a plausible mechanism for rho-induced increases in $[Ca^{2+}]_i$ sensitivity. It is also possible that the effects of inhibition of rho reflect actions on the cytoskeleton such as disruption of the links between the contractile machinery and the cytoskeleton at cytoplasmic dense bodies, though at present this possibility has not been investigated.

How agonists linked to G proteins might link into activation of ras or rho is uncertain. There is evidence that the $\beta\gamma$ subunit of some heterotrimeric G proteins can activate ras family members, although whether this mechanism also extends to rho is unknown. Alternatively a number of G protein linked agonists such as angiotensin II and endothelin have been reported to induce tyrosine phosphorylation of cell proteins probably by activating the non-receptor tyrosine kinase pp60[c-src], which could then induce activation of rho.

Actin-associated proteins: caldesmon and calponin

Two actin-associated proteins, caldesmon and calponin, are possible regulators of the actin–myosin interaction and could contribute to sensitization phenomena in vascular smooth muscle (Marston, 1995). Caldesmon is a 87 kDa protein which binds to actin and inhibits actin–myosin ATPase activity. In skinned smooth muscle caldesmon has been reported to shift the relation between MLC_{20} phosphorylation and force in a rightward direction (desensitization) and in permeabilized vascular smooth muscle cells displacement of caldesmon from actin by a peptide analogue caused contraction. The interaction between caldesmon and actin may be regulated by phosphorylation and recently mitogen-activated protein (MAP) kinase has been reported to phosphorylate caldesmon in vitro. MAP kinase is known to be activated in response to both growth factors and contractile agonists and could therefore link activation to sensitization of the contractile machinery.

Calponin is another putative modulator of actin–myosin activity. Calponin is a 34 kDa protein specifically found in smooth muscle in association with actin and tropomyosin, it also blocks actin-stimulated myosin ATPase activity and this action is inhibited by phosphorylation of calponin. Calmodulin-dependent protein kinase and PKC can phosphorylate calponin in vitro, though whether these represent physiological actions of these enzyme remains uncertain.

Tonic contraction and the 'latch' hypothesis

How smooth muscle maintains prolonged (tonic) contraction remains a complex and somewhat unresolved question. In addition to processes modulating the Ca^{2+} sensitivity of myosin LC_{20} phosphorylation there is evidence that vascular smooth muscle can maintain force in the face of low levels of myosin LC_{20} phosphorylation. This process bears some similarities to the 'catch state' described in mollusc muscles, consequently it has been termed a 'latch state' in smooth muscle. The biochemical mechanism of this effect is uncertain, but a kinetic model involving the existence of a dephosphorylated, attached cross-bridge termed a 'latch bridge' has been proposed by Murphy and collegues (Hai & Murphy, 1992).

Conclusions

The generation of arterial tone is a complex and highly regulated process. Many of the basic features and some of the modulators of the contractile process in vascular smooth muscle are now reasonably well understood, nevertheless there are a number of deficits in our knowledge. Hopefully future studies will provide better understanding of the relations between vascular smooth muscle structure and function; in particular precisely how the biochemical processes activated during contraction and relaxation are translated into force generation and the precise role of actin and actin-related proteins in this process. In addition the discovery that novel signalling molecules such as tyrosine phosphorylated proteins, ras-related monomeric G proteins, members of the MAP kinase pathway and phosphatases may play important, if as yet undefined, roles in contraction should ensure that there will be many new developments in this field in the near future.

References

The references cited below are in no way intended to be comprehensive. A number of key reviews and original papers are listed as a starting point.

Allen, B. G. & Walsh, M. P. (1994). The biochemical basis of the regulation of smooth muscle contraction. *TIBS*, **19**, 362–8.

Amedee T., Benham, C. D., Bolton, T. B., Byrne, N.G. & Large, W. A. (1990). Potassium, chloride and non-selective cation conductances opened by noradrenaline in rabbit ear artery cells. *J Physiol Lond*, **423**, 551–68.

Bagby, R. (1986). Towards a comprehensive three-dimensional model of the contractile system of vertebrate smooth muscle cells. *Int Rev Cytol*, **105**, 67–128.

Berk, B. C. & Alexander, R. W. (1989). Vasoactive effects of growth factors. *Biochem Pharmacol*, **38**, 219–25.

Bourne, H. R. (1995). GTPases: a family of molecular switches and clocks. *Philos Trans R Soc Lond B Biol Sci*, **349**, 283–9.

Brayden, J. E. & Nelson, M. T. (1992). Regulation of arterial tone by activation of calcium-dependent potassium channels. *Science*, **256**, 532–5.

Cross, R. A. Smooth Operators. The molecular mechanics of smooth muscle contraction. Bioessays 1989; **11**, 18–21.

Daub, H., Weiss, F. U., Wallasch, C. & Ullrich, A. (1996). Role of transactivation of the EGF receptor in signalling by G-protein-coupled receptors. *Nature*, **379**, 557–60.

Etter, E. F., Kuhn, M. A. & Fay, F. S. (1994). Detection of changes in near-membrane Ca^{2+} concentration using a novel membrane-associated Ca^{2+} indicator. *J Biol Chem*, **269**, 1041–9.

Gollasch, M., Hescheler, J., Quayle, J. M., Patlak, J. B. & Nelson, M. T. (1992). Single calcium channel currents of arterial smooth made at physiological calcium concentrations. *Am. J. Physiol.* **263**, 2948–52.

Hai, C. M. & Murphy, R. A. (1992). Adenosine 5'-triphosphate consumption by smooth muscle as predicted by the coupled four-state crossbridge model. *Biophys J*, **61**, 530–41.

Hermsmeyer, K. (1982). Electrogenic ion pumps and other determinants of membrane potential in vascular smooth muscle. *Physiologist*, **25**, 454–465.

Himpens, B., Missiaen, L. & Casteels, R. (1995). Ca^{2+} homeostasis in vascular smooth muscle. *J Vasc Res*, **32**, 207–19.

Hughes, A. D. (1995). Calcium channels in vascular smooth muscle cells. *J Vasc Res*, **32**, 353–70.

Katsuyama, H. & Morgan, K. G. (1993). Mechanisms of Ca^{2+}-independent contraction in single permeabilized ferret aorta cells. *Circ Res*, **72**,: 651–7.

Klockner, U. (1993). Intracellular calcium ions activate a low-conductance chloride channel in smooth-muscle cells isolated from human mesenteric artery. *Pflüger's Arch*, **424**, 231–7.

McCarron, J. G., Walsh, J. V. Jr & Fay, F. S. (1994). Sodium/calcium exchange regulates cytoplasmic calcium in smooth muscle. *Pflügers Arch*, **426**, 199–205.

Marston, S. (1995). Ca^{2+}-dependent protein switches in actomyosin based contractile systems. *Int J Biochem Cell Biol*, **27**, 97–108.

Moore, E. D., Etter, E. F., Philipson, K. D., Carrington, W.A., Fogarty, K.E., Lifshitz, L.M. & Fay, F. S. (1993). Coupling of the Na^+/Ca^{2+} exchanger, Na^+/K^+ pump and sarcoplasmic reticulum in smooth muscle. *Nature*, **365**, 657–60.

Mulvany, M. J. & Aalkjaer, C. (1990). Structure and function of small arteries. *Physiol Rev*, **70**, 921–61.

Nelson, M. T., Cheng, H., Rubart, M., Santana, L. F., Bonev, A. D., Knot, H. J, & Lederer,

W. J. (1995). Relaxation of arterial smooth muscle by calcium sparks. *Science*, **270**, 633–7.

Nelson, M. T. & Quayle, J. M. (1995). Physiological roles and properties of potassium channels in arterial smooth muscle. *Am J Physiol*, **268**, C799–C822.

Osol G. (1995). Mechanotransduction by vascular smooth muscle. *J Vasc Res*, **32**, 275–92.

Pacaud, P., Loirand, G., Gregoire, G., Mironneau, C. & Mironneau, J. (1992). Calcium-dependence of the calcium-activated chloride current in smooth muscle cells of rat portal vein. *Pflüger's, Arch*, **421**, 125–30.

Schlessinger, J. & Ulrich, A. (1992). Growth factor signaling by receptor tyrosine kinases. *Neuron*, **9**, 383–91.

Small, J. V. (1995). Structure–function relationships in smooth muscle: the missing links. *Bioessays*, **17**, 785–92.

Somlyo, A. P. & Somlyo, A. V. (1995). Signal transduction and regulation in smooth muscle. *Nature*, **372**, 231–6.

Stull, J. T., Gallagher, P. J., Herring, B. P. & Kamm, K. E. (1991). Vascular smooth muscle contractile elements. *Hypertension*, **17**, 723–32.

Symons, M. (1996). Rho family GTPases: the cytoskeleton and beyond. *TIBS*, **21**, 178–81.

Van Breemen, C., Chen, Q. & Laher, I. (1995). Superficial buffer barrier function of smooth muscle sarcoplasmic reticulum. *TIPS*, **16**, 98–104.

Van Breemen, C. & Saida, K. (1989). Cellular mechanisms regulating Ca^{2+} in smooth muscle. *Ann Rev Physiol*, **51**, 315–29.

Walsh, M. P., Andrea, J. E., Allen, B. G., Clement Chomienne, O., Collins, E. M. & Morgan, K. G. (1994). Smooth muscle protein kinase C. *Can J Physiol Pharmacol*, **72**, 1392–9.

Wilkinson, S. E. & Hallam, T. J. (1994). Protein kinase C: is its pivotal role in cellular activation over-stated. *TIPS*, **15**, 53–7.

5

Neurohumoral regulation of vascular tone

K. M. McCULLOCH and J. C. McGRATH

Introduction

The primary factors that govern blood flow to organs and tissues are perfusion pressure and the overall calibre of the small resistance arteries and arterioles, which together constitute the major resistance to blood flow. The total active tension of the vascular smooth muscle in a segment of blood vessel wall, i.e. vascular tone, is influenced in vivo by numerous factors which fall into two broad categories: (1) local or intrinsic control, which includes physical forces, myogenic responses, tissue metabolites and autocoids; and (b) extrinsic neurohumoral regulation, which involves the action of autonomic nerves and circulating endocrine secretions.

Since the start of the twentieth century the investigation of neurohumoral regulation of vascular tone has centred essentially on the action of catecholamines and acetylcholine (ACh) released from perivascular nerves, and catecholamine release from the adrenal medulla into the bloodstream (Bevan, et al, 1980; Burnstock, 1980). It took half a century before it was appreciated that these were actually the issues involved, transmission being referred to by the pseudo-physiological terms 'Sympathetic' and 'Parasympathetic' linked to the differing anatomical makeup of the two sets of non-somatic efferent nerves. Since the first decade of the century, adrenaline was known and chemically identified in the adrenal gland and blocking drugs were available, which turned out to be antagonists of adrenergic and cholinergic receptors. Identification of the neurotransmitters was delayed because identifying the very small concentrations of ACh and noradrenaline (NA) in the body took much longer. At that point the explanation of much research fell into place on the basis of the reciprocal 'noradrenergic' and 'cholinergic' systems.

Throughout the autonomic nervous system it was clear that there were many examples where blocking drugs were ineffective and thus transmission could not be explained by adrenergic or cholinergic hypotheses. The recent history of the study of neurohumoral vascular modulation has involved the gradual accrual of information on the roles of further endogenous substances as methods have emerged for their identification and localization, and as antagonists of their actions have been developed. This gives rise to a constantly emerging picture of the importance of nonadrenergic, non-cholinergic (NANC) components of the autonomic nervous system with a number of peptides, purines and amines being implicated in neurohumoral control of the vasculature.

Hormonal control of the vasculature

Several endocrine secretions have been shown to have acute effects on the vasculature (Fig. 5.1). It is a general belief that, in the normal subject, hormones are of less importance for short-term regulation of vascular tone in comparison to neural control. Circulating hormones and vasoactive agents modulate vascular tone via direct action on receptors present on the vascular smooth muscle cells, or via indirect action at the vascular endothelium, which releases secondary vasoconstrictor or vasodilator factors. As a result of such actions on both vascular and endothelial receptors, certain humoral agents may have either vasoconstrictor or vasodilator properties depending on species, preparation studied and the level of preexisting vascular tone. Care is therefore required

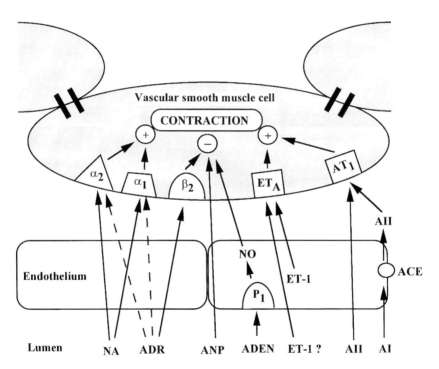

Fig. 5.1. Schematic representation demonstrating some of the important humoral regulators of vascular tone. Agents may act directly upon receptors present on the vascular smooth muscle, or through interaction with receptors present on the vascular endothelium to cause the release of a secondary factor. NA: noradrenaline; ADR: adrenaline; ADEN: adenosine; ANP: atrial natriuretic peptide; AII: angiotensin II; AI: angiotensin I; ACE: angiotensin converting enzyme; ET-1: endothelin-1 (? role of circulating ET-1 in control of vascular tone still controversial); NO: nitric oxide; P_1: P_1-purinoceptors; α_1, α_2 and β_2: α_1-, α_2-, and β_2-adrenoceptors; ET_A: endothelin type A receptor; AT_1: angiotensin type 1 receptor. Dashed lines indicate actions of adrenaline at high concentrations. For additional explanation see text.

in interpreting experimental data and in comprehending the past literature, as emphasis alters both with knowledge and with fashion.

The overall control of vascular tone centres on the regulation of intracellular free calcium ion concentration ($[Ca^{2+}]_i$) in the smooth muscle cells. Constriction occurs when $[Ca^{2+}]_i$ is increased. Therefore by altering the levels of $[Ca^{2+}]_i$, neurotransmitters and circulating hormones regulate the contractile state and hence vascular tone. They accomplish this through activation of cell surface receptors, which use various signalling cascades to release Ca^{2+} from intracellular stores, allow entry of extracellular Ca^{2+} by opening channels present in the cell membrane or do both. As time goes on, the number of endogenous substances appreciated to possess such actions, increases.

Localization of vascular receptors

A feature common to both neural and humoral control of the vasculature is the action of many vasoactive agents upon specific receptor proteins present on neuronal, smooth muscle and endothelial cells. Although receptors can be studied biochemically in purified preparations their cytological localization is an area of weakness, which can lead to erroneous interpretation. The reason for this, which has not yet been overcome, is that the cells of blood vessels are heterogeneous and collecting enough homogeneous tissue, particularly of the more interesting small resistance vessels, is technically very difficult. For example, if a substance changes the tone of a blood vessel, the first assumption is that it is acting on smooth muscle; however, it may be acting indirectly. The most striking example of this is the demonstration by Furchgott in the late 1970s that ACh relaxes vascular smooth muscle by releasing a vasodilator substance (later identified as nitric oxide (NO)) from the endothelium (Furchgott & Zawadzski, 1980). Rubbing off the endothelium abolished the response and attaching a piece of tissue with endothelium restored the response. Such multiple sites of action continue to bedevil this area of research. For example, there is great current interest in peptides such as vasopressin and endothelin which, with other examples, apparently act on both endothelium and smooth muscle. Going back even further, the ability of α-blockers to increase the nerve-induced release of NA was attributed for 40 years to an effect on the smooth muscle α-adrenoceptors, until the concept of pre-junctional (α_2) receptors was introduced in the 1970s. The localization and biology of vascular receptors thus remains an area awaiting full exploitation.

This has been facilitated by the development of novel and highly selective agonists and antagonists for vascular receptors, initially for functional studies, but of great value in the past 20 years for the study of isolated receptors and now, potentially, to provide visual evidence for the presence of receptors in blood vessels. First described by Young & Kumar in 1979, autoradiography has been used for localization of a wide range of receptors using reversibly binding radioligands. Spatial localization is not, however, high enough to be of value in small blood vessels. More recently, fluorescent receptor ligands have been developed, for example BODIPY fluorescent prazosin which can be utilized for visualisation of receptors in live vascular preparations (McGrath et al, 1996).

This has much higher spatial resolution than autoradiography, has the potential to localize receptors at the subcellular level and as it is a dynamic process can be used in pharmacological competition experiments to measure receptor binding properties.

At present, however, assumptions about the site of action of vascular modulators rely almost entirely on interpretation of functional responses.

Catecholamines

The major circulating hormones which play a role in the control of vascular tone are the catecholamines, NA and adrenaline. Central sympathetic activity will not only activate perivascular nerves but also stimulates exocrine secretions from the adrenal glands. The secretion of adrenaline, and to a lesser extent NA (in humans the adrenal gland contains approximately four times more adrenaline than NA, but this varies widely with species) is initiated by the release of ACh from preganglionic sympathetic nerve fibres. ACh depolarizes the adrenal medullary cells via nicotinic receptors facilitating Ca^{2+} entry into the cells and triggers the secretory process. The plasma levels of adrenaline and NA are 0.1–0.5 nM and 0.5–3.0 nM, respectively, at rest, with the higher levels of plasma NA arising from 'spillage' from the tonic activity of sympathetic perivascular nerves, rather than adrenal gland secretion. Experiments using electrical stimulation of the splanchnic nerve have shown that the relative amounts of NA and adrenaline released from the adrenal medulla depend on the pattern of stimulation (Bloom et al, 1988). Circulating NA is cleared as it passes through certain vascular beds, predominantly the pulmonary vasculature, and is also filtered in the kidney and excreted in the urine.

Adrenergic receptors have been classified into four main groups α_1, α_2, β_1, and β_2. In blood vessels the main adrenoceptors are of the α_1 and α_2 subtypes with β_2-adrenoceptors found mainly in coronary, cerebral and skeletal vascular smooth muscle. The vascular actions of circulating NA and adrenaline can have similar or differing effects depending on the vascular bed studied. In general these catecholamines mediate vasoconstriction via activation of α_1- and possibly α_2-adrenoceptors. The differing effects of the two major catecholamines is most apparent when studied *in vivo*. Intra-venous administration of NA produces sustained increases in systemic vascular resis-tance due to the activation of α-adrenoceptors. The administration of adrenaline has a less dramatic effect due to the compound being more efficacious on β_2-adrenoceptors in coronary, skeletal and cerebral vessels. At high concentrations adrenaline also evokes vasoconstriction through activation of α-adrenoceptors.

Although both α_1- and α_2-adrenoceptor mediated pressor responses could be clearly demonstrated in whole animals (McGrath et al, 1989), initially there were very few examples of α_2-adrenoceptor mediated contractions in vitro. It was found that by raising vascular tone in some preparations responses to α_2-adrenoceptor agonists could be uncovered showing facilitatory actions between vasoconstrictor agonists (for examples see MacLean & McGrath, 1990; Dunn et al, 1991).

Attenuation of the effects of catecholamines or strategies to prevent their release from nerves have long been issues for therapeutic intervention to reduce vasoconstriction and hence to lower blood pressure. Non-specific α-blockers were introduced from the 1950s and the first selective α_1-blocker, prazosin, was introduced in the 1970s.

Angiotensins

Angiotensin II is a circulating octapeptide with powerful vasoconstrictor properties. Its production is initiated by the enzyme renin, which cleaves the precursor angiotensinogen which is present in the plasma, to produce the peptide angiotensin I. The angiotensin I is then modified by angiotensin converting enzyme (ACE) present on the surface of endothelial cells to form angiotensin II, a process which takes place predominantly in the lungs. Angiotensin II elicits vasoconstriction by direct action of AT_1 receptors present on the vascular smooth muscle (Fig. 5.1) but will also act in vivo to enhance NA release from the sympathetic nerve fibres (Fig. 5.2). Angiotensin I also produces vasoconstriction being approximately 10–100 fold less potent than angiotensin II, and the actions of angiotensin I depends upon its cleavage into angiotensin II locally by the ACE present on the vascular endothelium (Fig. 5.3); in vivo this can involve a rise in plasma levels of angiotensin II but the importance of local conversion can be demonstrated by the blockade of the vasoconstrictor effects of angiotensin I by ACE inhibitors even in vitro in isolated blood vessels.

A knowledge of the importance of angiotensins in vascular control was greatly accelerated by the development of ACE inhibitors from the late 1970s and of angiotensin receptor antagonists in the late 1980s, resulting in the rapid spread of such agents in treating cardiovascular disease in the 1990s.

Vasopressin

Vasopressin is a peptide produced by the magnocellular neurons in the supraoptic and paraventricular nuclei of the hypothalamus and secreted from the posterior lobe of the pituitary gland. The secretion of vasopressin is regulated partly by hypothalamic cells sensitive to tissue fluid osmolarity and partly by cardiovascular pressure receptors. The cardiovascular effects of vasopressin are profound vasoconstriction in most tissues (Fig. 5.3), and it remains the most potent known endogenous vasoconstrictor. In contrast, cerebral and coronary vessels respond to vasopressin with an endothelium-derived relaxing factor (EDRF)-mediated vasodilatation. Assessment of vasopressin's importance relative to other agents in the physiological control of the vasculature has been held up by the lack of potent and selective antagonists. This is an area of current interest.

Endothelin

The endothelium-derived peptide endothelin-1 (ET-1) has been suggested to play a role in the maintenance of systemic vascular tone. This was demonstrated by Haynes & Webb (1994), whereby infusion of the ET_A receptor antagonist BQ-123 into the brachial artery of normal human subjects caused progressive forearm vasodilatation and an

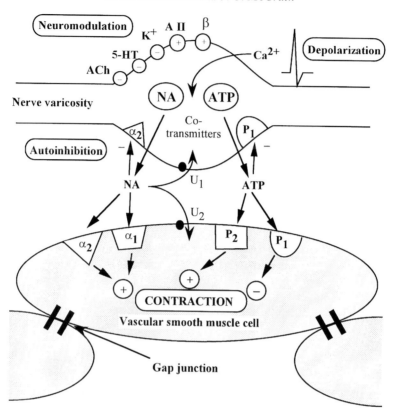

Fig. 5.2. Schematic representation of neural regulation of vasular tone by the two main neurotransmitters NA and ATP, which are released from some perivascular nerves as cotransmitters. Main points: (1) NA and ATP released from the varicosity act upon receptors present on the vascular smooth muscle cells initiating the mechanical response. (2) Autoinhibition: released NA and ATP can act prejunctionally to inhibit further transmitter release. (3) Neuromodulation: certain factors can inhibit (−) or enhance (+) transmitter release from the sympathetic nerve terminals, some examples of which are demonstrated. NA: noradrenaline; ATP: adenosine 5′ triphosphate; ACh: acetylcholine; 5-HT: 5-hydroxytryptamine; K^+: potassium ion; AII: angiotensin II; α_1, α_2 and β: α_1-, α_2-, and β-adrenoceptors; P_1 and P_2: P_1- and P_2-purinoceptors; U_1: uptake$_1$; U_2: uptake$_2$. For additional explanation see text.

increase in blood flow. Although this suggests the presence of endogenous ET-1 induced tone under normal physiological conditions, it is unclear whether plasma ET-1 levels are sufficiently high to act in an endocrine fashion; therefore the actions of ET-1 may be paracrine or autocrine in nature.

Endothelin was discovered in the 1980s and antagonists of its receptors have been developed during the early 1990s leading to rapidly accruing knowledge of its physiological and possible pathophysiological significance. There is a technical problem to its

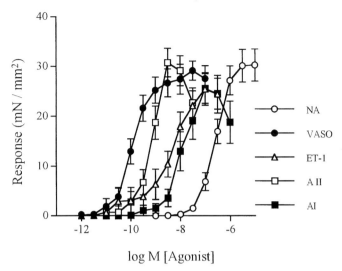

Fig. 5.3. Cumulative concentration responses curves to vasoconstrictor agents in rabbit cutaneous arteries (250 μm i.d.) mounted on Mulvany wire myograph indicating the broad range of potencies of vasoactive agents. NA: noradrenaline; VASO: vasopressin; ET-1: endothelin-1; AII: angiotensin II; AI: angiotensin I. After Macmillan et al (1996) with permission.

accurate pharmacological analysis as its contractile effect on vascular smooth muscle is essentially irreversible.

Atrial natriuretic peptide

Atrial natriuretic peptide (ANP), an amino acid peptide produced by specialized my-ocytes in the atria, has been shown to have vasodilator actions in some blood vessel preparations and vascular beds (Januszewicz, 1995). This peptide is secreted in response to increased cardiac filling pressures and mediates vasodilatation via direct action in the vascular smooth muscle, stimulating particulate guanylate cyclase activity leading to elevation of intracellular cyclic guanosine monophosphate levels. Study of its role awaits good antagonists but its levels can now be followed by radioimmunoassay. Recent work shows that a rise in its level is an early indication of heart failure and this is likely to lead to increased emphasis on studying its actions.

Purines

Circulating purines may play a role in controlling vascular tone. Purinoceptors have been subdivided into two main classes, P_1 and P_2, both of which may be present in the vasculature (Fig. 5.1 and 5.2). In general adenosine dilates most blood vessels by direct activation of P_1-purinoceptors present on the vascular smooth muscle or through endothelial release of nitric oxide (NO), although in some it may mediate vasoconstriction through indirect release of 5-hydroxytryptamine (5-HT) or angiotensin II. Adenosine triphosphate (ATP) has also been shown to mediate vasodilatation via activation of P_2-purinoceptors present on the vascular endothelium, activation of which releases the vasodilator NO. There is a long-standing literature on the study of the vascular effects of purines. Clarification of much of the controversy within this awaits good selective antagonists. Study of purinoceptors at the molecular biological level is a topic currently of great interest so developments may well follow.

Vascular nerves and neurotransmitters

The localisation of vascular nerves can be shown readily by electron microscopy but knowledge of the particular nerve type tends to rely on either a method for conversion of the neurotransmitter into something visible (NA can be converted to a fluorescent analogue), which is limited to a few compounds, or on immunocytochemistry, which depends on the specificity of the antibodies, and again is limited in practice to few examples. This limitation has been a major factor in many controversies in this field. For example, the ubiquity of ATP and the impossibility of demonstrating it satisfactorily by cytochemistry, long delayed its acceptance as a neurotransmitter by the scientific community. On the other hand the localization in blood vessels, in nerve-like structures, of antibodies to various peptides such as calcitonin-gene related peptide (CGRP) and neuropeptide Y (NPY) was a stimulus to their study as putative transmitters long before any useful pharmacological analysis was possible.

Localisation of vascular nerves

It has been observed histologically in a number of blood vessel preparations that the structure and degree of autonomic innervation of the vasculature varies with the size and the location of the blood vessel studied. Most large elastic arteries are sparsely innervated, but as the size of the vessel decreases the innervation density increases, with small arteries and large arterioles being richly innervated. Terminal arterioles are poorly innervated and are probably controlled by intrinsic mechanisms, chiefly tissue metabolites. Blood vessels may be innovated by up to three major classes of neurons; most common are the sympathetic vasoconstrictor neurons, with sympathetic or parasympathetic vasodilator neurons and peripheral fibres of small diameter sensory neurons less commonly observed. The postganglionic nerve fibres supplying blood vessels are unmyelinated and form a plexus of branching terminal axons (Fig. 5.4). In most blood vessels, the nerve plexus is situated in the outer adventitial layer with axons running along the adventitial–medial border (Devine & Simpson, 1967). There are some exceptions, for example in venous preparations, where axons have been reported to ramify the outer two or three layers of smooth muscle cells in the tunica media. Terminal axons widen at regular intervals into varicosities ($1-2\,\mu$m diameter) separated by intervaricose regions ($0.1-0.3\,\mu$m diameter) (Burnstock, 1986). Ultrastructural examination using

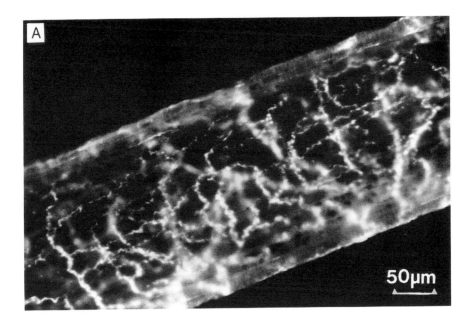

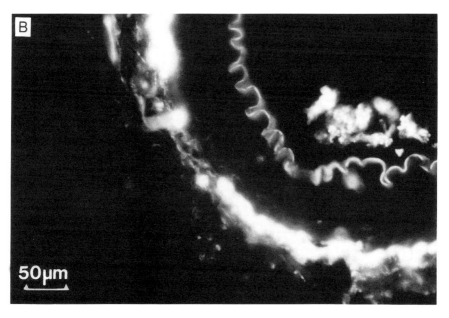

Fig. 5.4. (a) Segment of rabbit anterior cerebral artery stained using glyoxylic acid condensation technique in which axons containing catecholamines fluoresce when illuminated with UV light. The nerve fibres can be seen to form a branching varicose network around the vessel. Bar: 50 μm. (b) Cross-section of rabbit cutaneous artery stained using Falck technique, in which adrenergic nerve terminals display fluorescence when illuminated with UV light. Nerve fibres are restricted to the outer adventitial layer and do not penetrate the medial smooth muscle layer. The internal elastic lamina clearly visible due to the autofluorescent nature of elastic tissue. Bar: 50 μm.

electron microscopy and freeze fractionation shows that the varicosities contain numerous vesicles, some smooth endoplasm reticulum, mitochondria, neurofilaments and microtubules.

Localization of neurotransmitters

NA can be turned into a fluorescent compound by formaldehyde vapour (for a modified technique see Falck et al, 1982) or glyoxylic acid condensation (Axelsson et al, 1973). This provides a reliable and sensitive fluorescence histochemical technique for localizing and visualizing perivascular adrenergic nerves (Fig. 5.4). Noradrenergic nerves are probably the most important components involved in neural control of vascular tone, and most arteries and arterioles have been shown to be innervated by nerves which contain catecholamines. Cholinergic nerves fibres have been identified in some vascular beds (e.g. in the brain, tongue, skeletal muscle and external genitalia) using histochemical methods to detect acetylcholinesterase, an enzyme involved in the degradation of ACh, and also by immunohistochemical identification of choline acetyltransferase (Burnstock et al, 1980).

More recently immunohistochemical techniques have been utilized to identify not only adrenergic and cholinergic nerves, but also novel vascular neurotransmitters including peptides and purines. Substance P (Furness et al, 1982), vasoactive intestinal polypeptide (VIP) (Uddman et al, 1981), NPY (Uddman et al, 1982), and somatostatin (Forssmann et al, 1982) have all been identified in perivascular nerve terminals. A fluorescence histochemical technique using quinacrine has also been used to identify nerves containing purines such as ATP (Burnstock et al, 1979) which, next to NA, is the most-studied neurotransmitter contained in vascular nerves. Recently nitric oxide synthase (NOS)-containing fibres have also been identified using immunohistochemical techniques in some arterial preparations (e.g. cerebral arteries) which together with functional pharmacological evidence suggests that NO is an inhibitory vascular neurotransmitter in blood vessels (Nozaki et al, 1993). 5-HT immunofluorescent nerves have been detected in a number of vessels; however, it would appear that 5-HT is not synthesized within the nerve fibre, but is taken up, stored in and released as a false transmitter from sympathetic nerves (Jackowski et al, 1989). Three types of storage vesicles are found in sympathetic varicosities: many granular and agranular vesicles and a few dense cored large vesicles. Both large and small vesicles contain NA and ATP, the relative quantities of which may vary in different vessel types (Burnstock, 1990). Neuropeptides and other soluble proteins are found only in large dense-cored vesicles coexisting with NA and ATP (see Cotransmission).

Fluorescent histochemical and immunohistochemical techniques have also been used to provide semiquantitative analysis of the density of autonomic innervation. This has improved over the years with the development of more sophisticated image analysis techniques, and has been utilized for comparing the density of innervation of different vessel sizes and types, not to mention the effects of ageing and disease all which may affect the degree of innervation, and perhaps the levels of certain neurotransmitters (Griffith et al, 1982; Cowen et al, 1982).

Transmitter release and smooth muscle activation

Action potentials are propagated along the nerve fibre to the varicosities via the influx of Na^+ and Ca^{2+} into the neuroplasm. As a consequence of increased intraneuronal $[Ca^{2+}]$, the storage vesicles migrate towards and fuse with the neuronal cell membrane, emptying their contents into the synaptic cleft (Fig. 5.2). Once released the transmitter diffuses across the junctional gap, which can vary between 50 to 2000 nm depending on the size of the vessel. Upon reaching the vascular smooth muscle cells the neurotransmitter interacts with receptors on the postjunctional membrane leading to changes in the membrane potential and/or intracellular signalling mechanisms. Only vascular smooth muscle cells close to the varicosity are affected directly by the released transmitter; therefore in richly innervated arterioles most smooth muscle cells will be directly activated but in larger vessels the innervation is restricted to cells in the medio–adventitial border. To affect the deeper non-innervated layers electrical activity must be propagated from cell to cell. This occurs through specialized electrical coupling between neighbouring smooth muscle cells known as nexuses or gap junctions (Bevan et al, 1980); therefore although many vascular smooth muscle cells are not directly innervated they may still be influenced by nerves. This may also be a source of differences between the actions of different neurotransmitters. Those whose signalling includes depolarization of the cell membrane may transfer their effects further through the media than those with exclusively 'pharmaco-mechanical coupling' via non-depolarizing signalling pathways. For example, the effect of NA may stop at the first cell activated, whereas ATP-induced depolarization may propagate further afield. Teleologically this provides a rationale for different neurotransmitters.

Cotransmission

It was initially thought that each neuron synthesised and released only a single neurotransmitter, and this concept became known as Dale's Principle; however, there is now substantial evidence both in vitro and in vivo that nerves synthesise, store and release more than one neurotransmitter. An example of such evidence was illustrated by Su (1975), who demonstrated that after priming tissues with tritiated [³H]adenosine (a precursor in the synthesis of ATP) and then using tritium efflux as a measure of ATP release, electrical stimulation of the rabbit aorta and portal vein evoked the release of a [³H]purine together with NA. The same technique has also been shown to demonstrate cotransmission of ATP and NA in a variety of vascular preparations. To generalize, it would appear that ATP and NPY coexist with NA in sympathetic neurons, whereas VIP and ACh are cotransmitters in perivascular nerves (Burnstock, 1990).

Vascular modulation by neurotransmitters

In studying the effects of autonomic nerve activity on the vasculature, probably the most common preparations utilized are isolated blood vessels. These can be set up as perfused or wire mounted preparations, with the perivascular nerves being selectively stimulated

a

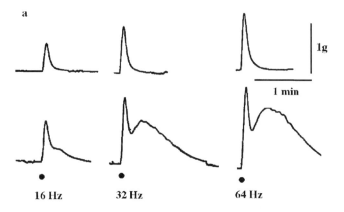

b

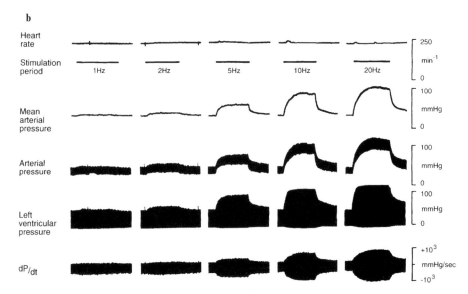

Fig. 5.5a. Representative trace showing frequency dependent contractions in the rabbit isolated saphenous vein in response to electrical field stimulation. Top panel shows control responses at 16, 32 and 64 Hz stimulation from left to right (stimulation parameters of 0.1 ms pulse width, 1 s train duration, 35 volts). Bottom panel shows responses at the same frequencies in the presence of 10 μM cocaine (which blocks U$_1$ mechanism, see Fig. 5.2). Note how response is prolonged in the presence of cocaine. Daly (1993) with permission. (b) Representative trace of heart rate and carotid arterial and left ventricular pressures in a pithed rabbit. The sympathetic outflows in the upper lumbar region were stimulated at different frequencies for 3 min periods via the pithing rod. At this level stimulation of the outflow produces direct stimulation of vasoconstrictor nerves without activation of sympathetic nerves to the heart or to the adrenal medulla. Pharmacological analysis showed that this vasoconstrictor response is mediated partly by α_1 and partly by α_2 adrenoceptors, from McGrath et al (1982).

by an electrical field consisting of pulses of short duration, typically 0.1–1 ms, too short to stimulate the smooth muscle cells directly. This elicits a functional response from the blood vessel, either a change in perfusion pressure, vessel width or isometric tension, according to the preparation (Fig. 5.5). Direct comparison can be made with the effects of exogenously applied agonists or putative transmitters and pharmacological analysis carried out.

A useful preparation which provides a bridge to the in vivo situation is the pithed animal. Here, the brain and spinal cord are physically destroyed to eliminate all central or reflex activity and the circulation remains functional providing that temperature and respiration are artificially controlled. This allows the study of the effects upon the intact circulation, in the absence of confounding effects of reflexes, of (1) autonomic nerve stimulation applied to selected spinal outflows via the pithing rod, and (2) their comparison with exogenously administered neurotransmitters and other substances by appropriate pharmacological analysis. This often enables the demonstration of phenomena which are resistant to study in vitro, perhaps due to the inaccessibility or impracticability of the particular vascular bed or vessels involved or because the in vitro medium lacks some vital characteristic such as the appropriate blood gas conditions or a facilitatory hormone or a necessary enzyme. For example, α_2-adrenoceptor-mediated vasoconstriction is difficult to demonstrate in vitro but was discovered, and is readily studied, in pithed animals. In principle the technique can be applied to any species, and has been used with rats, cats, ferrets and rabbits. The rat is by far the most common with the rabbit next (Fig. 5.5) McGrath et al, 1982), although some important very early studies at the turn of the nineteenth and twentieth centuries used pithed cats.

An important issue in analysing neurotransmission in general by pharmacological techniques, particularly comparing the effects of antagonists against nerves and putative neurotransmitters, is the non-equilibrium nature of the neurotransmission process. Each junctional release of neurotransmitter causes a rapid rise followed by a slower but still rapid fall in concentration of the transmitter at the region of its target receptors. Although there may be a gradual build up of transmitter level at high frequencies, the process is essentially one of repetitive rising and falling concentration. This is not appropriate for quantitative comparison with the equilibrium between agonists and antagonists. Indeed, because an antagonist must dissociate from the receptor before an agonist can occupy it, this gives antagonists greater ability to block agonist transmitters from nerves than to block the same agonist at equilibrium when administered exogenously. In practice this means that the identification of receptor subtypes involved in neurotransmission can never be as quantitative as might be expected versus agonists. Consequently, where the relative affinities of antagonists are crucial, controversy is likely.

Vasoconstrictor nerves

To generalize, sympathetic nerve stimulation produces vasoconstriction in most vascular beds. Depolarization of the vasoconstrictor sympathetic nerve terminal releases NA and/or ATP, which act upon postjunctional adrenoceptors and purinoceptors, respectively. Electrophysiological experimentation has shown that in a number of preparations the postjunctional electrical response to sympathetic nerve stimulation involves two distinct phases. The first is a rapid, transient depolarization or excitatory junction potential (e.j.p.) of which several must summate to produce depolarization of some 15–20 mV before threshold is reached for voltage dependent Ca^{2+} channels to be activated, initiating the contractile process (Hirst & Edwards, 1989). These e.j.p.s are rapid in onset, are resistant to the action of α-adrenoceptor antagonists, abolished by the blockade of P_2-receptors, and therefore would appear to be mediated by the actions of ATP (Vidal et al, 1986). This initial phase is followed by a slow prolonged depolarization, which is mimicked by the effects of exogenous NA and can be abolished by α-adrenoceptor antagonists (Sneddon & Burnstock, 1984). Postsynaptically the α_1-adrenoceptor is the predominant receptor mediating vasoconstriction, but there are also postsynaptic α_2-adrenoceptors which mediate vasoconstriction in some vascular preparations (McGrath et al, 1989).

Although a range of putative peptide neurotransmitters have been identified in perivascular nerves, their exact role in maintaining vascular tone is not well understood. The release of these peptides may produce persistent vasoconstriction in some vascular preparations (Wharton & Gulbenkian, 1987). The major role of NPY in the vasculature may be that of a pre or postjunctional modulator of sympathetic transmission (Lundberg et al, 1990).

Measurement of sympathetic nerve firing activity using electrical recordings from the skin of healthy human volunteers showed that sympathetic vasoconstrictor nerves discharge continually at about 1 Hz or less at rest, with the maximum frequency of approximately 8–10 Hz (Bini et al, 1980). Interruption of tonic sympathetic activity in vivo by nerve sectioning or pharmacological blockade results in vasodilatation, as can be demonstrated for example in pithed animals whereby destruction of spinal sympathetic outflow causes a fall in blood pressure partly due to systemic vasodilatation. The overall degree of vascular tone can be controlled by increasing or decreasing sympathetic nerve firing activity from basal levels to produce vasoconstriction or vasodilatation, respectively. The rate of firing of sympathetic neurons can be affected in vivo by a number of factors including rhythm of respiration, temperature and mental activity or stress.

Vasodilator nerves

In a limited number of tissues the arterioles are innervated by vasodilator fibres as well as by the ubiquitous sympathetic vasoconstrictor fibres. Unlike the vasoconstrictor fibres, they are not tonically active. Sympathetic vasodilator nerves are rare but have been suggested to be present in the arterioles of skeletal muscle in carnivores such as the dog and cat. This part of the sympathetic nervous system is activated solely as part of the 'alerting response' to fear and danger and when activated elicits a transient vasodilator response mediated via activation of muscarinic receptors by ACh. Evidence for this relies largely on pharmacological analysis using muscarinic antagonists and has long been controversial.

Parasympathetic vasodilator nerves are less widely distributed in comparison to the sympathetic vasoconstrictor fibres. Examples of some of the parasympathetic innervated tissues are blood vessels of the salivary glands and exocrine pancreas, the gastric and colonic mucosa and cerebral and coronary arteries. Most commonly parasympathetic vasodilatation is mediated via ACh release, hyperpolarizing the vascular smooth muscle; however, cotransmission of ACh and VIP may occur in some tissues, for example the rabbit lingual artery (Brayden & Large, 1986).

The ability of antidromic impulses in collateral branches of sensory nerves to cause vasodilatation, forming the flare component of the triple response to mild trauma in the human skin, is well documented. The sensory nerves mediating this response are the nociceptive C fibres which have been shown to contain substance P and CGRP (Gamse et al, 1980).

Modulation of sympathetic neurotransmission

Given a constant activity of the sympathetic neuron, the amount of transmitter released can be either augmented or attenuated by the actions of locally released or circulating factors (Fig. 5.2). Angiotensin II is considered to be an important facilitatory modulator of vascular adrenergic transmission. It acts to increase the release of NA from sympathetic nerve terminals. Activation of β-adrenoceptors present on the neuronal membrane can enhance exocytotic release of adrenergic transmitter evoked by nerve impulses. It has been suggested that these effects may play a role in certain forms of hypertension, with increased levels of adrenaline and/or angiotensin II reaching the adrenergic neuronal membrane, facilitating NA release and hence vasoconstriction. Autocoids such as histamine and 5-HT have inhibitory actions on NA release, as does activation of muscarinic receptors present on the neuronal membrane by ACh. Metabolic acidosis, increases in K^+ levels and hyperosmolarity all act to reduce the release of NA from sympathetic nerve terminals (Shepherd & Vanhoutte, 1985).

Released NA is removed from the synaptic cleft by uptake into nerve terminals (uptake$_1$) and / or uptake into nonneural cells (uptake$_2$), and will also seep into surrounding capillary networks clearing the released transmitter from the junctional cleft (Fig. 5.2). NA taken up into the nerve terminal cytoplasm may undergo further active uptake into the NA storage vesicles although most is broken down by enzymes present in the nerve fibres.

The neuronal membrane also senses the concentration of released NA and ATP via prejunctional receptors, which exert a negative feedback effect on vesicular exocytosis (Fig. 5.2). Pharmacological investigation has demonstrated that the receptors responsible for this autoinhibition are the α_2-adrenoceptor and the P_1-purinoceptor for NA and ATP, respectively. Feedback inhibition of transmitter release can also be initiated by exogenous circulating catecholamines and purines. Postjunctionally the effects of NA and ATP released as transmitters are generally cooperative as both typically act as vasoconstrictors. Their physiological roles may radically differ due to differences in their actions, both temporally (long and short acting, respectively) and spatially (due to non-propagating signalling and propagating action potentials, respectively; see previous section). This applies also to peptide neurotransmitters, which are expected to have long-lived actions. The nature and physiological and pathophysiological roles of purinergic and peptidergic transmission, although potentially of great importance, remains obscure. This could rapidly be clarified if good antagonists became available.

Summary

Vascular tone can be modulated by an ever growing number of endogenous substances, which can act directly to contract or relax vascular smooth muscle or indirectly by the release of other substances from the endothelium. Nerve terminals, mainly autonomic sympathetic or sensory release vasoactive substances which modulate smooth muscle tone. Translation of this knowledge of the capability of circulating substances or neurotransmitters to modulate vascular tone into information on the role of particular substances or phenomena in the physiological regulation of vascular tone is dependent on the following: (1) availability of appropriate selective antagonist drugs and in vitro preparations responsive to the appropriate stimuli, including nerve stimulation and allowing discrimination between direct (vascular smooth muscle) and indirect (endothelial) effects, (2) in vivo preparations amenable to these same manoeuvres. Proof of a role for a given phenomenon in humans requires the further feasibility of testing such antagonists in humans. Paradoxically this means that the phenomena best understood are those already taken to the level of developing therapeutic blockers rather than blockers having been developed on the basis of what is physiologically or pathophysiologically most appropriate. This useful symbiosis continues.

References

Axelsson, S., Bjorklund, A., Falck, B., Lindvall, O. & Svensson, L. A. (1973). Glyoxylic acid condensation: a new fluorescence method for the histological demonstration of biogenic monoamines. *Acta Physiologica Scandinavica*, **87**, 57–62.

Bevan, J. A., Bevan, R. D. & Duckles, S. P. (1980). Adrenergic regulation of vascular smooth muscle. In *Handbook of Physiology*. The cardiovascular system, vol. II. Vascular smooth muscle Section 2, ed. D. F. Bohr, A. P. Somlyo & H. V. Sparks, pp. 515–66. Bethesda: American Physiological Society.

Bini, G., Hagbarth, K. E., Hynninen, P. & Wallin, B. G. (1980). Regional similarities and differences in thermoregulatory vaso- and sudomotor tone. *Journal of Physiology*, **306**, 1553–565.

Bloom, S. R., Edwards, A. V. & Jones, C. T. (1988). The adrenal contribution to the neuroendocrine responses to splanchnic nerve stimulation in conscious calves. *Journal of Physiology*, **397**, 513–26.

Brayden, J. E. & Large, W. A. (1986). Electrophysiological analysis of neurogenic vasodilatation in the isolated lingual artery of the rabbit. *British Journal of Pharmacology*, **89**, 163–71.

Burnstock, G. (1980). Cholinergic and purinergic regulation of blood vessels. In *Handbook of Physiology*. The cardiovascular system, vol. II. Vascular smooth muscle Section 2, ed. D. F. Bohr, A. P. Somlyo & H. V. Sparks, pp. 567–612. Bethesda: American Physiological Society.

Burnstock, G. (1986). Autonomic neuromuscular junctions: current developments and future directions. *Journal of Anatomy*, **146**, 1–30.

Burnstock, G. (1990). Co-transmission. The Fifth Heymans Memorial Lecture. *Archives Internationales de Pharmacodynamie et de Therapie*, **304**, 7–33.

Burnstock, G., Crowe, R. & Wong, H. K. (1979). Comparative pharmacological and histological evidence for purinergic inhibitory innervation of the portal vein of the rabbit, but not guinea pig. *British Journal of Pharmacology*, **65**, 377–88.

Cowen, T., Haven, A. J., Wen Qin, C., Gallen, D., Franc, F. & Burnstock, G. (1982). Development and ageing of perivascular adrenergic nerves in the rabbit. A quantitative fluorescent histochemical study using image analysis. *Journal of the Autononomic Nervous System*, **5**, 317–36.

Daly, C. J. (1993). *The contribution of α2-adrenoceptors to sympathetic neuroeffector transmission in the rabbit isolated saphenous and plantaris veins*. MSc Thesis, University of Glasgow.

Devine, C. E. & Simpson, F. O. (1967). The fine structure of vascular sympathetic neuromuscular contacts in the rat. *American Journal of Anatomy*, **121**, 153–74.

Dunn, W. R., Daly, C. J., McGrath, J. C. & Wilson, V. G. (1991). A comparison of the effects of angiotensin II and Bay K 8644 on responses to noradrenaline mediated via postjunctional α_1- and α_2-adrenoceptors in rabbit isolated blood vessels. *British Journal of Pharmacology*, **103**, 1475–83.

Falck, B., Björklund, A. & Lindvall, O. (1982). Recent progress in aldehyde fluorescence histochemistry. *Brain Research Bulletin*, **9**, 3–10.

Forssmann, W. G., Hock, D. & Metz, J. (1982). Peptidergic innervation of the kidney. *Neuroscience Letters*, **10** (Suppl.), S183.

Furchgott, R. F. & Zawadzki, J. V. (1980). The obligatory role of endothelial cells in the relaxation of arterial smooth muscle by acetylcholine. *Nature*, **299**, 373–6.

Furness, J. B., Papka, R. E., Della, N. G., Costa, M. & Eskay, R. L. (1982). Substance P-like immunoreactivity in nerves associated with the vascular system of guinea pigs. *Neuroscience*, **7**, 447–59.

Gamse, R., Holzer, P. & Lembeck, F. (1980). Decrease of substance P in primary afferent neurones and impairment of neurogenic plasma extravasation by capsaicin. *British Journal of Pharmacology*, **68**, 207–13.

Griffith, S. G., Crowe, R., Lincoln, J., Haven, A. J. & Burnstock, G. (1982). Regional differences in the density of perivascular nerves and varicosities, noradrenaline content and responses to nerve stimulation in the rabbit ear artery. *Blood Vessels*, **19**, 41–52.

Haynes, W. G. & Webb, D. J. (1994). Contribution of endogenous generation of endothelin-1 to basal vascular tone. *Lancet*, **344**, 852–4.

Hirst, G. D. S. & Edwards, R. R. (1989). Sympathetic neuroeffector transmission in arteries and arterioles. *Physiological Reviews*, **69**, 546–604.

Januszewicz, A. (1995). The natriuretic peptides in hypertension. *Current Opinions in Cardioliology*, **10**, 495–500.

Jackowski, A., Crockard, A. & Burnstock, G. (1989). 5-Hydroxytryptamine demonstrated immunohistochemistry in rat cerebrovascular nerves largely represents 5-hydroxytryptamine uptake into sympathetic nerve fibres. *Neuroscience*, **29**, 453–62.

Lundberg, J. M., Franco-Cereceda, A., Hemsen, A., Lacroix, J. S. & Pernow, J. (1990). Pharmacology of noradrenaline and neuropeptide tyrosine (NPY)-mediated sympathetic co-transmission. *Fundamentals of Clinical Pharmacology*, **4**, 373–91.

MacLean, M. R. & McGrath, J. C. (1990). Effects of pre-contraction with endothelin-1 on α_2-adrenoceptor and (endothelium-dependent) neuropeptide Y-mediated contractions in the isolated vascular bed of the rat tail. *British Journal of Pharmacology*, **101**, 205–11.

MacMillan, J. B., Smith, K. M. & McGrath, J. C. (1996). Investigation of vasoconstriction responses of rabbit cutaneous resistance arteries. *Journal of Autonomic Pharmacology*, (abstract) in press.

McGrath, J. C., Arribas, S. & Daly, C. J. (1996). Fluorescent ligands for the study of receptors. *Trends Pharmacological Science*, **207**, 385–427.

McGrath, J. C., Brown, C. M. & Wilson, V. G. (1989). Alpha-adrenoceptors: a critical review. *Medical Research Reviews*, **9**, 407–533.

McGrath, J. C., Flavahan, N. A. & McKean, C. E. (1982). α_1 and α_2-adrenoceptor-mediated pressor and chronotropic effects in the rat and rabbit. *Journal of Cardiovascular Pharmacology* **4**, S101–S107.

Nozaki, K., Moskowitz, M. A., Maynard, K. I., Koketsu, N., Dawson, T. M., Bredt, D. S. & Snyder, S. H. (1993). Possible origins and distribution of immunoreactive nitric oxide synthase-containing nerve fibres in cerebral arteries. *Journal of Cerebral Blood Flow and Metabolism*, **13**, 70–9.

Shepherd, J. T. & Vanhoutte P. M. (1985). Local modulation of adrenergic neurotransmission in blood vessels. *Journal of Cardiovascular Pharmacology*, **7** (Suppl. 3), S167–S178.

Sneddon, P. & Burnstock, G. (1984). Inhibition of excitatory junction potentials in guinea-pig vas deferens by α,β-methylene ATP: further evidence for ATP and noradrenaline as cotransmitters. *European Journal of Pharmacology*, **100**, 85–90.

Su, C. (1975). Neurogenic release of purine compounds in blood vessels. *Journal of Pharmacology and Experimental Therapeutics*, **195**, 159–66.

Uddman, R., Alumets, J., Edvinsson, L., Hakanson, R. & Sundler F. (1981). VIP nerve fibres around peripheral blood vessels. *Acta Physiologica Scandinavica*, **112**, 65–70.

Uddman, R., Alumets, J., Edvinsson, L., Hakanson, R., Owman, C & Sundler F. (1982). Immunohistochemical demonstration of APP (avian pancreatic polypeptide) -immunoreactive nerve fibres around cerebral blood vessels. *Brain Research Bulletin*, **9**, 715–18.

Vidal, M., Hicks, P. E. & Langer, S. Z. (1986). Differential effects of α,β-methylene ATP on responses to nerve stimulation in SHR and WKY tail arteries. *Naunyn-Schmiedebergs's Archives of Pharmacology*, **332**, 384–90.

Wharton, J. & Gulbenkian, S. (1987). Peptides in the mammalian cardiovascular system. *Experientia Basel*, **43**, 821–32.

Young, W. S. III & Kumar, M. J. (1979). A new method for receptor autoradiography: [^{3}H]opioid receptors in rat brain. *Brain Research*, **179**, 255–70.

Part 2
Hypertension, atherosclerosis and diabetes

6

Vascular structure and function in hypertension

H. A. J. STRUIJKER-BOUDIER

Introduction

The vascular system is composed of a number of vascular segments coupled in series and in parallel. The structure of this system is determined relatively early during embryogenesis, but is subject to continuous modeling and remodeling throughout life. Its structure adapts to tissue requirements for nutrition and exchange as well as to physical forces imposed upon the vascular system. From this perspective, diseases characterized by major vascular abnormalities, such as hypertension, are based upon an abnormal pattern of vascular development or derangements in the physical and metabolic signal transduction in the vessel wall.

The segments coupled in series consist of large elastic arteries, different orders of large and small muscular arteries, arterioles, capillaries, venules and veins (Fig. 6.1). These segments all differ in their relative composition of the two major cell types – vascular smooth cells (VSMC) and endothelial cells (EC) – and the extracellular matrix that constitute the vessel wall. The functional consequences of structural vascular abnormalities differ per segment. In this contribution, I briefly review (1) major methodologies to study the various segments of the arterial tree, and (2) the functional consequences of structural vascular abnormalities in hypertension.

Large arteries

The large arteries comprise the aorta and its most proximal side branches. These arteries contain an endothelial cell layer, a medium consisting of a number of VSMC layers and a relatively large adventitial layer. From a functional point of view these arteries are regarded as elastic arteries, contributing importantly to the compliance properties of the arterial system.

Methodology

The most widely used approach to study large artery structure and function has been the use of isolated arterial segments. These can be mounted in organ baths to force transducers for elaborate mechanical analyses and to study mechanisms of contractility.

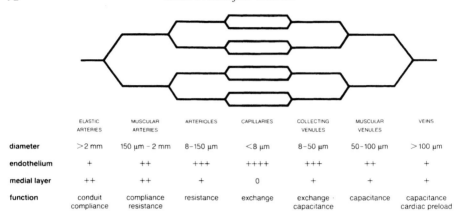

	ELASTIC ARTERIES	MUSCULAR ARTERIES	ARTERIOLES	CAPILLARIES	COLLECTING VENULES	MUSCULAR VENULES	VEINS
diameter	>2 mm	150 µm – 2 mm	8–150 µm	<8 µm	8–50 µm	50–100 µm	>100 µm
endothelium	+	++	+++	++++	+++	++	+
medial layer	++	++	+	0	+	+	+
function	conduit compliance	compliance resistance	resistance	exchange	exchange capacitance	capacitance	capacitance cardiac preload

Fig. 6.1. Schematic representation of the vascular tree and some of the anatomical and functional characteristics of its various segments.

A range of structural parameters can be determined in fixed isolated large artery segments. These pertain to geometry (wall thickness, media thickness, cross sectional area) and to molecular composition of the vessel wall. Immunohistochemistry and molecular biology have added a large number of tools to study the molecular make up of vessel walls. These developments are the focus of other chapters of this volume.

The second important approach to the study of vascular function and structure is the use of in situ preparations (Levy et al, 1990). Segments of large arteries are studied in their normal environment with this approach. A major advantage is that the longitudinal stress of the artery is maintained at its in vivo value. Thus, the in situ approach is particularly suited for mechanical studies. On the other hand, vascular segments have to be perfusion-fixed and analysed in vitro for structural analyses.

A relatively new development in the study of large artery properties has been the introduction of non-invasive in vivo ultrasound techniques. These were developed originally some 25 years ago to study arterial wall displacement in humans (Arndt et al, 1968; Hokanson et al, 1972). Later developments in the fields of echography and pulsed Doppler velocimetry gave significant improvements in the detection and processing methods, allowing accurate determination of arterial diameter and compliance, even in small experimental animals (Hoeks et al, 1990; Hayoz et al, 1992; Van Gorp et al, 1996) (Fig. 6.2). Present developments go in the direction of more sophisticated measurements of local physical forces, such as shear stress and vessel wall geometry (intima and media thickness).

Abnormalities in hypertension

There is considerable evidence for important structural and functional changes in large arteries in experimental models of hypertension. Less data are available for human hypertension. The general picture that emerges is that: (1) the diameter of large arteries

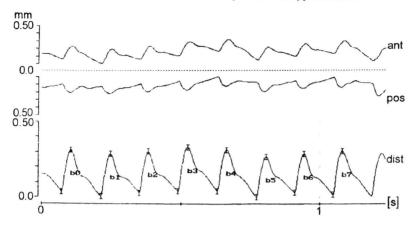

Fig. 6.2. Recording of displacement of anterior and posterior walls of aorta as a function of time during seven consecutive cardiac cycles in a conscious rat (above) and the difference between both, reflecting changes in aortic diameter during the heart cycle (below). Reproduced from Van Gorp et al (1996) with permission.

is increased in hypertensive individuals, (2) the wall mass of these arteries is increased, (3) this increase is caused by both hypertrophy and hyperplasia of VSMC, (4) the composition of the extracellular matrix shows distinct changes, and (5) in parallel to these structural changes the compliance of large arteries in hypertension is reduced (Struijker-Boudier, 1994). These observations trigger a number of mechanistic, pathophysiological and therapeutic questions. First, the cause of the VSMC hypertrophy and hyperplasia in large arteries from hypertensive individuals is still largely unknown. De Mey (1995) has recently reviewed the potential role of the endothelium, the renin–angiotensin system and the sympathetic nervous system as candidate mechanisms to cause large artery wall mass increase. Recent observations on renin-transgenic rats, overexpressing renin at the vascular level, support the view that the renin–angiotensin system is a powerful mechanism to induce large artery hypertrophy (Struijker-Boudier et al, 1996b). Whatever the mechanism that mediates large artery hypertrophy in hypertension, it seems to represent an adaptive process as a response to the rise in blood pressure. The nature of this adaptation remains to be established, but may well be related to a maintenance of a constant circumferential wall stress distribution in the vessel wall (Qiu et al, 1995).

The second important large artery abnormality in hypertension is altered composition of the extracellular matrix. The extracellular matrix of the arterial wall is an integrated system composed of collagen fibrils, elastic lamellae, proteoglycans and structural proteins that, together with the cells, determine the major properties of the vessel wall. Some investigators suggest an increase in collagen and elastin fibres in many forms of hypertension (Safar & London, 1994). Much less is known about changes in the extracellular matrix proteoglycans and glycoproteins. As the interaction

of these molecules with different integrin cell receptors may alter the phenotype characteristics of VSMC, they are potential candidate mechanisms of vascular hypertrophy.
In this regard, fibronectin may be of special interest as this extracellular matrix protein
can modify the phenotype of VSMC from contractile to synthetic state (Hedin et al,
1988; Schwartz & Mecham, 1995). Although it is not certain whether extracellular
matrix changes represent a primary or an adaptive phenomenon in hypertension, they
play an important role in the reduced compliance of the large arteries (Safar & London, 1994).

Small arteries

The small arteries have diameters that range from approximately 2 mm to 150 μm. They
include both the muscular arterial segments of the major branches of the aorta and the
most distal arterial branches just before entering the tissues. Their composition differs
from the elastic arteries by the relatively smaller contribution of an adventitial layer.
Functionally, they contribute both to the compliance and resistance properties of the
arterial system.

Methodology

In vitro studies using isolated small arterial segments mounted in organ baths to force
transducers have been the most widely used approach. The introduction of the myograph, allowing segments with diameters as small as 150–200 μm to be studied, has
been a major methodological advancement (Mulvany & Halpern, 1976). A more recent
approach entails in vitro cannulation of the vessel to allow control of the intraluminal
pressure, while monitoring lumen diameter (Duling et al, 1981). These approaches have
greatly enhanced the knowledge on mechanical and structural abnormalities of the
vascular tree in hypertension. Moreover, they are particularly well-suited techniques in
pharmacological studies on this segment of the vasculature. On the other hand, the in
vitro approach may create experimental artefacts, such as loss of longitudinal stress and
surgical trauma. These limitations can, at least partly, be overcome by in situ measurements (Qiu et al, 1995) (Fig. 6.3); however, the in situ approach is not suited for all
vascular beds and still involves an in vitro measurement of structural properties. A
pulsed Doppler, echo-tracking system has been introduced that allows the in vivo study
of the mechanics of medium-sized arteries, such as the radial artery (Hayoz et al, 1992;
Laurent et al, 1994).

Abnormalities in hypertension

Small muscular arteries contribute both to the resistance and compliance properties of
the vascular system. Increased vascular resistance is a uniform property of the circulation in almost all human and experimental forms of hypertension. The increased
resistance can – at least partly – be localized in the smallest branches of this segment of
the vascular tree. The mechanisms underlying the resistance increase in small arteries in

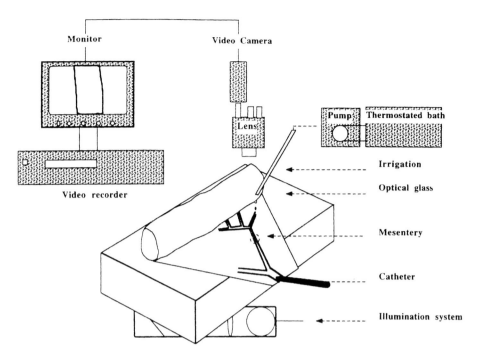

Fig. 6.3. Schematic representation of the experimental set-up used to study in situ segments of small mesenteric arteries (diameters 200–600 µm). Reproduced from Qiu et al (1995) with permission.

hypertension have been the subject of intensive research in the past decade, and the major evidence has been reviewed (Mulvany & Aalkjaer, 1990; Heagerty et al, 1993). At least part of the resistance increase in hypertension is maintained by a structural factor: the increased wall:lumen ratio.

Two major mechanisms have been implied in the increased wall:lumen ratio in small arteries from hypertensive individuals. One has been the hypertrophy of VSMCs and the other the remodeling of the same VSMC mass around a smaller diameter. The reader is referred to reviews by Mulvany & Aalkjaer (1990) and Heagerty et al (1993) for a critical discussion of the evidence for these mechanisms.

The nature of the change in compliance properties in this segment of the vasculature is still a matter of debate (Laurent et al, 1994). Studies in experimental models of hypertension in which static compliance was determined suggest an increased stiffness of small arteries (Qiu et al, 1995). Observations on radial arteries in human hypertensives, on the other hand, suggest that the dynamic compliance may be normal (Hayoz et al, 1992; Laurent et al, 1994). Clearly, differences in methodology and species may underlie some of these differences.

Microcirculation

The third segment of the vascular tree is the microcirculation, the collective name for the smallest components of the vascular channels. It compromises arterioles, capillaries and venules, each with their own characteristic structure and function. The arterioles are resistance vessels as a major fraction of total pressure dissipation occurs in this segment of the vascular tree.

Methodology

The reader is referred to a recent review for a critical discussion of methods to assess the microcirculation in hypertension (Struijker-Boudier et al, 1996a). Briefly, microcirculation methodology is based on histological (both morphometry and chemistry) and intravital microscopical techniques. Histomorphometry has been particularly helpful to study the architecture of the microcirculation. It is used more and more in combination with immunohistochemical markers to study the molecular basis of vascular function. Powerful new microscopy techniques (e.g. confocal microscopy, fluorescent imaging, atomic force microscopy) have facilitated the study of cellular and subcellular control of microvessel wall function.

The central methodology in the past three decades of microcirculation studies has been intravital microscopy. It allows the direct observation of microcirculatory dynamics in a range of tissues, such as skeletal muscle, mesentery, brain and kidney (Struijker-Boudier et al, 1996a). A particularly helpful development for hypertension research has been the introduction of chronic window techniques to observe the microcirculation in conscious animals. Such chambers now exist for use in rats, the most common species for present models of experimental hypertension, and mice, the species of choice in the age of animal models based on genetic alterations (Fig. 6.4).

Abnormalities in hypertension

The central concept of microcirculatory abnormalities in hypertension is that of 'rarefaction'. Rarefaction refers to the disappearance of blood vessels, in particular arterioles and capillaries. Indeed, a smaller number of arterioles and capillaries have been observed in many tissues in most human and experimental forms of hypertension (Struijker-Boudier et al, 1992, 1996a; Shore & Tooke, 1994). Functionally, rarefaction of small arterioles and capillaries can contribute significantly to the resistance and pressure increase in hypertension (Greene et al, 1989).

The cause of microvascular rarefaction in hypertension is still largely unknown. Three major views have been advanced. The first involves a gradual shift from functional to structural disappearance of small vessels (Prewitt et al, 1990). Functional rarefaction is the result of arteriolar constriction to the point of non-perfusion of the vessel, whereas structural rarefaction represents the actual disappearance of the vessel. According to Prewitt et al (1990) functional rarefaction is caused by an increased sensitivity of small arterioles to vasoconstrictor stimuli, with subsequent chronic vasoconstriction. Han-

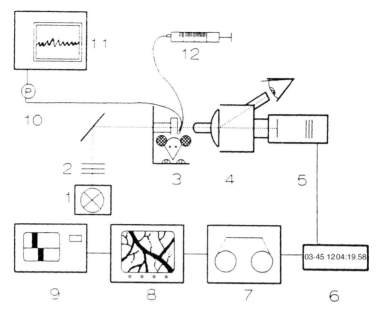

Fig. 6.4. Schematic representation of the experimental set-up used in chronic dorsal microcirculatory (DMC) experiments in conscious rats. 1: xenon lamp; 2: filter-set; 3: microscope stage with rat; 4: microscope; 5: video camera; 6: video timer; 7: video recorder; 8: video monitor; 9: shearing monitor; 10: pressure transducer; 11: recorder; 12: syringe for drug administration.

sen-Smith et al (1991) have indeed found evidence for atrophy and degeneration of both endothelial cells and VSMC's in the cremaster muscle of rats made hypertensive by renal mass reduction.

The second hypothesis regards rarefaction as an adaptive response to the altered local haemodynamics in hypertension. It would represent structural autoregulation to a chronically increased tissue blood flow (Hogan & Hirschmann, 1984) or circumferential wall stress (Price & Skalak, 1994). These two hypotheses provide attractive explanations for microvascular rarefaction in several models for secondary hypertension; however, they are difficult to reconcile with data that microvascular rarefaction may exist already before pressure elevations in animals or humans prone to develop hypertension. We have suggested that in these situations microvascular rarefaction is not the result of an actual disappearance of vessels, but represents a hampered angiogenic mechanism (Struijker-Boudier et al, 1992, 1994).

Conclusion

Vascular changes are a main aspect of hypertensive disease. The major complications of hypertension are related to both macro- and microvascular pathology. Adequate

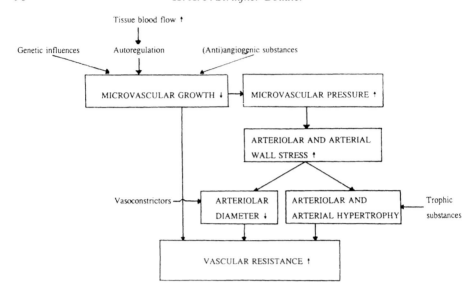

Fig. 6.5. Outline of hypothesis on how vascular growth contributes to the development of hypertension. Reproduced from Struijker-Boudier et al (1992) with permission.

methodology is available now to assess vascular function and structure in hypertension. Available evidence points to abnormalities in vascular growth mechanisms as an important pathogenic mechanism in hypertension. Figure 6.5 gives an outline of how vascular growth mechanisms could contribute to the development of hypertension.

References

Arndt, J. O., Klauske, J, & Mersch, F. (1968). The diameter of the intact carotid artery in man and its change with pulse pressure. *Pfluegers Archives*, **301**, 230–40.

De Mey, J. G. R. (1995). Smooth muscle cell proliferation in hypertension. In *The Vascular Smooth Muscle Cell*, ed. S. M. Schwartz & R. P. Mecham, pp. 361–401. New York: Academic Press.

Duling, B. R., Gore, R. W., Dacey, R. G. & Damon, D. N. (1981). Methods for isolation, cannulation and in vitro study of single microvessels. *American Journal of Physiology*, **241**, H108–H116.

Greene, A. S., Tonellato, P. J., Lui, J., Lombard, J. H. & Cowley, A. W. (1989). Microvascular rarefaction and tissue vascular resistance in hypertension. *American Journal of Physiology*, **256**, H126–H131.

Hansen-Smith, F., Greene, A. S., Cowley, A. W. Jr., Lougee, L. & Lombard, J. H. (1991). Structural alterations of microvascular smooth muscle cells in reduced renal mass hypertension. *Hypertension*, **17**, 902–8.

Hayoz, D., Tardy, Y., Perret, F. Waeber, B. Meister, J.-J. & Brunner, H. R. (1992). Non-invasive determination of arterial diameter and distensibility by echo-tracking techniques in hypertension. *Journal of Hypertension*, **10** (Suppl. 6), S95–S100.

Heagerty, A. M., Aalkjaer, C., Bund, S. J., Korsgaard, N. & Mulvany, M. J. (1993). Small artery structure in hypertension. Dual processes of remodeling and growth. *Hypertension*, **21**, 391–7.

Hedin, U., Bottger, B. A., Forsberg, E., Johansson, S. & Thyberg, J. (1988). Diverse effects of fibronectin and laminin on phenotype properties of cultured arterial smooth muscle cells. *Journal of Cellular Biology*, **107**, 307–19.

Hoeks, A. P. G., Brands, P. J., Smeets, F. A. M. & Reneman, R. S. (1990). Assessment of the distensibility of superficial arteries. *Ultrasound Medical Biology*, **16**, 121–8.

Hogan, R. D. & Hirshmann, L. (1984). Arteriolar proliferation in the rat cremaster muscle as a long-term autoregulatory response to reduced perfusion. *Microvascular Research*, **27**, 290–6.

Hokanson, D. E., Mozersky, D. J., Summer, D. S. & Strandness, D. E. (1972). A phase locked echo-tracking system for recording arterial diameter changes in vivo. *Journal of Applied Physiology*, **32**, 728–33.

Laurent, S., Girerd, X., Mourad, J.-J., Lacolley, P., Beck, L., Boutouyrie, P., Mignot, J.-P. & Safar, M. (1994). Elastic modulus of the radial artery wall material is not increased in patients with essential hypertension. *Arteriosclerosis Thrombosis*, **14**, 1223–31.

Lévy, B. I., Benessiano, J., Poitevin, P. & Safar, M. E. (1990). Endothelium-dependent mechanical properties of the carotid artery in WKY and SHR, role of angiotensin converting enzyme inhibition. *Circulation Research*, **66**, 321–8.

Mulvany, M. J. & Halpern, W. (1976). Mechanical properties of vascular smooth muscle cells in situ. *Nature*, **260**, 617–19.

Mulvany, M. J. & Aalkjaer, C. (1990). Structure and function of small arteries. *Physiological Review*, **70**, 921–61.

Price, R. J. & Skalak, T. C. (1994). Circumferential wall stress as a mechanism of arteriolar rarefaction and proliferation in a network model. *Microvascular Research*, **47**, 188–202.

Prewitt, R. L., Hashimoto, H. & Stacy, D. L. (1990). Structural and functional rarefaction of microvessels in hypertension. In *Blood Vessel Changes in Hypertension: Structure and Function*, ed. R. Lee, pp. 71–90. Florida: Boca Raton, CRC Press.

Qiu, H. Y., Valtier, B., Struijker-Boudier, H. A. J. & Levy, B. I. (1995). Mechanical and contractile properties of in situ localized mesenteric arteries in normotensive and spontaneously hypertensive rats. *Journal of Pharmacological and Toxicological Methods*, **33**, 159–70.

Safar, M. E. & London, G. M. (1994). The Arterial System in Human Hypertension. In *Textbook of Hypertension*, ed. J. D. Swales, pp. 85–103, Oxford: Blackwell Scientific.

Schwartz, S. M. & Mecham R. P. Ed. (1995). *The Vascular Smooth Muscle Cell*. New York: Academic Press, pp. 1–410.

Shore, A. C. & Tooke, J. E. (1994). Microvascular function in human essential hypertension. *Journal of Hypertension*, **12**, 712–28.

Struijker-Boudier, H. A. J., le Noble, J. L. M. L., Messing, M. W. J., Huijberts, M. S. P., le Noble, F. A. C. & Van Essen, H. (1992). The microcirculation and hypertension. *Journal of Hypertension*, **10** (Suppl. 7), S147–S156.

Struijker-Boudier, H. A. J. (1994). Vascular growth and hypertension. In: *Textbook of Hypertension*, ed. J. D. Swales, pp. 200–12. Oxford: Blackwell Scientific.

Struijker-Boudier, H. A. J., Crijns, F. R. L., Stolte, J. & Van Essen, H. (1996a). Assessment of the microcirculation in cardiovascular disease. *Clinical Science*, **91**, 131–9.

Struijker-Boudier, H. A. J., Van Essen, H., Fazzi, G., De Mey, J. G. R., Qiu, H. Y. & Levy, B. I. (1996b). Disproportional arterial hypertrophy in hypertensive mREN-2 transgenic rats. *Hypertension*, **28**, 779–84.

Van Gorp, A., Van Ingen Schenau, D., Willigers, J., Hoeks, A. P. G., De Mey, J. G. R., Struijker-Boudier, H. A. J. & Reneman, R. S. (1996). A technique to assess aortic distensibility and compliance in anesthetized and awake rats. *American Journal of Physiology*, **270**, H780–H786.

7

Pulmonary hypertension

J. R. GOSNEY

Introduction

When the mean pulmonary arterial pressure exceeds 25 mmHg at rest, a state of pulmonary hypertension exists. This simple haemodynamic definition belies the wide range of causes of the condition as well as the diversity of structural changes which occur in the pulmonary blood vessels and which themselves may act to further elevate pulmonary intravascular pressure. The purpose of this chapter is to summarize the causes of pulmonary hypertension and its pathology and to review recent advances in our knowledge of the pathogenetic mechanisms involved.

Causes of pulmonary hypertension

It is useful, if somewhat empirical, to recognize three broad groups of conditions causing pulmonary hypertension: those causing pulmonary venous congestion, those which obstruct the flow of blood by narrowing or obstructing the pulmonary vessels, and those characterized by a particular pattern of morphological changes known as plexogenic pulmonary arteriopathy or PPA (Hatano & Strasser, 1975).

In congestive pulmonary hypertension, the cause of the elevated pressure lies outwith the lungs, in the pulmonary veins or, more often, in the left side of the heart. Examples include profound left ventricular failure, mitral stenosis and incompetence and left atrial myxoma. The elevation of pressure first affects the pulmonary veins and is then transmitted to the arterial side of the circulation, although the mechanisms involved are poorly understood. It is not clear, for example, why the arterial pressure under such circumstances is often considerably greater than the venous pressure (Wagenvoort, 1995).

Obstructive pulmonary hypertension develops when there is physical obstruction to the flow of blood through the pulmonary blood vessels as a consequence of their narrowing. The commonest cause of this is alveolar hypoxia, which leads to vasoconstriction and structural remodelling. This is discussed in detail below. Other causes include recurrent pulmonary embolism, which is usually thrombotic, pulmonary veno-occlusive disease, pulmonary vascular parasitosis, pulmonary capillary haemangio-

100

matosis and lymphangioleiomyomatosis, all of which lead to physical occlusion of pulmonary blood vessels.

Plexogenic pulmonary arteriopathy has a characteristic morphology (described below). It occurs in only a small group of conditions causing severe pulmonary hypertension but is not, of itself, specific other than as a marker of a severe elevation in pulmonary arterial pressure.

Most often, it is seen when blood is forced into the lungs at increased pressure due to structural abnormalities of the heart or great vessels which lead to shunting from the systemic to the pulmonary circulations (Wagenvoort, 1995). Examples of such conditions, the great majority of which are congenital, are ventricular or atrial septal defects, patent ductus arteriosus, and anomalous pulmonary venous drainage. Rarely, it arises in association with portal venous hypertension (Hadengue et al, 1991), the acquired immune deficiency syndrome (Speich et al, 1991) or may be caused by certain drugs or toxins (Gurtner, 1990). Finally, it may develop for no apparent reason, usually in young or middle-aged women, when it forms the pathological basis of the disease known as primary pulmonary hypertension or PPH (Rubin, 1995).

This term PPH causes confusion because it has been used inconsistently. For example, some use it to refer to all cases of pulmonary hypertension in which an underlying cardiopulmonary cause has been excluded by clinical and laboratory investigation (Rich et al, 1986). Inevitably, such a group is heterogeneous in terms of the underlying pathology. In a recent prospective pathological study of patients chosen by these criteria (Pietra et al, 1989), for example, some had thromboembolic lesions and veno-occlusive disease as well as PPA.

Others use the term PPH more narrowly to refer to only those cases in which all possible causes have been excluded by histopathological examination as well as clinical and other laboratory investigation effectively excluding those with thromboembolic and veno-occlusive disease as well as patients with rare causes of pulmonary hypertension such as lymphangioleiomyomatosis and pulmonary capillary haemangiomatosis. By these criteria, the term PPH describes only those cases characterized by inexplicable plexogenic arteriopathy, which is the sense in which it will be used in this review.

Pathology of pulmonary hypertension

Structure of the normal pulmonary vasculature

To understand the pathology of pulmonary hypertension, some knowledge of the structure of the normal pulmonary vasculature is necessary. Unlike the systemic circulation, the adult human pulmonary circulation is a low pressure high flow system, so that its component vessels are wide with thin walls. The extrapulmonary arteries and intrapulmonary arteries down to a diameter of about 1 mm are elastic vessels, but the elastic laminae are regular only in the latter, being disrupted and fragmented in the extrapulmonary vessels. The arterial vessels between 1 and 0.5 mm, the so-called muscular pulmonary arteries, have a distinct muscular media which is sandwiched between

internal and external elastic laminae and comprises about 5% of the external arterial
diameter (Fig. 7.1a). As the vessels decrease further in diameter, the arteries becoming
arterioles, the muscular media spirals out so that, immediately before breaking up into
alveolar capillaries, they are devoid of muscle and indistinguishable in cross-section
from venules (Fig. 7.1c). As venules become veins, they acquire an irregular arrangement
of muscle, elastic and collagen, but do not develop a definable media.

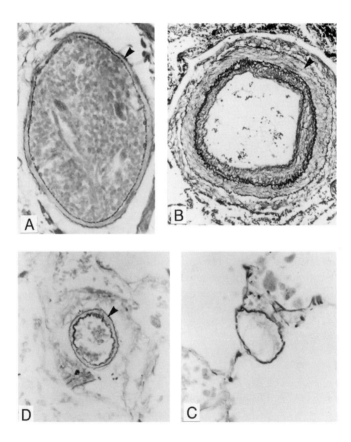

Fig. 7.1. Muscular hypertrophy and fibroelastosis in pulmonary hypertension. The vessels
shown are all stained with the elastic van Gieson method which stains elastin black.
Photographed at medium (A,B) and high (C,D) magnification. The media of each vessel is
delineated by an arrowhead. When the pulmonary arterial pressure rises, the normally thin
muscular media of muscular pulmonary arteries (A) undergoes hypertrophy (B) and arterioles, normally devoid of a muscular media (C), become muscularised (D). Fibroelastosis is
a predominantly intimal process shown well in (B), where it forms a sheath internal to the
media.

Pathology of hypertensive pulmonary vascular disease

The pathological changes in the pulmonary blood vessels in pulmonary hypertension are, of course, dependent on the precise cause, and may well be diagnostic for it, but the general non-specific response of the pulmonary blood vessels to increased pressure is that of muscularization and fibroelastosis. The first of these involves medial hypertrophy of muscular pulmonary arteries (Fig. 7.1b) and development of a muscular media in arterioles and veins (Fig. 7.1d), but muscle fibres may also appear in the intima. The second is a predominantly intimal process (Fig. 7.1b), but may also occur in the media in some instances.

These basic processes vary in pattern and severity according to the cause of the elevated pressure. In congestive pulmonary hypertension, for example, there is medial thickening of muscular arteries due to muscular hypertrophy, fibrosis and an increase in ground substance, and they undergo marked intimal fibrosis. Arterioles and veins become muscularized (Wagenvoort, 1975). In obstructive pulmonary hypertension due to alveolar hypoxia, medial hypertrophy and muscularization involves predominantly the smallest arteries and arterioles, medial and adventitial collagen and elastic tissue is increased and smooth muscle bundles develop in the intima (Reid, 1979). In PPA, as already mentioned, a unique pattern of histopathology is seen, the hallmark of which is the plexiform lesion (Fig. 7.2a). These develop in dilated branches of muscular pulmonary arteries and comprise a plexus of narrow vascular channels separated by narrow septa into which myofibroblasts migrate to become embedded in an acid proteoglycan matrix (Smith & Heath, 1979). They are classically accompanied by other lesions of muscular arteries, including localized dilatation lesions (Fig. 7.2b), sometimes 'angiomatoid' in appearance, foci of fibrinoid necrosis (Fig. 7.2c), and a particularly striking concentric laminar fibroelastosis of the intima (Fig. 7.2d) which, like the plexiform lesion, is characterized by myofibroblasts. These characteristic lesions are accompanied, as might be expected, by non-specific medial hypertrophy of muscular arteries and muscularization of arterioles.

Pathogenesis of pulmonary hypertension

The pulmonary vascular pressure is maintained as a dynamic equilibrium between opposing forces of vasoconstriction and vasodilatation. Part of this control is, of course, neurally mediated, but the nature of the humoral factors responsible for local control was unclear until relatively recently. Over the past decade, however, research into the biology of a variety of agents with vasoactive and trophic effects on the pulmonary vasculature has led to a rapid increase in knowledge. This new information is enlightening not only the physiological control of the pulmonary blood pressure, but also is providing new insights into the pathogenesis of pulmonary hypertensive disease. Two substances in particular, the endothelins and nitric oxide (NO), have generated considerable interest.

Before going on to discuss the possible role of these mediators in pulmonary hypertension, the current understanding of their biology will be briefly reviewed.

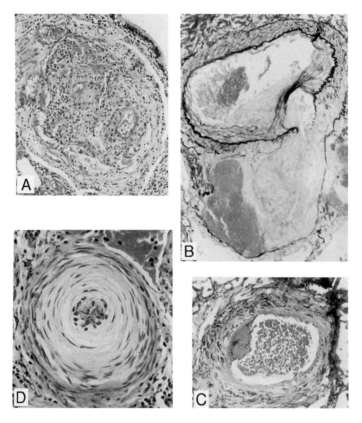

Fig. 7.2. Morphological changes which characterize plexogenic pulmonary arteriopathy (PPA). (A) Plexus of narrow vascular channels separated by narrow septa containing myofibroblasts constitutes the plexiform lesion. (B) Example of a localized dilatation lesion, where the parent vessel is on the top and the thin-walled balloon-like dilatation beneath it. (C) Muscular pulmonary artery containing a nodular focus of fibrinoid necrosis. (D) Similar vessel almost occluded by concentric laminar fibroelastosis. The vessel in (B), is stained by the elastic and van Gieson method. The other three lesions are in sections stained by haemotoxylin and eosin. All are photographed at medium magnification.

Endothelins

The endothelins, ET-1, ET-2 and ET-3, are a group of separately encoded but closely similar 21 amino acid peptides with a widespread distribution in human lungs (Barnes, 1994). Although first described in endothelium, ETs are secreted by a variety of epithelial cells in the airways and submucous glands (Giaid et al, 1991; Marciniak et al, 1992) as well as alveolar macrophages (Ehrenreich et al, 1990). They have at least two effects on human airways, a sustained bronchoconstriction, which appears to be a direct effect on smooth muscle (Advenier et al, 1990) and a trophic effect on myofibroblasts (Brewster et al, 1990). Such effects might play a role in a variety of pulmonary conditions, including asthma, the adult respiratory distress syndrome and pulmonary fibrosis (Barnes, 1994).

The effects of ETs on the pulmonary vasculature are similar (Brink et al, 1991), ET-1 producing a powerful, sustained vasoconstriction, especially of small pulmonary arteries (Loach et al, 1990), and stimulating proliferation of vascular smooth muscle and fibroblasts (Muldoon et al, 1989). Such effects inevitably provoke the question of whether ETs might play a role in the pathogenesis of pulmonary hypertension.

ETs are probably not important in mediating the rapid pulmonary vasoconstriction such as occurs in acute hypoxia, but more so in mediating persistent, sustained vasoconstriction and stimulating vascular remodelling. The vasoconstrictive effects of ETs are slow to develop and very sustained, and levels of endothelial ET-1 are particularly high in vessels where remodelling is marked (Giaid et al, 1993). Patients with pulmonary hypertension have elevated levels of ET-1mRNA and ET-1 itself in their pulmonary endothelium (Giaid et al, 1993) and elevated levels of ET-1 in their plasma (Steward et al, 1991).

Nitric oxide

NO is a simple gas with an important role in the regulation of smooth muscle activity in the lung. The enzyme which generates it from arginine, NO synthase, may be either constitutive, in which case the NO produced acts as a physiological transducer, or inducible, in which case it forms in response to endotoxin and cytokines (Adnot et al, 1995) There are many types of cell in which NO synthase is inducible, but the constitutive form is found in endothelium, certain neurons and some epithelial cells.

In pulmonary blood vessels, NO is generated as either a direct response to the physical effect of blood flow or by activation of receptors in response to a variety of stimuli, to induce smooth muscle relaxation and vasodilatation. It is unclear whether it is responsible for maintaining the natural state of low vascular tone when the level of oxygen in the airways is normal (Frostell et al, 1991; Adnot et al, 1995), but it undoubtedly resists the vasoconstrictive effects of hypoxia and ET (Frostell et al, 1991). In addition, it has the effect of inhibiting platelet activity and proliferation of vascular smooth muscle (Garg & Hassid, 1989).

Arachidonic acid derivatives

Substances derived in the pulmonary vascular endothelium from arachidonic acid via the cyclo-oxygenase pathway have potent effects on the pulmonary vasculature; they are active in maintaining normal pulmonary vascular tone and may be an important factor in pulmonary vascular remodelling (Voelkel & Tuder, 1995). Thromboxane is a powerful vasoconstrictor and promoter of platelet aggregation and prostacyclin has potent opposing effects, so that the balance between them may be crucial. For example, the ratio of metabolites of thromboxane to those of prostacyclin is increased in subjects with PPH (Christman et al, 1992), and 5-lipoxygenase inhibitors attenuate development of pulmonary hypertension in animals (Morganroth et al, 1985). Damage to endothelial cells resulting in imbalance between these substances would lead to vasoconstriction, smooth muscle cell proliferation and thrombosis, events which might be significant in the pathogenesis of PPA in particular (Voelkel & Tuder, 1995).

Growth factors

A variety of growth factors may play a role in stimulating cell growth and activity in the pulmonary vessels (Gossage & Christman, 1994). Insulin-like growth factor (IGF)-I stimulates proliferation of bovine pulmonary vascular smooth muscle cells (Dempsey et al, 1990) and increases in the lungs of sheep in which pulmonary hypertension is induced by air embolization (Perkett et al, 1992a). Transforming growth factor (TGF)-β is similarly increased in the lungs of such sheep (Perkett et al, 1990) in which both it and its mRNA are detectable in remodelled pulmonary arteries (Perkett et al, 1992b). Platelet-derived growth factor (PDGF) is a powerful mitogen for aortic smooth muscle cells (Kourembanas et al, 1990), although its role in mediating pulmonary vascular remodelling is presently uncertain (Gossage & Christman, 1994). Epidermal growth factor (EGF) is also powerfully mitogenic to vascular smooth muscle cells, its infusion into rat lungs leading to medial muscular hypertrophy when it can be found in the remodelled vessels (Gillespie et al, 1989). Pulmonary neuroendocrine cells containing gastrin-releasing peptide (GRP), also a smooth muscle mitogen, are greatly increased in number in lungs from patients with PPA, although the significance of this observation is unclear (Gosney et al, 1989). Finally, a variety of vasoactive agents has been shown to have some degree of trophic effect on the pulmonary vasculature in vitro. These include certain arachidonic acid derivatives, serotonin and angiotensin, although whether these effects are significant in vivo in either the maintenance of the pulmonary vasculature in health or the pathogenesis of pulmonary hypertension is unknown (Gossage & Christman, 1994).

Mediation of pulmonary hypertension

As the knowledge of these mediators has increased, their possible roles in the pathogenesis of two forms of pulmonary hypertension in particular has attracted considerable interest. These are pulmonary hypertension due to chronic alveolar hypoxia and pulmonary hypertension characterized by PPA, especially PPH. It is likely that the changes provoked in the pulmonary vasculature by other causes of pulmonary hypertension, such as those causing pulmonary venous congestion and obstruction of the pulmonary vessels, are likely to be mediated by the same or similar mechanisms. The pathogenesis of these forms of pulmonary hypertension has not been closely studied and they will not be considered further in this review.

Hypoxic pulmonary vascular disease

The acute and chronic pulmonary vascular responses to hypoxia probably have separate mechanisms (Vender, 1994). The former is rapid in onset, purely vasoconstrictive and immediately reversible when oxygen tension normalizes (Voelkel, 1986). The latter is sustained and much less readily reversible (Anthonisen, 1983) and has, as its basis, not only vasoconstriction but also structurally altered vessels. As described above, this latter process involves predominantly the smallest arteries and arterioles. Medial and adventitial collagen and elastic tissue is increased and there is proliferation and migration of smooth muscle cell precursors leading to arteriolar medial muscularization and, sometimes, development of smooth muscle bundles in the intima (Reid, 1979). The hypoxic pulmonary hypertension these processes lead to is common, because it arises whenever alveolar hypoxia causes pulmonary arterial hypoxaemia, such as occurs in hypoventilatory states, in chronic bronchitis and emphysema, and at high altitude.

Deficient synthesis of NO is probably an important factor in the persistent vasoconstriction caused by chronic alveolar hypoxia. In hypoxic pulmonary hypertension associated with vascular remodelling in rats, NO activity is impaired (Adnot et al, 1991) and the same appears to be the case in hypoxic human lungs (Dinh Xuan et al, 1991). This does not appear to be due to any barrier to its diffusion from endothelium to smooth muscle, an increase in its breakdown, or to a lack of smooth muscle sensitivity to it, but to reduced expression of NO synthase (Adnot et al, 1995). This lack of NO would remove not only a force opposing vasoconstriction, but also an inhibitory effect on intraluminal platelet aggregation and smooth muscle proliferation. As might be expected, inhalation of NO by rats with hypoxic pulmonary hypertension produces vasodilatation and attenuates pulmonary arteriolar muscularization and right ventricular hypertrophy (Adnot et al, 1995).

The neatness of these observations makes the idea attractive that hypoxic inhibition of NO synthase is the basis of hypoxic pulmonary hypertension, but other factors may also be important. For example, direct mechanical stimulation itself appears to play a key role (Rabinovitch et al, 1983) and decreased oxygen tension is a stimulus to secretion of ET; chronic hypoxia increases levels of ET mRNA and ET secretion from human pulmonary endothelium (Kourembanas et al, 1991) and the same effect occurs in rats (Elton et al, 1992), where it can be blocked by specific antagonism of the appropriate ET receptor (Bonvallet et al, 1993).

Arachidonic acid derivatives may be important also. Decreased production of prostacyclin and prostaglandin E2 has been described in pulmonary arterial rings from neonatal calves with hypoxic pulmonary hypertension (Badesch et al, 1989) and infusion of angiotensin II prevents pulmonary vascular remodelling in hypoxic rats, probably by stimulating vasodilator prostaglandins (Rabinovitch et al, 1988). Platelet-activating factor (PAF) and vasoconstrictor eicosanoids have also been implicated (Richalet et al, 1991), as have polyamines (Shiao et al, 1990) and PDGF (Katayose et al, 1993).

Plexogenic pulmonary arteriopathy

Although not the commonest of those forms of pulmonary hypertension characterized by PPA, the pathogenesis of PPH has attracted most interest, probably because it is so intriguing (Rubin, 1993, 1995; Gossage & Christman, 1994; Voelkel & Tuder, 1995).

There seems little doubt that the disease is triggered in genetically predisposed individuals by stimuli which injure the pulmonary endothelium (Rubin, 1993; Gossage & Christman, 1994; Voelkel & Tuder, 1995). Such injury may be mechanical, hypoxic, chemical, immune-mediated or inflammatory. The resulting endothelial dysfunction probably then leads to vasoconstriction, which is an important and to some extent reversible component of the disease. A variety of mechanisms may underlie this vasoconstriction, two of which have already been mentioned, namely imbalance between thromboxane and prostacyclin (Christman et al, 1992) and increased synthesis of ET (Giaid et al, 1993). Other substances which have been implicated in mediating the vasoconstrictive component of PPH include serotonin, angiotensin II and catecholamines (Gossage & Christman, 1994).

The gross remodelling which characterizes PPA probably involves similar agents stimulating proliferation and migration of smooth muscle cells which assume a myofibroblastic phenotype and contribute to the concentric laminar intimal fibrosis and plexiform lesions which are typically seen (Smith et al, 1990). Important in this process, in addition, are likely to be one or more of a variety of growth factors, including IGF, TGF-β and PDGF. Such substances could be released by not only injured endothelium, but also by aggregated platelets in the focal thrombotic lesions which frequently accompany PPA, and the cells which make up the inflammatory infiltrate which is often present in and around plexiform lesions (Voelkel & Tuder, 1995).

When PPA is caused by excessive flow of blood into the lungs due to left-to-right intra- or extra cardiac shunting, it presumably is due to mechanical damage to the endothelium which initiates the same sequence of events.

References

Adnot, S. B., Raffestin, S., Eddahibi, P., Braquet, P. & Chabrier, P. E. (1991). Loss of endothelium-dependent relaxant activity in the pulmonary circulation of rats exposed to chronic hypoxia. *Journal of Clinical Investigation*, **87**, 155–62.

Adnot, S., Raffestin, B. & Eddahibi, S. (1995). NO in the lung. *Respiration Physiology*, **101**, 109–20.

Advenier, C., Sarria, B., Naline, E., Puybasset, L. & Lagente, V. (1990). Contractile activity of three endothelins (ET-1, ET-2 and ET-3) on the human isolated bronchus. *British Journal of Pharmacology*, **100**, 168–72.

Anthonisen, N. R. (1983). Long term oxygen therapy. *Annals of Internal Medicine*, **99**, 519–27.

Badesch, D. B., Orton, E. C. & Zapp, L. M. (1989). Decreased arterial wall prostaglandin production in neonatal calves with severe chronic pulmonary hypertension. *American Journal of Respiratory Cell and Molecular Biology*, **1**, 489–98.

Barnes, P. J. (1994). Endothelins and pulmonary diseases. *Journal of Applied Physiology*, **77**, 1051–9.

Bonvallet, S. T., Morris, K. G., Yano, M., Zamora, M. R., McMurty, I. F. & Stelzner, T. J.

(1993). A selective ET_A receptor antagonist (BQ 123) attenuates the development of hypoxic pulmonary hypertension in vivo (abstract). *American Review of Respiratory Diseases*, **147**, A493.

Brewster, C. E. P., Howarth, P. H., Djukanovic, R., Wilson, J., Holgate, S. T. & Roche, W. R. (1990). Myofibroblasts and subepithelial fibrosis in bronchial asthma. *American Journal of Respiratory Cell and Molecular Biology*, **3**, 507–11.

Brink, C., Gillard, V. & Roubert, J. M. (1991). Effects and specific binding sites of endothelin in human lung preparations. *Pulmonary Pharmacology*, **4**, 54–9.

Christman, B. W., McPherson, B. D., Newman, J. H., King, G. A., Bernard, G. R. & Loyd, J. E. (1992). An imbalance between the secretion of thromboxane and prostacyclin metabolites in pulmonary hypertension. *New England Journal of Medicine*, **327**, 70–5.

Dempsey, E. C., Stenmark, K. R., McMurtry, I. F., O'Brien, R. F., Voelkel, N. F. & Badesch, D. B. (1990). Insulin like growth factor I and protein kinase C activation stimulate pulmonary artery smooth muscle cell proliferation through separate but synergistic pathways. *Journal of Cell Physiology*, **144**, 159–65.

Dinh Xuan, A. T., Higenbottam, T. W., Clelland, C. A., Pepke-Zaba, J., Cremona, G., Butt, A. Y., Large, S. R., Wells, F. C. & Wallwork, J. (1991). Impairment of endothelium-dependent pulmonary artery relaxation in chronic obstructive lung disease. *New England Journal of Medicine*, **324**, 1539–47.

Ehrenreich, H., Anderson, R. W., Fox, C.H., Rieckmann, P., Hoffman, G. S., Travis, W. D., Coligan, J. E., Kehrl, J. H. & Fauci, A. S. (1990). Endothelins, peptides with potent vasoactive properties, are produced by human macrophages. *Journal of Experimental Medicine*, **172**, 1741–8.

Elton, T. S., Oparil, S., Taylor, G. R., Hicks, P. H., Yang, R. H., Jin, H. & Chen, Y. F. (1992). Normobaric hypoxia stimulates endothelin-1 gene expression in the rat. *American Journal of Physiology*, **263**, R1260–R1264.

Frostell, C., Fratacci, M. D., Wain, J.C., Jones, R. & Zapol, W. M. (1991). Inhaled nitric oxide, a selective pulmonary vasodilator reversing hypoxic pulmonary vasoconstriction. *Circulation*, **83**, 2038–47.

Garg, U. C. & Hassid, A. (1989). Nitric oxide-generating vasodilators and 8-bromocyclic guanosine monophosphate inhibit mitogenesis and proliferation of cultured rat vascular smooth muscle cells. *Journal of Clinical Investigation*, **83**, 1774–7.

Giaid, A., Polak, J.M., Gaitonde, V., Hamid, Q. A., Moscoso, G., Legon, S., Uwanogho, D., Roncalli, M., Shinmi, O., Sawamura, T., Kimura, S., Yanagisawa, M., Masaki, T. & Springall, D. R. (1991). Distribution of endothelin-like immunoreactivity and mRNA in the developing and adult human lung. *American Review of Respiratory Diseases*, **4**, 50–8.

Giaid, A., Yanagisawa, M., Langleben, D., Michel, R. P., Levy, R., Shennib, A., Kimura, S., Masaki, T., Duguid, W. P. & Stewart, D. J. (1993). Expression of endothelin in the lungs of patients with pulmonary hypertension. *New England Journal of Medicine*, **328**, 1732–9.

Gillespie, M. N., Rippetoe, P. E. & Haven, C. A. *et al.* (1989). Polyamines and epidermal growth factor in monocrotaline-induced pulmonary hypertension. *American Review of Respiratory Diseases*, **140**, 1463–6.

Gosney, J., Heath, D., Smith, P., Harris, P. & Yacoub, M. (1989). Pulmonary endocrine cells in pulmonary arterial disease. *Archives of Pathology and Laboratory Medicine*, **113**, 337–41.

Gossage, J. R. & Christman, B. W. (1994). Mediators of acute and chronic pulmonary hypertension: Part II. *Seminars in Respiratory and Critical Care Medicine*, **15**, 453–62.

Gurtner, H. P. (1990). Aminorex pulmonary hypertension. In *The Pulmonary Circulation: Normal and Abnormal*, ed. A. P. Fishman, pp. 397–412. Philadelphia: University of Pennsylvannia Press.

Hadengue, A., Behayoun, M. K. & Lebrec, D. & Benhamou, J. P. (1991). Pulmonary hypertension complicating portal hypertension: prevalence and relation to splanchnic hemodynamics. *Gastroenterology*, **100**, 520–8.

Hatano, S. & Strasser, T. (eds) (1975). *Primary Pulmonary Hypertension*. WHO: Geneva.

Katayose, D., Ohe, M., Yamauchi, K., Ogata, M., Shirato, K. & Fujita, M. (1993). Increased expression of PDGF A- and B- chain genes in rat lungs with hypoxic pulmonary hypertension. *American Journal of Physiology*, **264**, L100–L106.

Kourembanas, S., Hannan, R. L. & Faller, D. V. (1990). Oxygen tension regulates the expression of the platelet-derived growth factor-beta chain gene in human endothelial cells. *Journal of Clinical Investigation*, **86**, 670–4.

Kourembanas, S., Marsden, P. A., McQuillan, L. P. & Faller, D. V. (1991). Hypoxia induces endothelin gene expression and secretion in cultured human endothelium. *Journal of Clinical Investigation*, **88**, 1054–7.

Loach, R. M., Twort, C. H. C. & Cameron, I. R. & Ward, J. P. T. (1990). The mechanisms of action of endothelin-1 on small pulmonary arterial vessels. *Pulmonary Pharmacology*, **3**, 103–9.

Marciniak, S. J., Plumpton, C., Barker, P. J., Huskisson, N. & Davenport, A. P. (1992). Localization of immunoreactive endothelin and proendothelin in the human lung. *Pulmonary Pharmacology*, **5**, 175–82.

Morganroth, M. L., Stenmark, K. R., Morris, K. G., Murphy, R. C., Mathias, M. & Reeves, J. T. (1985). Diethylcarbamazine inhibits acute and chronic hypoxic pulmonary hypertension in awake rats. *American Review of Respiratory Diseases*, **131**, 488–92.

Muldoon, L., Rodland, R. D., Forsythe, M. L. & Magun, B. E. (1989). Stimulation of phosphatidylinositol hydrolyso, diacylglycerol release, and gene expression in response to endothelin, a potent new agonist for fibroblasts and smooth muscle cells. *Journal of Biological Chemistry*, **264**, 8529–36.

Perkett, E. A., Badesch, D. B., Roessler, M. D., Stenmark, K. R. & Meyrick, B. (1992a). Insulin-like growth factor I and pulmonary hypertension induced by continuous air embolization in sheep. *American Journal of Respiratory Cell and Molecular Biology*, **6**, 82–7.

Perkett, E. A., Lyons, R. M. & Moses, H. L. (1990). Transforming growth factor-beta activity in sheep lung lymph during the development of pulmonary hypertension. *Journal of Clinical Investigation*, **86**, 1459–64.

Perkett, E. A., Pelton, R. W. & Gold, L. I. (1992b). Expression of transforming growth factor (TGF)-beta I, -beta 2 and -beta 3 in sheep lungs during the development of pulmonary hypertension secondary to air embolization: immunohistochemistry and in situ hybridization. *American Review of Respiratory Diseases*, **145**, A478.

Pietra, G. G., Edwards, W. D., Kay, J. M., Rich, S., Kernis, J., Schloo, B., Ayres, S. M., Bergofsky, E. H., Brundage, B. H., Detre, K. M., Fishman, A. P., Goldring, R. M., Groves, B. M., Levy, P. S., Reid, L. M., Vreim, C. E. & Williams, G. W. (1989). Histopathology of primary pulmonary hypertension: a qualitative and quantitative study of pulmonary blood vessels from 58 patients in the National Heart, Lung and Blood Institute, Primary Pulmonary Hypertension Registry. *Circulation*, **80**, 1198–206.

Rabinovitch, M., Konstam, M. A., Gamble, W. J., Paponicolaou, N., Aronovitz, M. J. & Treves, S. (1983). Changes in pulmonary blood flow effect vascular response to chronic hypoxia in rats. *Circulation Research*, **54**, 432–41.

Rabinovitch, M., Mullen, M. & Rosenberg, H. C. (1988). Angiotensin II prevents hypoxic pulmonary hypertension and vascular changes in rats. *American Journal of Physiology*, **254**, H500–H508.

Reid, L. (1979). The pulmonary circulation: remodeling in growth and disease. *American Review of Respiratory Diseases*, **119**, 531–46.

Rich, S., Pietra, G. G., Kieras, K., Hart, K. & Brundage, B. H. (1986). Primary pulmonary hypertension: radiographic and scintigraphic patterns of histologic subtypes. *Annals of Internal Medicine*, **105**, 499–502.

Richalet, J. P., Hornych, A. & Rathat, C. (1991). Plasma prostaglandins, leukotrienes and thromboxane in acute high altitude hypoxia. *Respiration Physiology*, **85**, 205–15.

Rubin, L. J. (1993). ACCP consensus statement: primary pulmonary hypertension. *Chest*, **104**, 236–50.

Rubin, L. J. (1995). Pathology and pathophysiology of primary pulmonary hypertension. *American Journal of Cardiology*, **75**, 51A–54A.

Shiao, R.-T., Kostenbauder, H. B., Olson, J. W. & Gillespie, M. N. (1990). Mechanisms of lung polyamine accumulation in chronic hypoxic pulmonary hypertension. *American Journal of Physiology*, **259**, L351–L358.

Smith, P. & Heath, D. (1979). Electron microscopy of the plexiform lesion. *Thorax*, **34**, 177–86.

Smith, P., Heath, D., Yacoub, M., Madden, B., Caslin, A. W. & Gosney, J. R. (1990). The ultrastructure of plexogenic pulmonary arteriopathy. *Journal of Pathology*, **160**, 111–21.

Speich, R., Jenni, R., Opravil, M., Pfab, M. & Russi, E. W. (1991). Primary pulmonary hypertension in HIV infection. *Chest*, **100**, 1268–71.

Stewart, D. J., Levy, R. D., Cernacek, P. & Langleben, D. (1991). Increased plasma endothelin-1 in pulmonary hypertension: marker or mediator of disease? *Annals of Internal Medicine*, **114**, 464–9.

Vender, R. L. (1994). Chronic hypoxic pulmonary hypertension. *Chest*, **106**, 236–43.

Voelkel, N. F. (1986). Mechanisms of hypoxic pulmonary vasoconstriction. *American Review of Respiratory Diseases*, **133**, 1186–95.

Voelkel, N. F. & Tuder, R. M. (1995). Cellular and molecular mechanisms in the pathogenesis of severe pulmonary hypertension. *European Respiratory Journal*, **8**, 2129–38.

Wagenvoort, C. A. (1975). Pathology of congestive pulmonary hypertension. *Progress in Respiratory Research*, **9**, 195–202.

Wagenvoort, C. A. (1995). Pulmonary vascular disease. In *Practical Pulmonary Pathology*, ed. M. N. Sheppard, pp. 145–64. London: Edward Arnold.

8

Mechanisms of atherosclerosis

I: Introduction and current concepts

M. SCHACHTER

Introduction

The importance of atherosclerosis in cardiovascular medicine needs no emphasis. Although the pathological appearance and clinical implications of this process have been known for at least a century, understanding of the cellular and molecular mechanisms has been very largely a product of the past 20 years. Much of it has derived from the work of Russell Ross and his colleagues at the University of Washington in Seattle. In 1973 Ross proposed the hypothesis that atherosclerosis is a 'response to injury' (Ross & Glomset, 1973), in particular to injury to the vascular endothelium. The hypothesis has been repeatedly revised and modified in the light of new findings, and is now accepted at least as a useful working concept by most researchers in this area (Ross, 1993). In recent years there has been recognition of an increasing number of potentially injurious agents, which can of course be regarded as 'risk factors' for atherogenesis.

The response to injury hypothesis

In its most recent form the hypothesis can be summarized as follows:

1. Many factors can damage or activate the endothelium. Table 8.1 lists those currently recognised but the list will certainly grow. To these agents must also be added the very important role of mechanical influences. The clearest demonstration of this is the fact that some parts of the vascular tree are much more prone to atheroma than others. These are areas of low shear stress and reversing blood flow, where the residence times of cells and lipoproteins are increased (Nerem & Sprague, 1993). Aspects of endothelial activation, especially the role of adhesion molecules, will be discussed in detail in Section II of this chapter.
2. Endothelial dysfunction and activation leads to increased permeability so that lipoprotein particles, and circulating cells (particularly monocytes which become macrophages in the vessel wall, and T lymphocytes) adhere to endothelial cells

Table 8.1. *Causes of endothelial injury or dysfunction*

Hyperlipidaemia (esp. low-density lipoproteins, lipoprotein (a))
Diabetes (hyperglycaemia, dyslipidaemia)
Hypertension
Smoking
Hyperhomocystinaemia
Ischaemia/reperfusion (e.g. thrombolysis)
Viruses, *Chlamydia*, other infective agents (?)

(Section II) and then enter the sub endothelial space and form the initial lesion of atherosclerosis, the fatty streak.

3. Increasing cellular and lipid infiltration may lead to increased endothelial disruption leading to the exposure of thrombogenic surfaces to which platelets adhere.

4. Platelets, macrophages, endothelial cells, as well as smooth muscle cells themselves, can all release growth modulatory factors interacting with smooth muscle and potentially leading to the proliferation of these cells and of fibroblasts.

5. This process leads to the formation of the fibrous plaque and ultimately to the complex advanced lesion of atherosclerosis containing all the cell types mentioned above , as well as large quantities of extracellular matrix proteins, such as collagens, and of free and esterified extracellular cholesterol. Lesions with large amounts of such lipids are considered to be particularly unstable and liable to rupture, leading to thrombosis and vessel occlusion.

The hypothesis is shown in highly schematic form in Fig. 8.1 and the possible interrelations of the stages of the lesion in Fig. 8.2. There is still considerable uncertainty and controversy about the latter issue although it is likely that all the stages of this process are at least potentially reversible, but perhaps not completely. Ross' concept of atherosclerosis is as an 'inflammatory fibroproliferative process', in fact a repair mechanism which becomes harmful. At least in part this is due to the chronic and unremitting nature of the injury or indeed multiple injuries, for instance hyperlipidaemia, hypertension or smoking.

Cellular mechanisms
Endothelium (considered in greater detail in Section II)

Increasing knowledge about atherosclerosis has been paralleled by an explosion of interest in the endothelium arising from the realization that it is far more than an inert cellular barrier. Among the vital functions of endothelium is to maintain a non-thrombogenic non-adherent surface for platelets, one which is also non-adherent for neutrophils (Gimbrone, 1976) . It is certainly a permeability barrier, but one which is highly dynamic and closely regulated. Endothelial cells are also sources of many growth-modulatory molecules (Ross,1995; Oemar et al, 1995), interacting mostly with

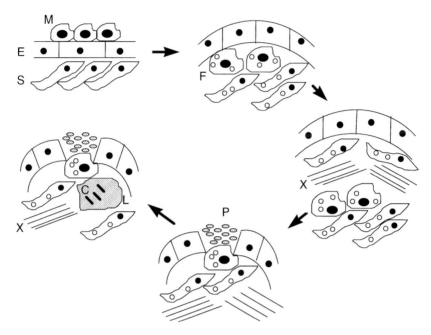

Fig. 8.1. Schematic representation of the stages and progression of atherosclerosis, broadly based on the response to injury hypothesis. M: monocyte/macrophage; E: endothelium; S: smooth muscle cell (later stages with lipid droplets); F: foam cell; P: platelet; L + C: core of extracellular lipid with calcification; X: collagen and other extracellular matrix proteins. Progression may *not* necessarily follow a linear sequence (see Fig. 8.2).

smooth muscle cells, as well as agents regulating vascular tone (Cohen, 1995), notably nitric oxide (NO), prostacyclin and the endothelins. There is substantial overlap between the two groups, with most molecules possessing activity in both areas. As a broad generalization, growth-promoting agents are vasoconstrictor while vasodilators inhibit smooth muscle proliferation. A recently defined, and very probably undesirable, property of the endothelium is its capacity to oxidize low-density lipoproteins (LDL) (Parthasarathy et al, 1989).

Monocytes/macrophages

The macrophage, in other words, the monocyte which has become 'resident' in the vascular wall, is the principal inflammatory cell of the atherosclerotic lesion (Hansson et al, 1989). These cells acts as scavengers, internalizing lipoproteins (Goldstein et al, 1979), especially oxidized LDL (oxLDL), forming foam cells. In fact, macrophages may be the main mediators of oxidation (Parthasarathy et al, 1986), but the exact mechanisms involved remain obscure. Macrophages replicate within atheromatous plaques and are also rich sources of growth modulators for the smooth muscle cells (see also Section II).

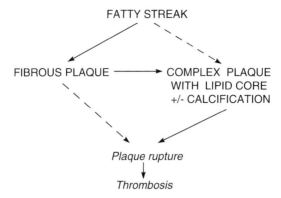

Fig. 8.2. Interrelations between stages of the atheromatous plaque. There is likely to be reversibility at each stage, but this is not proven in human disease.

Smooth muscle

In the normal blood vessel the smooth muscle cell is the only cell type found in the media, while very few if any smooth muscle cells are found in any other vessel layer. Despite this apparent uniformity in their distribution these cells are heterogeneous with distinct embryonic origins and variable responses to atherogenic stimuli (Schwartz et al, 1990). They are the main proliferative cell within the plaque and are also largely responsible for the synthesis of extracellular matrix (Wight, 1989). Smooth muscle cells are often described as existing in two phenotypic states: 'contractile' or quiescent, their usual healthy condition, and 'synthetic' or proliferative, where the cells replicate as well as synthesizing matrix proteins (Thyberg et al, 1990). While there is considerable evidence for such a distinction, it is of course an oversimplification (Owens, 1995). It is also uncertain how this concept relates to the long-established observations that smooth muscle cells within a particular plaque are monoclonal (Benditt, 1977), although it is now generally believed that the capacity for phenotypic modulation may not be found in all smooth muscle cells. In addition to the above activities smooth muscle cells must migrate from the media to the intima in response to chemotactic stimuli because the plaque is exclusively an intimal lesion (Stary et al, 1992).

T lymphocytes

Although the T lymphocyte is found in abundance within plaques its role remains obscure. The numbers of these cells in the plaque will be enhanced by proliferative cytokines secreted by adjacent macrophages (Hansson et al, 1989; Watanabe et al, 1995). It has recently been proposed that T lymphocytes within plaques are specifically responding to the presence of oxLDL (Zhou et al, 1996).

Oxidized LDL

Almost everyone now accepts that high circulating levels of LDL are strongly associated with atherosclerosis. In the past decade it has also been established that these particles become modified to more atherogenic forms in the vessel wall, mostly by oxidation (Witztum, 1994; Berliner et al, 1995). It is believed that the macrophage is a key element in this process, as is the endothelial cell, but the precise details remain to be unravelled: it is uncertain whether this is primarily an enzyme catalyzed process (e.g. by a lipoxygenase) or one mediated by oxygen free radicals generated by neighbouring cells (Sparrow & Olszewski, 1992). The extent of the oxidation has important functional implications. Highly oxidized LDL is cytotoxic to endothelium, macrophages and smooth muscle (Cathcart et al, 1991) but less extensively damaged lipoprotein also has multiple biological effects, although their relevance in vivo is uncertain: a mitogenic and chemotactic effect on smooth muscle cells (Auge et al, 1995); chemotactic activity for monocytes; activation of endothelial cells, with increased expression of adhesion molecules for leukocytes (see Section II); and the activation of monocytes/macrophages themselves (Holvoet & Collen, 1994). OxLDL is therefore very likely to play a central role in the inflammatory fibroproliferative process described by Ross. It is taken up by scavenger receptors on macrophages, and probably also by a specific receptor, leading to foam cell formation (Goldstein et al, 1979). This also occurs in smooth muscle cells (Raines & Ross, 1993).

LDL oxidation is constantly opposed by endogenous enzymatic and non-enzymatic antioxidants, even though some of these probably do not have access to the parts of the vessel wall where the lipoprotein particles are located and oxidation takes place. A particularly interesting if mainly indirect antagonist of oxidation is high-density lipoprotein (HDL) (Gordon et al, 1989), and it is tempting to suppose that this may be one mechanism by which HDL is protective in atherosclerotic cardiovascular disease.

Growth modulators

It has already been noted that growth modulators are produced by the various cell types involved in atherogenesis. The smooth muscle cell is their main target, although macrophage replication is also affected by some of the molecules (see Section II). Table 8.2 includes the major factors currently recognized, but is not meant to be comprehensive. Ross' discovery of platelet-derived growth factor (PDGF), the most potent known smooth muscle mitogen and chemotactic agent, dates from the same time as the original version of his response to the injury hypothesis (Ross et al, 1974). In the succeeding 20 years there has been a huge proliferation of potential positive and negative growth regulators (Ross, 1993; Raines & Ross, 1993; Oemar et al, 1995), together with a mass of information on the expression of genes both for the factors themselves and for their receptors (Wilcox et al, 1988). There has also been a parallel increase in interest in genes involved in proliferative processes, such as the proto-oncogenes c-*fos* and c-*myc* (Parkes et al, 1991). It is not possible at present to produce a coherent scheme which contains the multitude of possible interactions between all these molecules and it may be years before

Table 8.2. *Factors modulating vascular smooth muscle growth*

Positive	Negative
PDGF * (P, E, S, M)	IL-1
bFGF * (E, S, M)	TGF-β
IGF-1 (P, E, S, M)	IFNγ (M, T)
EGF/TGFα (P, M)	Nitric oxide (E, M, S)
IL-1 (E, S, M, T)	Prostacyclin (E)
TGF-β* (P, E, S, M, T)	Adenosine (E, S)
VEGF * (M)	Heparan sulphates (E, S)
oxLDL * (E, M)	
Angiotensin II (E)	
Endothelin (E)	

Note: PDGF: platelet-derived growth factor; bFGF: basic fibroblast growth factor; IGF-1: insulin like growth factor; EGF: epidermal growth factor; TGF-α, β: transforming growth factor α, β; VEGF: vascular endothelial growth factor; ox-LDL: oxidized LDL; IFNγ: interferon γ.
Cells of origin: P: platelet; E: endothelium; S: smooth muscle; M: macrophage; T: T lymphocyte.
* Also possess known chemotactic activity.

a convincing picture emerges. The complexity is emphasized by the fact that two molecules, interleukin 1 and transforming growth factor β, appear as both growth stimulants and inhibitors, depending on the circumstances. It is more than likely that other modulators will also prove to be bidirectional. (See also Chapter 13).

Aortic aneurysms: a special type of atherosclerosis?

The pathogenesis of abdominal aortic aneurysms is a controversial issue (Chapter 11). It was long believed that they were just one manifestation of generalized atherosclerosis; however, this seems increasingly unlikely (MacSweeney et al, 1994; Patel et al, 1995). Patients with aneurysms are generally older than those with coronary atheroma or other occlusive arterial disease and often have little or no atherosclerosis elsewhere. Furthermore, aneurysms are often associated with a strong family history. More recent research has focused on the disruption of extracellular matrix proteins, particularly elastin, which always occurs in aneurysms. It now appears that vascular smooth muscle cells within the aneurysmal wall secrete significantly increased quantities of metalloproteinases which degrade elastin and the other matrix proteins (Patel et al, 1996). Aneurysms also contain large numbers of inflammatory cells in their walls, and these secrete similar proteolytic enzymes (Newman et al, 1994). Both aneurysmal and atherosclerotic disease can therefore be considered as varieties of inflammatory process, and can indeed co-exist in the same vessel.

Problems and prospects

Although we know a great deal about the mechanisms of atherosclerosis many details remain sketchy and contentious. For instance, has the importance of cell proliferation been overstated and should we be more interested in remodelling, where the vessel lumen is reduced but the mass of the vessel wall does not increase? This may have greater relevance for the problem of restenosis following coronary angioplasty than for primary atherosclerosis (Lafont et al, 1995). As indicated above, we do not know which growth factors really matter. Even more importantly from a clinical standpoint, there are outstanding therapeutic questions. It is evident that reducing levels of circulating lipids, notably LDL cholesterol and triglycerides, reduces cardiovascular morbidity and mortality (Scandinavian Simvastatin Study Group, 1994; Shepherd et al, 1995), but what else would be helpful? There has been much interest in antioxidants, especially in the hope that they may prevent LDL oxidation, but the issue is very far from being resolved (Hoffman & Garewal, 1995). There is also the proposition that existing cardiovascular drugs, such as calcium channel blockers (Borcherding et al, 1993) and angiotensin converting enzyme (ACE) inhibitors (Sharpe, 1993), may have additional anti atherosclerotic effects. Furthermore, should we literally *treat* atherosclerosis as an inflammatory condition? Irrespective of these considerations, it is clear that the techniques of molecular genetics such as the use of transgenic models of atherosclerosis e.g. as apolipoprotein E knockout mice; will make immense contributions to our understanding of this complex process (Nakashima et al, 1994).

II: Relations between monocytes, macrophages and the endothelium

R. POSTON

Atherosclerosis as a self-perpetuating process

It is a universal feature of atherosclerotic disease that it develops in localized lesions termed plaques. As this is true of animal models and human disease, it seems likely that this morphology reflects basic mechanisms involved in it (Fig. 8.3). Many factors can initiate atherosclerosis, as described in Section I, however the plaque morphology can be explained by the hypothesis that the atherosclerotic plaque represents a self-perpetuating focus of chronic inflammation which is dependent on elevated lipid levels in the arterial wall. Evidence for a self-perpetuating nature of atherosclerosis was first obtained some years ago when Albrecht & Schuler (1965) fed rabbits a high cholesterol diet for 6 weeks. Early atherosclerotic lesions were initiated in the aorta, and in rabbits that were then put back onto a normal diet, lipid continued accumulating in the aortic lesions, despite low levels in the blood. Such a mechanism can explain the near random local development of atheroma in suceptible arteries, as minor damaging stimuli would be capable of initiating it at a particular point and, once started, it would tend to develop spontaneously there to become a mature plaque. This view is an extension to the classic response to injury hypothesis, as the endothelium has been considered a major target for injury, and also is likely to be at the centre of the self-regenerative process (Table 8.3). Although there has been limited success in human trials of low-lipid diets, human atherosclerosis is clearly also very difficult to reverse.

Macrophage morphology

It can be proposed that monocyte–macrophage traffic into the arterial intima is the critical and rate limiting process in atherogenesis. Immunohistology of atherosclerotic human arteries shows that the great majority of atherosclerotic plaques contain large numbers of macrophages in the intima. Indeed, the earliest lesions, the fatty streaks, consist of little else but sub-endothelial collections of macrophages that have accumu-lated lipids to become foamy cells. Fibro-fatty plaques usually have macrophages on the outer aspect of the fibrous cap in the central part of the lesion, i.e. separated by the fibrous cap from the lumen, while at the peripheral shoulders of the lesion, they remain near the endothelium. A particular significance has been attached to the presence of macrophages close to the lumen, as the macrophages produce matrix-degrading metal-loproteinases, and it is in these regions that the plaque is particularly liable to crack, and thrombosis to be initiated (Galis 1995).

Within the plaque huge masses of macrophages can often accumulate, and the individual cells also can become very large, particularly on the outer aspect of the cell groups. In this region, the cells may die, and release their lipid contents into pools of extracellular gruelly material, from which the name atheroma is derived - porridge in Greek. The gradual enlarging of the cells towards the outer side of the intima suggests that there is a slow outward movement accompanied by lipid accumulation. Further support for this view comes from the smallest macrophages closest to the endothelium having monocyte-specific cell markers that are not expressed by mature macrophages (Poston & Hussain 1993). These observations correlate well with evidence that mono-cytes cross the arterial endothelium into the plaques, which will be discussed below.

By contrast with the atherosclerotic plaques, few macrophages are seen within the relatively normal areas of the arterial wall. There may be some differences in various arterial sites, as we have seen negligible numbers in coronary arteries, whilst a few scattered cells may be present in the non-atherosclerotic intima of carotid arteries and aortas which elsewhere have severe disease. There can be no doubt that monocyte–macrophage traffic is specific to the atherosclerotic lesions, and in a recent unpublished quantitative image analysis study on seven carotid arteries, we found a mean of 32% of atherosclerotic intima stained by the CD68 macrophage marker compared with 2% of normal regions ($p < 0.001$). Furthermore, many authors have commented on the

Table 8.3. *Adhesion molecules in endothelial-leukocyte adhesion*

Addressin (endothelium) binds	Homing receptor (leukocyte)	Notes
Selectins		
E-selectin	Sialyl-Lewis x carbohydrate in glycoproteins	Homing receptors on most leukocytes. E-selectin normally low, increased with inflammation.
P-selectin	Sialyl-Lewis x in glycoprotein PSGL-1	P-selectin binds polymorphs and monocytes. Present on platelets
Gly-CAM-1 (mucin) CD34 (mucin) MAD-CAM-1 (mucin)	L-selectin	L-selectin in present on most leukocytes, the addressins are selectively distributed on endothelia.
Immunoglobulin supergene family intercellular adhesion molecules		
ICAM-1	Beta-2 integrins:- LFA-1, Mac-1 (LFA-1 is on most leukocytes)	ICAM-1 is increased with inflammation but is normally present on small vessels
ICAM-2	LFA-1	ICAM-2 is normally present, but is not regulated with endothelial activation
Vascular cell adhesion molecule	Beta-1 integrin: VLA-4	VCAM-1 is not normally expressed, appears with inflammation
Platelet-endothelial adhesion Molecule (PECAM)	Homophilic (PECAM-PECAM) and other unidentified ligands	PECAM is present on endothelial cells, platelets and leukocytes
Other adhesion molecules		
Not identified	CD14 (on monocytes)	Major role in adhesion of monocytes to activated endothelium
Vascular adhesion protein-1 (VAP-1)	Not identified	Found in rheumatoid arthritis joints

See text for references to atherosclerosis.

selective adhesion of blood monocytes to the surface of atherosclerotic regions of the arterial wall. In areas of active monocyte traffic into plaques, monocytes are also often found within the endothelial layer, or even occasionally forming a pseudoendothelium composed mostly of monocytes.

T lymphocytes and immune responses

The resemblance of atherosclerosis to chronic inflammation is increased by the presence of some T lymphocytes in addition to macrophages in the plaques. This is typical of the

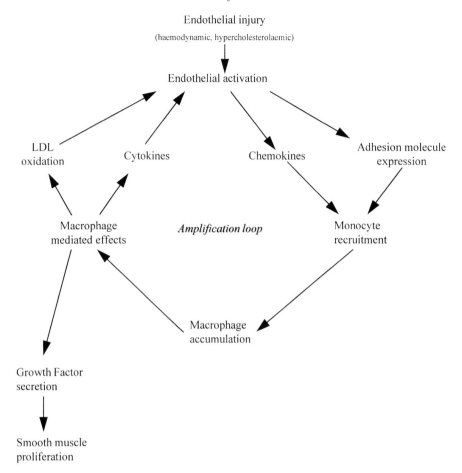

Fig. 8.3. Positive feedback model for atherosclerosis, based on endothelial activation, consequent monocyte traffic, and feedback activation of the endothelium by macrophage products.

mononuclear leukocytes of chronic inflammation, which consist mainly of a mixture of these cell types. It is not clear what the role of these T cells may be, but it is worth noting that their presence does not necessarily imply that a specific immune response is taking place, because in chronic inflammation it is known that they are recruited without regard to their immune specificity. Indeed it is possible that they could play a role in a non-immune fashion, as ox-LDL is capable of activating them (Frostegard et al, 1992). On the other hand, it is quite possible that immune responses against plaque constituents may contribute to the disease process. In particular, the recent demonstration of *Chlamydia pneumoniae* organisms in the plaque, and the presence of circulating antibodies, gives exciting new evidence in favour of such a mechanism (Mlot, 1996). In addition, it is now established that immune reactivity can develop to oxLDL and to heat shock proteins, both of which are present in the plaques (Salonen et al. 1992; Xu et al., 1993). It seems unlikely that immune reactivity is essential for atherogenesis, as the disease can be induced in mice with a congenital lack of immune responsiveness (Fyfe et al, 1994).

Cellular adhesion mechanisms

Endothelial activation forms a central concept to the understanding of atherosclerosis and vascular biology in general. It can take an acute form, discussed in a later section, and a chronic form. The chronic form shows metabolic alterations, including changes involved in leukocyte adhesion. The mechanisms for leukocyte recruitment to foci of inflammation have been studied extensively, particularly by Springer in Boston (Springer, 1994). The leukocyte traffic is induced by adhesion between the surfaces of the circulating leukocytes and the endothelial cells, which causes the arrest of the leukocytes and subsequent migration into the tissues. The adhesion is induced by the expression of adhesive molecules on the surfaces of the endothelium and the leukocytes. The expression and activation of these adhesion molecules is greatly increased by metabolic activation of either cell type. Endothelial cells in a focus of inflammation are activated by inflammatory mediators, such as interleukin (IL-1), and the leukocytes by molecules best known as chemotactic factors, such as the complement component C5a. The adhesion molecules involved in inflammation are listed in Table 8.1. Endothelial cells are also sensitive to blood flow and can, for example, be activated to increased expression of ICAM-1, even by shear stresses within the physiological range (Nagel et al, 1994).

Recent work has strongly suggested a role for adhesion mechanisms in atherosclerosis. Expression of the endothelial adhesion molecules VCAM-1 and ICAM-1 has been found to be increased in the endothelium over rabbit atherosclerotic plaques (Cybulsky & Gimbrone, 1991) Likewise ICAM-1 has been detected in human atherosclerosis, whereas reports on VCAM-1 have been variable (Wood et al, 1993, Duplaa et al, 1996). Furthermore, the normal arterial endothelium differs from that of small vessels in that it expresses little or no ICAM-1, whereas the small vessels have high levels. A similar set of findings have been made for P-selectin in human arteries, no normal expression, but greatly increased cytoplasmic and surface expression in the endothelial cells of atherosclerotic plaques (Johnson-Tidey et al, 1994). E-selectin is also moderately increased.

It is possible to test for adhesion reactions in vitro, by an assay originally devised by Stamper & Woodruff (1976), which uses histological sections and leukocyte suspensions. The cells are incubated with the tissue section on a gently rotating slide. With such an assay, selective binding of monocytes to human atherosclerotic plaques has been observed. Quite unexpectedly, binding was found not only to the endothelium, but also to large areas of atherosclerotic intima. Inhibition of the adhesion by antibodies was used to analyse the adhesion molecules involved, and demonstrated a dependence on ICAM-1 and β-2 integrins, and on the monocyte surface molecule CD14 (Poston & Johnson-Tidey, 1996).

Chemoattractants and mediators activating the endothelium

As mentioned above, it is important that chemoattractant and activating substances are available to synergize with adhesion molecules in inducing leukocyte traffic. In atherosclerosis, the monocyte chemoattractant-1 molecule (MCP-1), a chemotactic cytokine, has been identified in plaque macrophages (Nelken et al, 1991). Thus it seems possible that macrophages, once resident in the arterial intima, may attract more monocytes to migrate and join in the process. There are further mechanisms by which the same effect may be produced. Plaque macrophages produce the cytokine tumour necrosis factor (TNF), and possibly IL-1, which are capable of inducing adhesion molecules in endothelial cells. In addition, macrophages and other cells of the lesion are capable of oxidizing LDL, and macrophages are highly efficient at it (Morgan et al, 1993). Ox-LDL is present in the plaques, and has also been found capable of inducing monocyte–endothelial adhesion in vitro (Kim et al, 1994). This implies that endothelial activation is induced, and one mechanism in particular that may be mediating the adhesion is the induction of the P-selectin adhesion molecule (Gebuhrer et al, 1995). Ox-LDL is also able to induce macrophages to release factors that stimulate adhesion molecule expression on endothelial cells. If these potential mechanisms can be shown to have a function in vivo, then an understanding is possible of the self-perpetuating focal atherosclerotic plaque – as a focus where these processes have set up a positive feedback loop, allowing a massive self-perpetuating accumulation of macrophages to occur. It seems likely that the endothelium itself may have a self-perpetuating role, as the feeding of an atherogenic diet to rabbits induced the focal expression of VCAM-1 in the aorta before any macrophages infiltrated or other changes developed (Li et al, 1993). Again oxidative changes to LDL could be involved, as endothelial cells are capable of oxidizing LDL. Another significant factor is that the induction of adhesion molecules in areas of haemodynamic stress may explain the well-known presence of atherosclerosis at those sites (Nagel et al, 1994).

Smoking is an exogenous factor that may influence monocyte-endothelial interaction. Lehr et al (1994) showed that exposure of hamsters to smoke increased leukocyte adhesion to the aorta, and the exposure of monocytes and endothelial cells to tobacco extracts in vitro induces adhesion molecules (Kalra et al, 1994). Recent evidence has shown that human smokers have increased levels of circulating soluble ICAM-1 (Koundouros et al, 1996). Adhesion molecules are shed from cell surfaces after expression, so their appearance in the circulation suggests that elevated levels or increased numbers of cells bearing them are present in the vascular system. Both endothelial cells and leukocytes express ICAM-1, and the increase could relate to inflammatory events in the lung. The hamster data suggest that there is a systemic adhesive effect, and the interesting possibility arises that activated monocytes might leave the lung and subsequently bind more readily in the arteries, or that smoking might exert a direct effect on the arterial endothelium. As no other mechanism has emerged for the profound atherogenic effects of smoking, these possibilities deserve serious consideration.

Much interest has developed recently in the clinical measurement of endothelial dysfunction, a state in which acetylcholine (ACh) injected into a subject induces vasoconstriction, rather than vasodilatation. This is thought to be due to a reduction in the the induced production of nitric oxide (NO), a vasodilator, from the endothelium, exposing the inherent constrictor effect of ACh itself. Endothelial dysfunction is present in hypercholesterolaemia (Celermajer et al, 1992) and it is interesting to speculate whether this is a clinical correlate of the ox-LDL induced experimental endothelial activation described above.

The endothelium and thrombosis

Endothelial activation or injury is also an important mechanism leading to thrombosis, and is included in one of Virchow's classic triad of predisposing factors, injury to the vessel wall. Endothelial cells exposed to mediators of acute inflammation show an acute form of activation, and mobilize their cytoplasmic Weibel–Palade bodies to the luminal surface, releasing their contents to it. They contain von Willebrand factor, which is a ligand for platelets via their GP1b receptor, and thus aids platelet aggregation on the endothelial surface, an important factor in arterial thrombosis (Roth, 1992). The adhesion molecule P-selectin is also released onto the surface in the same way to promote leukocyte adhesion, and our studies have shown surface P-selectin on the endothelial cells over human atherosclerotic plaques. Cytokine activated endothelium expresses more plasminogen activator inhibitor, and less of the activator itself. It has been shown in vitro to produce more tissue factor, although this has not been detected in the endothelium of atherosclerotic lesions in vivo (Wilcox et al, 1989).

Denuding endothelial injury exposes connective tissue collagen to which platelet integrin receptors can bind directly, and also via deposited von Willebrand factor and its platelet receptor. Antithrombotic subtances from the endothelium, such as prostacyclin and NO will be lost. These mechanisms are of potential significance in atherosclerosis, as the endothelium over atherosclerotic plaques is often ulcerated or cracked.

The possibility that adherent monocytes might induce thrombosis has been considered recently. Tissue factor is induced in monocytes binding to activated endothelium, and a collaboration between leukocytes, platelets and the P-selectin adhesion molecule can induce experimental thrombosis (Lewis et al, 1995; Palabrica et al, 1992). Furthermore, a recent specimen in our laboratory supports this idea, as surface adherent monocytes on an atherosclerotic plaque were seen gradually thickening into a thrombus across the lesion. Despite this plethora of possible mechanisms, there is still a considerable uncertainty about the pathways leading to thrombosis complicating atherosclerosis.

Macrophage expression of growth factors

A study of the distribution of growth factors in the atherosclerotic plaque gives a further facet to the role of the macrophage. Recent studies at UMDS (Poston et al, 1996) have demonstrated that a wide range of growth factors are present in atheroma macrophages. These include PDGF-A, PDGF-B, IGF-1, EGF and basic FGF. Large quantities of some, particularly PDGF-B and IGF-1, are present (Table 8.2). It seems possible that PDGF-B and IGF-1 have a role in stimulating the growth of smooth muscle cells in the intima, as the relevant receptors can be demonstrated on the smooth muscle cells. In this way, the characteristic smooth muscle proliferation of the fibrous cap may be secondary to the macrophage infiltration into the intima. Interestingly, the receptors for the other growth factors listed were not seen on the smooth muscle cells, but on macrophages themselves. This suggests the possibility of autocrine stimulation that might play a part in the maintenance of macrophage viability. Other potential sources of growth factors are the endothelium, adherent platelets and the smooth muscle cells themselves. The atherosclerotic endothelium does produce growth factors, but the bulk of the synthesizing tissue compared with plaque macrophages is small. Platelet thrombi are not invariably present in atherosclerosis, so have a restricted role at most. Smooth muscle cells produce a similar range of growth factors to the macrophages, but probably in lower quantity. Moreover, our observations on atherosclerotic tissues suggest that the levels of these growth factors in smooth muscle cells are largely similar to those in normal tissues. Hence it seems likely that the macrophages are the major source of additional growth factors in atherosclerosis.

Another molecule demonstrated recently in plaque macrophages is endothelin, which acts on smooth muscle cells via a specific receptor to cause contraction (Ihling et al, 1996). It is interesting to speculate that this might be a source of spasm in diseased arteries, and that smooth muscle growth might also result.

Conclusion

Although we now know much about the mechanisms of atherosclerois, many details remain sketchy and contentious, and no quantitative information is available. For example, it is unclear which growth factors really matter, and it is even possible that the importance of cell proliferation has been overstated, and remodelling is the significant event. This may apply particularly in post angioplasty restenosis (Lafont et al, 1995). The present state of the art gives reason for hope. Treatment of elevated LDL cholesterol and triglyceride by simvastatin reduces cardiovascular morbidity and mortality (Scandinavian Simvastatin Study Group, 1994; Shepherd et al, 1995). Antioxidant therapy with tocopherol has given encouraging results, but unequivocal benefit has not yet been demonstrated with any antioxidant. Maybe we should await a trial on red wine! Some existing cardiovascular drugs, such as calcium channel blockers and ACE inhibitors may have additional anti atherosclerotic effects (Borcherding et al, 1993; Sharpe, 1993).

There is further hope for the future. The remarkable technology of gene deletion in mice has allowed the development of murine atherosclerosis models by deletion of the LDL receptor and of apo-lipoprotein E genes. This promises an early acceleration in research productivity. Atherosclerosis is fortunately a relatively uniform disease, and it seems most unlikely that it will have the variable and complex pathogenesis that tumours exhibit. Hence one effective therapeutic agent may suffice for most of the affected population. The second part of this chapter has stressed the importance of the monocyte–macrophage axis in atherosclerosis, and the interaction of the monocyte with the endothelium. These may provide new targets for intervention, and if the hypothesis is proved, inhibition of monocyte traffic may reap major therapeutic rewards through the breaking of the self-perpetuating feedback loop. What is now required is a set of simple experimental models for the critical processes of the disease, once those processes are accurately defined. They can then be delivered to the pharmaceutical industry to aid in the discovery of suitable therapeutic inhibitors.

References

Albrecht, W. & Schuler, W.(1965). The effect of short-term cholesterol feeding on the development of aortic atheromatosis in the rabbit. *Journal of Atherosclerosis Research*, **5**, 353–68.

Auge, N., Pieraggi, M. T., Thiers, J. C., Negre-Salvayre, A. & Salvayre, R. (1995). Proliferative and cytotoxic effects of mildly oxidized low-density lipoproteins on vascular smooth-muscle cells. *Biochemical Journal*, **309**, 1015–20.

Benditt, E. P. (1977). Implications of the monoclonal character of human atherosclerotic plaques. *American Journal of Pathology*, **86**, 693–702.

Berliner, J A., Navab, M., Fogelman, A. M., Frank, J. S., Demer, L. L., Edwards, P. A., Watson, A. D. & Lusis, A. J. (1995). Atherosclerosis: basic mechanisms. Oxidation, inflammation and genetics. *Circulation*, **91**, 2488–96.

Borcherding, S. M., Meeves, S. G., Klutman, N. E. & Howard, P. A. (1993). Calcium-channel antagonists for the prevention of atherosclerosis. *Annals of Pharmacotherapy*, **27**, 61–7.

Cathcart, M. K., McNally, A. K. & Chisholm, G. M. (1991). Lipoxygenase-mediated transformation of human low-density lipoprotein to an oxidized and cytotoxic complex. *Journal of Lipid Research*, **32**, 63–70.

Celermajer, D. S., Sorensen, K. E., Gooch, V. M., Spiegelhalter, D. J., Miller, O. I., Sullivan, I. D., Lloyd, J. K. & Deanfield, J. E. (1992). Non-invasive detection of endothelial dysfunction in children and adults at risk of atherogenesis. *Lancet*, **340**, 1111–15.

Cohen, R. A. (1995). The role of nitric oxide and other endothelium-derived vasoactive substancesin vascular disease. *Progress in Cardiovascular Disease*, **38**, 105–28.

Cybulsky, M. I. & Gimbrone, M. A. (1991). Endothelial expression of a mononuclear leukocyte adhesion molecule during atherogenesis. *Science* **251**, 788–91.

Duplaa, C., Couffinhal, T., Labat, L., Moreau, C., Petit-Jean, M.-E., Doutre, M.-S., Lamaziere, J.-M. D. & Bonnet, J. (1996). Monocyte-macrophage recruitment and expression of endothelial adhesion proteins in human atherosclerotic lesions. *Atherosclerosis* **121**, 253–66.

Frostegard, J., Wu, R., Giscombe, R., Holm, G., Lefvert, A. K., Nilsson, J. (1992). Induction of T-cell activation by oxidized low density lipoprotein. *Arteriosclerosis and Thrombosis*, **12**, 461–7.

Fyfe, A. I., Qiao, J. H. & Lusis, A. J. (1994) Immune-deficient mice develop typical atherosclerotic lesions when fed an atherogenic diet. *Journal of Clinical Investigation*, **94**, 2516–20.

Galis, Z. S., Sikrova, G. K., Kranzhofer, R., Clark, S., Libby, P. (1995). Macrophage foam cells from experimental atheroma, constitutively produce matrix-degrading enzymes. *Proceedings of the National Academy of Sciences of the USA* **92**, 402–6.

Gebuhrer, V., Murphy, J., Bordet, J. C., Reck, M. P. & McGregor, J. L. (1995). Oxidised LDL induces the expression of P-selectin on human endothelial cells. *Biochemical Journal*, **306**, 293–8.

Gimbrone, M. A. (1976). Culture of vascular endothelium. *Progress in Hemostasis and Thrombosis*, **3**, 1–28.

Goldstein, J. L., Ho, Y. K., Basu, S. K. & Brown, M. S. (1979). Binding site of macrophages that mediates uptake and degradation of acetylated low-density lipoprotein, producing massive cholesterol deposits. *Proceedings of the National Academy of Sciences of the USA* , **76**, 333–37.

Hansson, G. K., Jonasson, L., Seifert, P. S. & Stemme, S. (1989). Immune mechanisms in atherosclerosis. *Arteriosclerosis*, **9**, 567–78.

Hoffman, R. M. & Garewal, H. S. (1995). Antioxidants and the prevention of coronary heart disease. *Archives of Internal Medicine*, **155**, 241–6.

Holvoet, P. & Collen, D. (1994). Oxidized lipoproteins in atherosclerosis and thrombosis. *FASEB Journal*, **8**, 1279–84.

Ihling, C., Gobel, H. R., Lippoldt, A., Wessels, S., Paul, M., Schaefer, H. E. & Zeiher, A. M. (1996). Endothelin-1-like immunoreactivity in human atherosclerotic coronary tissue: a detailed analysis of the distribution of endothelin-1. *Journal of Pathology* **179**, 303–8.

Johnson-Tidey, R. R., McGregor, J. L., Taylor, P. R., Poston, R. N. (1994). Increase in the adhesion molecule P-selectin in endothelium overlying atherosclerotic plaques. *American Journal of Pathology*, **144**, 952–61.

Kalra, V. K., Ying, Y., Deemer, K., Natarajan, R., Nadler, J. L. & Coates, T. D. (1994). Mechanisms of cigarette smoke condensate-induced adhesion of monocytes to cultured endothelial cells. *Journal of Cell Physiology*, **160**, 154–62.

Kim, J. A., Territo, M. C., Wayner, E., Carlos, T. M., Parhami, F., Smith, C. W., Haberland, M. E., Fogelman, A. M. & Berliner, J. A. (1994). Partial characterisation of the leukocyte binding molecules on endothelial cells induced by minimally oxidised LDL. *Arteriosclerosis and Thrombosis*, **14**, 427–33.

Koundouros, E., Odell, E., Coward, P., Wilson, R. & Palmer, R. M. (1996) Soluble adhesion molecules in serum of smokers and non-smokers with and without periodontitis. *Journal of Periodontal Research*, **31**, 596–9.

Lafont, A., Guzman, L. A., Whitlow, P. L., Goormastic, M., Cornhill, J. F. & Chisolm, G. M. (1995). Restenosis after experimental angioplasty. Intimal, medial, and adventitial changes associated with constrictive remodeling. *Circulation Research*, **76**, 996–1002.

Lehr, H.-A., Frei, B. & Arfors, K.-E. (1994). Vitamin C prevents cigarette smoke-induced leukocyte aggregation and adhesion to endothelium in vitro. *Proceedings of the National Acedemy of Sciences of USA*, **91**, 7688–92.

Lewis, J. C., Jones, N. L., Hermanns, M. I., Rohrig, O., Klein, C. L. & Kirkpatrick, C. J. (1995). Tissue factor expression during coculture of endothelial cells and monocytes. *Experimental and Molecular Pathology*, **62**, 207–18.

Li, H., Cybulsky, M. I., Gimbrone, M. A. & Libby, P. (1993). An atherogenic diet rapidly induces VCAM-1, a cytokine regulatable mononuclear leukocyte adhesion molecule, in rabbit aortic endothelium. *Arteriosclerosis and Thrombosis*, **13**, 197–204.

MacSweeney, S. T., Powell, J. T. & Greenhalgh, R. M. (1994). Pathogenesis of abdominal aortic aneurysm. *British Journal of Surgery*, **81**, 935–41.

Mlot, C. (1996). *Chylamydia* linked to atherosclerosis. *Science*, **272**, 1422.

Morgan, J., Smith, J. A., Wilkins, G. M. & Leake, D. S. (1993). Oxidation of low density lipoprotein by bovine and porcine aortic endothelial cells and porcine endocardial cells in culture. *Atherosclerosis*, **102**, 209–16.

Nagel, T., Resnick, N., Atkinson, W. J., Dewey, C. F. & Gimbrone, M. A. (1994). Shear stress selectively upregulates intercellular adhesion molecule-1 expression in cultured endothelial cells. *Journal of Clinical Investigation*, **94**, 885–91.

Nakashima, Y., Plump, A. S., Raines, E. W., Breslow, J. L. & Ross, R. (1994). ApoE-deficient mice develop lesions of all phases of atherosclerosis throughout the arterial tree. *Arteriosclerosis and Thrombosis*, **14**, 133–40.

Nelken, N. A., Coughlin, S. R., Gordon, D. & Wilcox, J. N. (1991). Monocyte chemoattractant protein-1 in atherosclerotic plaques. *Journal of Clinical Investigation*, **88**, 1121–27.

Nerem, R. M. & Sprague, E. A. (1993). Hemodynamic determinants of the development and distribution of lesions. In *New Horizons in Coronary Heart Disease*, ed. G. V. R. Born & C. J. Schwartz, pp. 1–10. London: Current Science.

Newman, K., Jean-Claude, J., Li, H., Scholes, J. V., Ogata, Y., Nagase, H. & Tilson, M. D. (1994). Cellular localization of matrix metalloproteinases in the abdominal aortic aneurysm wall. *Journal of Vascular Surgery*, **20**, 814–20.

Oemar, B. S., Yang, Z. & Luscher, T. F. (1995). Molecular and cellular mechanisms of atherosclerosis. *Current Opinion in Nephrology and Hypertension*, **4**, 82–91.

Owens, G. K. (1995). Regulation of differentiation of vascular smooth muscle cells. *Physiological Reviews*, **75**, 487–517.

Palabrica, T., Lobb, R., Furie, B. C., Aronovitz, M., Benjamin, C., Hsu, Y.-M., Sajer, S. A. & Furie, B. (1992). Leukocyte accumulation promoting fibrin deposition is mediated in vivo by P-selectin on adherent platelets. *Nature*, **359**, 848–52.

Parkes, J. L., Cardell, R. R., Hubbard, F. C., Hubbard, D., Meltzer, A. & Penn, A. (1991). Cultured human atherosclerotic plaque smooth muscle cells retain transforming potential and display enhanced expression of the *myc* protooncogene. *American Journal of Pathology*, **138**, 765–75.

Parthasarathy, S., Printz, D. J., Boyd, D., Joy, L. & Steinberg, D. (1986). Macrophage oxidation of low-density lipoprotein generates a modified form recognized by the scavenger receptor. *Arteriosclerosis*, **6**, 505–10.

Parthasarathy, S., Wieland, E. & Steinberg, D. (1989). A role for endothelial cell lipoxygenase in the oxidative modification of low-density lipoprotein. *Proceedings of the National Academy of Sciences of the USA*, **86**, 1046–50.

Patel, M. I., Hardman, D. T. A., Fisher, C. M. & Appleberg, M. (1995). Current views on the pathogenesis of abdominal aortic aneurysms. *Journal of the American College of Surgeons*, **181**, 371–82.

Patel, M. I., Melrose, J., Ghosh, P. & Appleberg, M. (1996). Increased synthesis of matrix metalloproteinases by aortic smooth muscle cells is implicated in the etiopathogenesis of abdominal aortic aneurysms. *Journal of Vascular Surgery*, **24**, 82–92.

Poston, R. N. & Johnson-Tidey, R. R. (1996). Localized adhesion of monocytes to human atherosclerotic plaques demonstrated in vivo. *American Journal of Pathology*, **149**, 73–80.

Poston, R. N., Britten, K., Nitkunan, T., Wilson, V., Ward, J., Thomas, C. & Burnand, K. (1996). Macrophage-associated growth factor and growth factor receptor expression in human atherosclerosis. *IX International Vascular Biology Symposium*, Seattle.

Raines, E. W. & Ross, R. (1993). Smooth muscle cells and the pathogenesis of the lesions of atherosclerosis. *British Heart Journal*, **69** (Suppl. 1), S30–S37.

Ross, R. & Glomset, J. A. (1973). Atherosclerosis and the arterial smooth muscle cell. *Science*, **180**, 1332–9.

Ross, R., Glomset, J., Kariya, B. & Harker, L. (1974). A platelet-dependent serum factor that stimulates the proliferation of arterial smooth muscle cells in vitro. *Proceedings of the National Academy of Sciences of the USA* , **71**, 1207–10.

Ross, R. (1993). The pathogenesis of atherosclerosis: a perspective for the 1990s. *Nature*, **362**, 801–9.

Ross, R. (1995). Cell biology of atherosclerosis. *Annual Review of Physiology*, **57**, 791–804.

Roth, G. J. (1992). Platelets and blood vessels: the adhesion event. *Immunology Today*, **13**, 100–5.

Salonen, J. T., Yla-Herttuala, S., Yamamoto, R., Butler, S., Korpela, H., Salonen, R., Nyyssonen, K., Palinski, W. & Witzum, J. L. (1992). Autoantibody against oxidised LDL and progression of carotid atherosclerosis. *Lancet*, **339**, 883–7.

Scandinavian Simvastatin Study Group. (1994). Randomised trial of cholesterol lowering in 4444 patients with coronary heart disease: the Scandinavian simvastatin survival study (4S).*Lancet*, **344**, 1383–9.

Schwartz, S. M., Heimark, R. L. & Majesky, M. W. (1990). Developmental mechanisms underlying pathology of arteries. *Physiological Reviews*, **70**, 1177–209.

Sharpe, N. (1993). The effects of ACE inhibition on progression of atherosclerosis. *Journal of Cardiovascular Pharmacology*, **22** (Suppl. 9), S9–S12.

Shepherd, J., Cobbe, S. M., Ford, I., Isles, C. G., Lorimer, A. R., Macfarlane, P. W., McKillop, J. H. & Packard, C. J. (1995). Prevention of coronary heart disease with pravastatin in men with hypercholesterolemia. *New England Journal of Medicine*, **333**, 1301–7.

Sparrow, C. P. & Olszewski, J. (1992). Cellular oxidative modification of low density lipoproteins does not require lipoxygenases. *Proceedings of the National Academy of Sciences of the USA*, **89**, 128–31.

Springer, T. A. (1994). Traffic signals for lymphocyte recirculation and leukocyte emigration: the multistep paradigm. *Cell* , **76**, 301–14.

Stamper, H. B. & Woodruff, J. J. (1976). Lymphocyte homing to lymph nodes: in vitro demonstration of the selective affinity of recirculating lymphocytes for high endothelial venules. *Journal of Experimental Medicine* , **144**, 828–33.

Stary, H. C., Blankenhorn, D. H., Chandler, A. B., Glagov, S., Insull, W., Richardson, M., Rosenfeld, M. E., Schaffer, S. A., Schwartz, S. J. & Wagner, W. D. (1992). A definition of the intima of human arteries and its atherosclerosis-prone regions. A report from the Committee on Vascular Lesions of the Council on Arteriosclerosis. *Arteriosclerosis*, **12**, 120–34.

Thyberg, J., Hedin, U., Sjöplund, M., Palmberg, L. & Bottger, B. A. (1990). Regulation of differentiated properties and proliferation of arterial smooth muscle cells. *Arteriosclerosis*, **10**, 966–90.

Watanabe, T., Shimokama, T., Haraoka, S. & Hishikawa, H. (1995). T lymphocytes in atherosclerotic lesions. *Annals of the New York Academy of Sciences*, **748**, 40–56.

Wight, T. N. (1989). Cell biology of arterial proteoglycans. *Arteriosclerosis*, **9**, 1–20.

Wilcox, J. N., Smith, K. M., Williams, L. T., Schwartz, S. M. & Gordon, D. (1988). Platelet-derived growth factor mRNA detection in human atherosclerotic plaques by *in situ* hybridization. *Journal ofClinical Investigation*, **82**, 1134–43.

Wilcox, J. N., Smith, K. M., Schwartz, S. M. & Gordon, D. (1989). Localisation of tissue factor in the normal arterial wall and in the atherosclerotic plaque. *Proceedings of the National Academy of Sciences of USA* , **86**, 2839–43.

Witztum, J. L. (1994). The oxidation hypothesis of atherosclerosis. *Lancet*, **344**, 793–5.

Wood, K. M., Cadogan, M. D., Ramshaw, A. L. & Parums, D. V. (1993). The distribution of adhesion molecules in human atherosclerosis. *Histopathology*, 22, 437–44.

Xu, Q., Willeit, J., Marosi, M., Kleindienst, R., Oberhollenzer, F., Kiechl, S., Stulnig, T., Luef, G. & Wick, G. (1993). Association of serum antibodies to heat-shock protein 65 with carotid atherosclerosis. *Lancet*, **341**, 255–9.

Zhou, X., Stemme, S. & Hansson, G. K. (1996). Evidence for a local immune response in atherosclerosis. CD4[+] T cells infiltrate lesions of apolipoprotein E-deficient mice. *American Journal of Pathology*, **149**, 359–66.

9

Vascular matrix proteins and their remodelling in atherosclerosis

S. YE and A. M. HENNEY

Introduction

Atherosclerosis is an example of a complex trait, i.e. a disease in which the effects of common variation in a constellation of genes combine with a wide range of environmental variables to develop the phenotype. One of the earliest events in the formation of an atherosclerotic lesion is the adherence of circulating monocytes to the vascular endothelium through which they gain entry to the subintimal tissue. The atherosclerotic plaque then evolves over a number of years through the migration and proliferation of cells, the accumulation of lipid in the vessel wall and, more pertinent to this discussion, through the extensive deposition and modification of a connective tissue matrix. This process of vascular connective tissue remodelling, where matrix macromolecules are both deposited and degraded, is controlled by a complex network of cell–cell and cell–matrix interactions, involving the secretion of a wide variety of growth factors and cytokines. Pathological studies have described a wide spectrum of structural architecture in atherosclerotic plaques which suggests that, with time, the vascular connective tissue matrix is extensively modified during atherogenesis. This brief overview describes the major vascular matrix constituents and discusses how matrix degradation is important in the pathogenesis of the complex atherosclerotic lesion.

Extracellular matrix remodelling and atherosclerosis

During the evolution of atherosclerotic lesions, there is continual reshaping and reconstruction of the vessel wall, which will inevitably affect both its cellular and extracellular components. The extracellular matrix constitutes up to 60% of the intimal volume and is thought to undergo continuous remodelling during atherogenesis (Stary et al, 1992). Such remodelling involves the deposition and removal of extracellular matrix macromolecules and is likely to be one of the major mechanisms underlying progression of atherosclerosis (for reviews see Newby et al, 1994; Dollery et al, 1995; Libby, 1995).

The connective tissue matrix not only provides the blood vessels with structural support, but also has multiple biological functions. It is an important medium through which essential nutrients are transported across the vessel wall, and a site for accumulation of products secreted by various cells and for accumulation of cell debris. It also

131

plays a role in regulating cell migration and proliferation (Stary et al, 1992). This vascular matrix consists of proteoglycans, collagen and elastin, as well as smaller amounts of fibronectin, laminin and various plasma components (Stary et al, 1992; Libby, 1995).

Proteoglycans (PGs)

Proteoglycans are a diverse group of macromolecules, each of which possesses one or more linear glycosaminoglycan chains attached to serine residues along a core protein (Wight et al, 1995). There are four types of proteoglycans present in the extracellular matrix of the vessel wall: chondroitin sulphate PG, heparan sulphate PG, dermatan sulphate PG and keratan sulphate PG (Wight et al, 1995), all of which are likely to be synthesized by endothelial cells and smooth muscle cells (SMCs) (Stary et al, 1992). Proteoglycans are important in the organization of the extracellular architecture. In addition, they function in arterial permeability, filtration, ion exchange, as well as transport and deposition of plasma materials such as low density lipoprotein (LDL) (Stary et al, 1992; Camejo et al, 1993, 1995). It has been suggested the proteoglycans also play a role in regulating cellular metabolism (Stary et al, 1992).

During atherogenesis, there is a significant increase in the content of chondroitin sulphate and dermatan sulphate PGs (Stary et al, 1994). In vitro studies have also shown that transforming growth factor-β (TGF-β) stimulates production of chondroitin sulphate by SMCs (Rabinovitch, 1995). Both chondroitin sulphate and dermatan sulphate PGs can bind plasma LDL and thus enhance its retention in the intima (Camejo et al, 1995). It has been shown that the amount of chondroitin sulphate PG is positively correlated with intimal accumulation of apolipoprotein B, a major component of the LDL particle (Hoff & Wagner, 1986; Ylä-Herttuala et al, 1987).

In contrast to chondroitin sulphate and dermatan sulphate PGs, heparan sulphate PG is reduced in lesions with increasing severity of atherosclerosis (Stary et al, 1994). Based on the possible role of cell surface heparan sulphate in the regulation of cell replication, it is suggested that changes in heparan sulphate content might affect the control over cell proliferation during lesion progression (Castellot et al, 1981; Fritze et al, 1985).

Collagens

Collagens are a large family of related proteins. Typically, fibrillar collagens are composed of three polypeptide chains (called α chains) wound around each other to confer the characteristic feature of long, stiff, triple helical structure (Olsen, 1995). Some 25 distinct collagen α chains have been identified, which constitute about 15 types of collagen molecules (Alberts et al, 1994a).

In the normal artery wall, the bulk of collagen exists in the form of two interstitial collagens, types I and III (Stary et al, 1992). In children, type III collagen which is probably secreted by the endothelium is the predominant form in the subendothelial space of the intima (Sage et al, 1979). With ageing, there is a change in the ratio of the two types of collagen in favour of type I (Stary et al, 1992). SMCs synthesise both types I and III collagen, so the increase in proportion of type I collagen probably reflects the increase in the number of SMCs in the intima, and a change in their metabolic properties (Morton & Barnes, 1982).

In addition to types I and III, other collagen types including types IV, V and VI are also present in the normal arterial wall, but in a much smaller amount, accounting for only 0.5–1.0% of the total arterial collagen content (Stary et al, 1992).

Apart from lipid, collagen is the major extracellular component of atherosclerotic lesions, comprising 30–60% of the total protein content (Stary et al, 1995). Both fibrillar collagen types I and III increase significantly in advanced lesions and account for the majority of collagen in the plaque (type I represents about 70% of the total collagen). There is also a significant increase in the minor collagen types such as types IV and V, with type V collagen prominent in advancing fibrotic lesions (Stary et al, 1995).

Studying the distribution of collagen in atherosclerotic lesions, Burleigh et al (1992) found that in ulcerated (fissured or ruptured) plaques, the collagen content in the centre of the plaque cap is lower than that in the periphery, whereas in the mechanically stable, non-ulcerated lesions, the enhanced content of collagen is uniform throughout the plaque.

As SMCs are the major cell type responsible for collagen generation in the vessel wall in adult, the increasing accumulation of collagen in atherosclerosis is likely to be related to SMC hyperplasia and phenotypic alteration (Stary et al, 1994). The stimuli for collagen deposition in atherosclerotic lesions have yet to be characterised; however, there is evidence suggesting that growth factors such as TGF produced by macrophages and platelets upregulate collagen gene expression (Roberts et al, 1986). An enhancement of collagen production attributed to the effects of high blood pressure has also been observed (Jaeger et al, 1990). Furthermore, mechanical stresses are likely to be redistributed and modulated as lesions develop, which may also play a role in inducing changes in matrix production (Stary et al, 1995).

Elastin

Elastin is the main component of the elastic fibres which give blood vessels their elasticity. Elastin molecules are secreted into the extracellular space where they become highly cross-linked, and then assemble with microfibrils into elastic fibres on the cell surface (Alberts et al, 1994b). The normal vascular wall contains a substantial amount of elastin, which is mainly located in the media and the musculoelastic layer of intima (Stary et al 1992). With increasing age, the relative elastin content as compared with collagen is decreased (Hosoda et al, 1984).

In the early stages of atherosclerosis, there are few changes in the elastin content (Stary et al, 1994). In contrast, advanced lesions contain an increased amount of subendothelial, medial and adventitial elastin; however, integration of the newly synthesized protein into a functional elastic fibre may be impaired (Stary et al, 1995). In addition, the elastic fibres in atherosclerotic lesions are split or frayed, and often appear to be closely associated with lipid and calcium deposits (Guyton & Klemp, 1995). It is suggested that lipid bound to elastic fibres may affect the elasticity of tissue by modifying the conformation of the elastin through hydrophobic interactions, and also increase the sensitivity of elastin to elastinolysis by elastases (Guantieri et al, 1983).

Fibronectin and laminin

Fibronectin is a high molecular weight, multifunctional, adhesive glycoprotein and is present on cell surfaces, in extracellular matrices and in blood (Alberts et al, 1994c). It plays important roles in cell–cell adhesion, cell–substrate adhesion, and cell–matrix interactions due to its multiple specialized domains, such as the collagen-binding, heparin-binding and cell membrane-binding domains (Stary et al, 1992). Laminin is another major non-collagenous glycoprotein. Along with heparan sulphate PG and type IV collagen, laminin is a major component of the basement membrane which underlies the endothelium and surrounds each SMC (Newby et al, 1994).

Fibronectin and laminin are present in the extracellular matrix of normal intima, and are increased in atherosclerotic lesions (Clausell et al, 1993, 1994). In vitro studies have demonstrated that fibronectin production by SMCs is enhanced by interleukin 1 and TNF-β (Molossi et al, 1995). It has been suggested that fibronectin may induce neointima formation by promoting SMC migration, as well as monocyte and T lymphocyte infiltration (Rabinovitch, 1995).

Extracellular matrix remodelling during atherogenesis

Extracellular matrix remodelling, involving the synthesis and degradation of matrix components, is a normal phenomenon that occurs, for example, during angiogenesis, tissue morphogenesis, growth and wound healing (Matrisian & Hogan, 1990; Alexander & Werb, 1991; Murphy & Reynolds, 1993). The normal operation of such processes requires tightly controlled, complex cell–cell and cell–matrix interactions involving the production of resident connective tissues, enzymes, activators, inhibitors and regulatory agents such as growth factors and cytokines (Murphy & Reynolds, 1993). Disruption of these regulatory processes is thought to contribute to various pathological states. For instance, unregulated expression of the matrix-degrading enzymes is partially the cause of the accelerated breakdown of extracellular matrix in arthritic disease, tumour invasion and metastasis while, on the other hand, inadequate production of these enzymes is associated with the excessive accumulation of connective tissue in systemic sclerosis (Birkedal-Hansen et al, 1993; Murphy & Reynolds, 1993; Bou-Gharios et al, 1994).

Connective tissue remodelling is an important physiological process associated with the maintenance of blood vessel integrity. The components of the extracellular matrix in the vessel wall interact to form a complex network which confers on blood vessels their elastic physical characteristics. As a functional component of the circulatory system, the blood vessel is under continual mechanical stress. In response to such haemodynamic conditions, the vessel wall is continually remodelling to repair and replace proteins that have become worn. It has been estimated that extracellular turnover of collagen in the normal adult canine cardiovasculature is approximately 0.6% per day (Bonnin et al, 1981).

Remodelling of the extracellular matrix occurs during all phases of human atherosclerosis.

Lesion initiation

This is by the infiltration of circulating monocytes into the vessel wall, and migration and proliferation of SMCs. In order to migrate and multiply, the cells must traverse major extracellular barriers including the basal lamina and a dense mesh of interstitial proteoglycans and collagen. A prerequisite of such cell migration is the degradation of the extracellular matrix surrounding the migrating cells (Newby et al, 1994).

Lesion development and growth

Once in the intima, the proliferating SMCs synthesize extracellular matrix components, whose accumulation in turn alters the intimal structure and increases its volume. In the early stages, growth of the atherosclerotic plaque occurs by outward, abluminal expansion, a phenomenon referred to as 'compensatory enlargement', to accommodate the increasing intimal volume. Later, growth of the atherosclerotic plaque outstrips the compensatory potential of the vessel, causing arterial stenosis (Ross, 1993; Libby, 1995).

Advanced and complex lesions

Excess degradation of extracellular matrix may occur at certain locations such as the 'shoulders' of the plaque, the regions in which plaques rupture most frequently. As a result of this focal destruction of extracellular matrix, the plaque becomes less resistant to the mechanical stresses imposed during systole and, hence, becomes vulnerable to rupture (Richardson et al, 1989). In complicated lesions, plaque rupture results in intraluminal thrombosis. As part of the repair process, the thrombi may become organized. This will involve the migration of SMCs into the clot where they lay down a large amount of extracellular matrix, further increasing the bulk of the lesion (Fuster et al, 1992).

Extracellular matrix degrading enzymes and their natural inhibitors

The key enzymes contributing to extracellular matrix turnover are endopeptidases from three major classes: the metalloproteinases, the serine proteinases and the lysosomal proteinases (Matrisian & Hogan, 1990; Alexander & Werb, 1991; Murphy & Reynolds, 1993). Matrix degradation initially takes place extracellularly. Except in special circumstances such as bone resorption, extracellular matrix degradation is thought to occur at neutral pH values, and is catalyzed primarily by the metallo- and serine proteinase families, both of which have neutral pH optima. The fragments generated by these initial

proteolytic attacks may then be phagocytosed by local cells for intracellular degradation, or digested further extracellularly. The lysosomal proteinases favour more acidic
pH values and their function appears to be confined to the subsequent degradative
events within the phagosome, although in some circumstances they may be secreted and
act within local acidic environments (Murphy & Reynolds, 1993).

The metallo- and serine proteinase classes are linked in an activation cascade, with
the metalloproteinases being downstream of the serine proteinases (Fig. 9.1) (Murphy &
Reynolds, 1993). In general, the serine enzymes have broader substrate specificities than
the metalloproteinases which tend to be more specialized. The major serine proteinase,
namely plasmin, is also responsible for the dissolution of fibrin clots, thus making a
connection with another process relevant in atherosclerotic disease - fibrinolysis. Under
normal conditions, the lytic potential of these enzymes is held in check by their specific
activators and inhibitors (Birkedal-Hansen, 1995). Disruption of the normal control
processes can contribute to various pathologies as mentioned above. Recently, both of
these classes of proteinase have been implicated in the pathogenesis of atherosclerosis.
For the purposes of this review, the discussion will focus exclusively on the matrix
metalloproteinase family; broader discussions can be found in reviews by Murphy &
Reynolds (1993) and Birkedal-Hansen (1995).

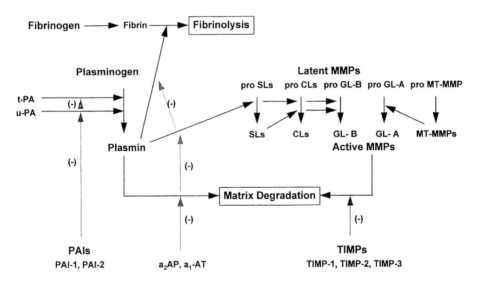

Fig. 9.1. Diagram showing intersecting protease cascade. Black lines denote activatory
pathways; grey lines indicate inhibitory pathways. Abbreviations: t-PA: tissue-type plasminogen activator; u-PA: urokinase-type plasminogen activator; PAI: plasminogen activator inhibitor; MMPs: matrix metalloproteinases; SL: stromelysin; CL: collagenase; GL:
gelatinase; MT-MMP: membrane-type MMP; TIMP: tissue inhibitor of metalloproteinases; a_2AP: a_2-antiplasmin; a_1-AT: a_1-antitrypsin. Adapted from Murphy and
Reynolds (1993).

Matrix metalloproteinases
Biochemistry and molecular biology

The matrix metalloproteinases (MMPs) constitute a family of 12 or more zinc-dependent endopeptidases which are generally expressed at low levels in normal adult tissue but are upregulated during normal and pathological remodelling processes. All MMPs share the following common features that allow their classification as a family: (1) they are secreted as latent zymogens requiring activation for proteolytic activity; (2) they degrade extracellular matrix components; (3) they function at neutral pH; (4) they contain Zn^{2+} at their active sites and require Ca^{2+} for stability; and (5) they are inhibited by specific tissue inhibitors of metalloproteinases (TIMPs).

The MMP family has been divided into three main subgroups, mainly based on their substrate preferences: the interstitial collagenases, the gelatinases and the stromelysins; however, two membrane-type MMPs (MT-MMPs) have been discovered recently and may be classified as a fourth group. As summarised in Table 9.1, each subgroup consists of two or more enzymes with similar substrate specificity. The collagenases are relatively specific, mainly degrading the interstitial collagen types I, II and III at a single locus within the native helical structure at about three-quarters of the distance from the N-terminus. The gelatinases have high affinity for gelatins (denatured collagen that has lost the typical triple helix) and thus may have a role in the further extracellular degradation of denatured collagen. The gelatinases are also named type IV collagenases because they are active against type IV collagen, a major component of basement membrane. In addition, they also degrade elastin actively.

The stromelysins have broad substrate specificities, capable of degrading a wide spectrum of extracellular matrix components, including proteoglycan core proteins, non-helical regions of type IV collagen, elastin (limited), gelatins, fibronectin, laminin, and collagen types II, V and IX (Murphy & Reynolds, 1993). Furthermore, the stromelysins can activate other members of the MMP family: stromelysin-1 is a potent activator of interstitial and neutrophil procollagenases, progelatinase A and B, and promatrilysin (Murphy et al, 1987; Miyazaki et al, 1992; Ogata et al, 1992; Knauper et al, 1993; Imai et al, 1995; Shapiro et al, 1995); stromelysin-2 can also activate the precursor for the neutrophil procollagenase (Knauper et al, 1994); matrilysin can activate interstitial procollagenase, and progelatinases A and B (Crabbe et al, 1994; Imai et al, 1995; Sang et al, 1995). The stromelysins may therefore indirectly control the degradation of other extracellular matrix components such as the fibrillar collagen types I, II and III.

The MT-MMPs have only been identified recently, and their substrate specificities remain to be defined. It has been suggested that they are capable of cleaving gelatin and type IV collagen, and may also be involved in the activation of gelatinase A (Sato et al, 1994; Cao et al, 1995).

A cluster of five genes encoding MMPs is located on chromosome 11, while other single MMP loci are found on chromosomes 16, 20 and 22 (Table 9.1). The MMP genes share a high degree of homology. Each of the genes encoding the collagenases, and stromelysins 1 and 2 contains ten exons and nine introns, spanning 8–12 kb of DNA (Collier et al, 1988; Muller et al, 1988). The matrilysin gene lacks four exons corresponding to exons 7–10 of

Table 9.1. *Matrix metalloproteinases*

Subgroup	Name	MMP No.	Gene location	Substrate
Collagenases	Interstitial collagenase (fibroblast-type collagenase)	MMP-1	Chr. 11q22.3	Collagen types I, II, III, (III > > I),VI, X, gelatins, proteoglycan
	Neutrophil collagenase (PMN-type collagenase)	MMP-8	Chr. 11q21	Same as interstitial collagenase (I > > III)
	Collagenase-3	MMP-13	Chr. 11q22.3	
Gelatinases	Gelatinase A (72 kD type IV collagenase)	MMP-2	Chr. 16q21	Gelatins, collagen types IV, V, VII, X and XI, elastin, fibronectin, proteoglycan
	Gelatinase B (92 kDa type IV collagenase)	MMP-9	Chr. 20q11.2-13.1	Gelatins, collagen types IV, V, elastin, proteoglycan
Stromelysins	*Stromelysin 1*	MMP-3	Chr. 11q22.3	Proteoglycan, fibronectin, laminin, elastin, gelatin, collagen types II, IV, V, IX and X
	Stromelysin 2	MMP-10	Chr. 11q22.3	Same as stromelysin 1
	Stromelysin 3	MMP-11	Chr. 22q11.2	Gelatin, fibronectin, proteoglycans
	Matrilysin (PUMP-1)	MMP-7		Gelatin, fibronectin, laminin, collagen type IV, proteoglycan
	Metalloelastase	MMP-12	Chr. 11q22.2-22.3	Elastin
Membrane- type MMPs	MT-MMP-1	MMP-14		Collagen type IV, gelatin
	MT-MMP-2	MMP-15		

Note: MMP: Matrix metalloproteinases.
Source: Murphy & Reynolds (1993) and Birkedal-Hansen (1995).

the collagenase and stromelysin genes (Gaire et al, 1994). In comparison with those for the collagenases and stromelysins, the genes coding for gelatinases A and B are considerably larger (26–27 kbp) and contain three additional exons, which encode the fibronectin-like inserts. The amino acid sequences of MMPs deduced from cDNA data show extensive homology, with about 70% identity between the enzymes within a subgroup, and about 50% among the subgroups (Alexander & Werb, 1991).

Each member of the collagenase and stromelysin subgroups (except matrilysin) consists of five domains, including a signal peptide, a propeptide containing a cysteine residue bonded to the active site Zn^{2+}, which is lost on activation, a catalytic domain that contains the catalytic machinery including the Zn^{2+} binding site, a so-called 'hinge region' that bridges the catalytic domain and the COOH-terminal domain, and a hemopexin- or vitronectin-like COOH-terminal domain that appears to be responsible for conferring substrate specificity.

The two gelatinases also have this five domain structure; however, within the catalytic domain of the gelatinases, there are three fibronectin type II repeats which are absent in the other MMPs and are thought to facilitate binding of gelatinases to their substrate (Huhtala et al, 1990, 1991). The MT-MMPs possess not only the five domains common to other MMPs, but also a unique transmembrane domain which anchors MT-MMPs to the cell surface (Sato et al, 1994). Matrilysin is the smallest MMP, containing only the signal peptide, propeptide and catalytic domains (Gaire et al, 1994).

MMP expression

In general, the MMPs are expressed by a wide variety of cell types and are synthesised in response to a range of growth factors and cytokines. There are some specific exceptions: while fibroblast-type collagenase is synthesised and secreted by cells, the polymorphonuclear (PMN) type collagenase (neutrophil collagenase) is synthesised and pre-packaged in specific granules of PMN leukocytes. The expression of the fibroblast-type is regulated by stimuli such as growth factors and cytokines and the enzyme is secreted from the cell after synthesis, but the PMN-type is instantly released from granule storage sites of triggered PMNs and it is unclear whether its expression is subject to transcriptional control. Like the fibroblast-type collagenase, gelatinase B responds to growth factors and cytokines, but gelatinase A does not: it is expressed constitutively by most cells in culture and is only moderately responsive to 12-O-tetradecanoylphorbol-13-acetate (TPA) and other growth factors which induce gelatinase B. Evidence also exists for differential expression of stromelysins 1 and 2, where the latter is the less responsive of the two.

MMP activation

All MMPs are secreted as inactive zymogens which are subsequently activated in the pericellular and extracellular environment. It is suggested that the latency of the proenzymes is, at least in part, due to the interaction between a cysteine thiol group within the propeptide and the Zn^{2+} atom at the active site, which displaces the molecule that is necessary for catalysis (Darlak et al, 1990; Van Wart & Birkedal-Hansen, 1990). The MMPs can be activated in vitro by physical (chaotropic agents), chemical (HOCl, mercurials, SDS) and enzymatic (trypsin, plasmin) treatments that separate the cysteine residue from the zinc atom (for a review see Birkedal-Hansen et al, 1993). This critical step in the activation process, described as opening of the 'cysteine switch', is followed by a series of autocatalytic cleavages resulting in the complete excision of the propeptide and activation of the enzyme (Van Wart & Birkedal-Hansen, 1990; for a review see Woessner, 1991).

Although the precise mechanism for MMP activation in vivo is still not fully resolved, a number of studies have shown that plasmin can cleave the propeptide sequences of the fibroblast-type collagenase and stromelysin 1, resulting in the activation of these MMPs (Goldberg et al, 1990; Suzuki et al, 1990; Baricos et al, 1995). The pro-MMPs may also be activated by 'superactivation' mechanisms as described above. In in vitro systems, stromelysins 1 and 2 are required for the efficient activation of collagenase, which otherwise has low activity (Suzuki et al, 1990). It has also been found that collagenase activated by stromelysins has up to 12-fold higher specific activity than the autotypically processed form (Murphy et al, 1987; Goldberg et al, 1990).

Recent research suggests that gelatinase A can be activated on the cell surface through the assembly of a ternary complex consisting of progelatinase A, TIMP-2 and activated MT-MMP (Cao et al, 1995; Strongin et al, 1995). It is unclear whether other MMPs are activated at the surface of the cell by similar, MT-MMP-dependent mechanisms, but most other MMPs do not appear to possess the same plasma membrane binding properties as gelatinase A (Birkedal-Hansen, 1995).

Tissue inhibitors of metalloproteinase (TIMPs)

The activity of the MMPs is counteracted by their natural inhibitors, TIMPs. To date, three TIMPs have been identified, which are encoded by three separate genes located on chromosomes X11p11.23-11.4, 17q23-q25 and 22q12.1-13.2, respectively (Willard et al, 1989; DeClerck et al, 1992; Apte et al, 1994). All TIMPs act effectively against MMPs of the collagenase, stromelysin and gelatinase groups, by forming inhibited, non-covalent, 1:1 stoichiometric complexes with MMPs and blocking access to their substrate (Stetler-Stevenson et al, 1992; Baragi et al, 1994; Bodden et al, 1994; Apte et al, 1995). It has been suggested that gelatinases A and B can form complexes with TIMPs in their zymogen forms as well as active forms, whereas collagenase-type and stromelysin-type MMPs only form complexes after exposure of the active site (Birkedal-Hansen, 1995).

TIMP-1 is synthesized and secreted by most connective tissue cells as well as by macrophages, and its expression is regulated by a variety of agents including growth factors (EGF, TNF-α, IL-1, TGF-β), phorbol esters and retinoids (Murphy et al, 1985; Clark et al, 1987; Edwards et al, 1987; Colige et al, 1992; Mackay et al, 1992). TIMP-2 is frequently colocalized with gelatinase A, and its expression is largely constitutive and is downregulated by TGF-β (Stetler-Stevenson et al, 1990). TIMP-3 is a new member of the TIMP family and its expression remains to be determined.

There is evidence that in particular cell types, some stimuli exert opposite effects on the transcription of TIMP-1 and some members of the MMP family. For instance, in human fibroblasts, TGF-β and retinoic acid increase TIMP-1 expression and reduce production of collagenase and stromelysin 1 (Edwards et al, 1987; Bizot-Foulon et al, 1995); therefore, such agents may have larger effects on the balance between active MMPs and their inhibitors. In contrast, other stimuli, such as EGF, IL-1 and PDGF, increase the expression of TIMP-1 as well as collagenase and stromleysin 1 (Colige et al, 1992; Mackay et al, 1992).

Matrix metalloproteinases: implication in the pathogenesis of atherosclerosis

Over the past few years, the MMPs have been implicated in the extracellular matrix remodelling during atherogenesis. This group of enzymes is thought to be involved in a number of important events in the atherogenic process.

The migration of vascular SMCs into and within the intima is a phenomenon associated with the development and progression of atherosclerosis (Hassler, 1970; Clowes & Schwartz, 1985; Pauly et al, 1992). In vivo, vascular SMCs are surrounded by and embedded in a variety of extracellular matrices that must be traversed during movement. Such barriers include the basement membrane (consisting of collagen type IV, laminin, and heparan sulphate proteoglycans), which surrounds each SMC. Pauly et al (1994) used a Boyden chamber to monitor the ability of rat vascular SMCs to degrade a barrier of reconstituted basement membrane as they migrated toward a chemoattractant (PDGF-B/B) and to study the role of MMPs in this process. They found that vascular SMCs in a proliferating or 'synthetic' state readily migrated across the basement membrane barrier and this ability was inhibited by synthetic peptides that inhibited MMP activity, suggesting that MMPs are required for cell migration. By Northern blotting and zymographic analyses, they found that gelatinase A (72 kDa type IV collagenase) was the only detectable MMP expressed and secreted by these cells, and that antisera capable of selectively neutralizing gelatinase A inhibited SMCs migration across the barrier. Newby et al (1994) studied rabbit SMCs and reported very similar findings. These data suggest that degradation of basement membrane by gelatinase is required for cell migration and may be one of the important mechanisms in pathogenesis.

Plaque disruption frequently occurs in the 'shoulder' regions where there is macrophage accumulation (Richardson et al, 1989; Lendon et al, 1991; Davies et al, 1993). As macrophages produce a number of matrix-degrading proteases, their presence in large numbers may weaken the plaque and lead to lesion disruption as a result of destabilisation of the supporting connective tissue matrix. By in situ hybridization, Henney et al (1991) demonstrated the presence of stromelysin 1 transcripts in coronary atherosclerotic lesions. Extensive expression of the stromelysin 1 gene was localized to large clusters of macrophages that contained intracellular lipid deposits, particularly in the regions considered prone to rupture, such as the plaque shoulders. These observations were supported subsequently by other investigators (Galis et al, 1994, 1995a,b; Brown et al, 1995; Nikkari et al, 1995).

By immunocytochemistry, Galis et al (1994, 1995a) found that non-atherosclerotic arteries contained ubiquitous immunoreactive gelatinase A, TIMP-1 and TIMP-2, which were localized to SMCs in all layers of the arteries. These lesion-free arteries stained weakly or not at all for the other three MMP studied (gelatinase B, interstitial collagenase and stromelysin). In contrast to the normal arteries, atheromata stained for all MMPs and TIMPs tested. Increased immunoreactivity of interstitial collagenase, gelatinase B and stromelysin 1 were colocalized in macrophages, SMCs, lymphocytes and endothelium, particularly in the fibrous cap, the shoulders of the lesions, and the base of the lesions' lipid core. As all MMPs are secreted in zymogen forms and require activation, increase in MMP immunoreactivity does not necessarily correspond to augmented enzymatic activity. Moreover, MMP containing areas in the plaques also contain TIMPs. To investigate whether atherosclerotic plaques contained activated MMPs, these investigators modified the technique of in situ zymography, which allows direct detection and microscopic localization of MMP activity in tissue sections. Using this technique, they detected both gelatinolytic and caseinolytic activity in atheros-clerotic tissues in the same areas of increased expression of immunoreactive interstitial collagenase, gelatinase B and stromelysin 1, which suggests the presence of the active forms of these enzymes. In contrast to the affected areas, non-atherosclerotic arteries and uninvolved regions of atherosclerotic specimens did not exhibit enzymatic activity determined by this method.

More recently, Tyagi et al (1995) studied the MMP levels in relation to the extracellu-lar matrix contents in normal and atherosclerotic arteries as wall as in restenotic vessels after angioplasty. In this study, they showed that weight-for-weight atherosclerotic vessels contained more collagen and proteoglycans but lower collagenolytic and elas-tinolytic activities than normal vascular tissues.

In summary, studies over the past two decades have provided substantial evidence implicating expression and activity of MMPs in connective tissue remodelling as well as in the pathogenesis of a number of chronic diseases. There is now substantial informa-tion to suggest that the MMPs are also involved in a number of events associated with the development and progression of atherosclerosis, where the overall effect on the vascular extracellular matrix is a balance between synthesis and degradation. In the early stages, pericellular gelatinase A activity is probably involved in SMC migration into and within the vascular intima. Evolution of the plaque is likely to arise from increased synthesis of both extracellular matrix proteins and proteinases, with produc-tion of the former exceeding the latter, resulting in matrix accumulation and a thickened intima. In the advanced stages, locally overexpressed MMPs in the rupture-prone areas may play a role in the weakening of plaque and thus lesion disruption.

Despite the amount of evidence implicating these proteins in pathogenesis, until relatively recently there has been no evidence showing a direct causal relationship between defects in MMP/TIMP genes and disease. This is a little surprising, given that maintenance of the normal balance of tissue turnover depends on tight control of enzyme activity at the level of transcription, activation of latent proenzymes, and inhibition of proteolytic activity. Disruption of the normal control in any of these steps could potentially lead to pathological consequences resulting from excessive accumulation or overdegradation of the extracellular matrix. We have speculated that genetic variants which disrupt this control may contribute to the pathogenesis of multifactorial diseases in which deficiencies in connective tissue remodelling is a feature, focusing on our attentions on atherosclerosis. The recent discovery of mutations in the TIMP-3 gene in patients with the ocular condition, Sorsby's fundus, dystrophy is the first evidence linking a rare mutation in an MMP/TIMP gene to a disease caused by defective connective tissue remodelling (Weber et al, 1994). This paper provides a 'proof of principle', albeit in a rare disorder rather than a common complex trait, that correct maintenance of the balance between active enzyme and inhibitor is crucial to preserving the function of the extracellular matrix. We have recently described a common genetic variant in the stromelysin 1 promoter which affects transcription of the gene in vitro and which is associated with the progression of atherosclerosis (Ye et al, 1995, 1996). This suggests that other common genetic variants may exist which modify, rather than drastically disrupt the function of the proteins, and which may be important to the pathogenesis of complex disease traits such as atherosclerosis.

References

Alberts, B., Bray, D., Lewis, J., Raff, M., Roberts, K. & Watson, J. (1994a). Collagens are the major proteins of the extracellular matrix. In *Molecular Biology of the Cell*, 3rd edn, ed. B. Alberts, D. Bray, J. Lewis, M. Raff, K. Roberts & J. Watson, pp. 978–80. New York: Garland Publishing, Inc.

Alberts, B., Bray, D., Lewis, J., Raff, M., Roberts, K. & Watson, J. (1994b). Elastin gives tissues their elasticity. In *Molecular Biology of the Cell*, 3rd edn, ed. B. Alberts, D. Bray, J. Lewis, M. Raff, K. Roberts & J. Watson, pp. 984–6. New York: Garland Publishing.

Alberts, B., Bray, D., Lewis, J., Raff, M., Roberts, K. & Watson, J. (1994c). Fibronectin is an extracellular adhesive protein that helps cells attach to the matrix. In *Molecular Biology of the Cell*, 3rd edn, ed. B. Alberts, D. Bray, J. Lewis, M. Raff, K. Roberts & J. Watson, pp. 986–7. New York: Garland Publishing.

Alexander, C. M. & Werb, Z.(1991). Extracellular matrix degradation. In *Cell Biology of Extracellular Matrix*, 2nd edn, ed. E. D. Hay, pp. 255–302. New York: Plenum Press.

Apte, S. S., Mattei, M. G. & Olsen, B. R. (1994). Cloning of the cDNA encoding human tissue inhibitor of metalloproteinases-3 (TIMP-3) and mapping of the TIMP-3 gene to chromosome 22. *Genomics*, **19**, 293–7.

Apte, S. S., Olsen, B. R. & Murphy, G. (1995). The gene structure of tissue inhibitor of metalloproteinases (TIMP)-3 and its inhibitory activities define the distinct TIMP gene family. *Journal of Biological Chemistry*, **270**, 14313–18.

Baragi, V. M., Fliszar, C. J., Conroy, M. C., Ye, Q. Z., Shipley, J. M. & Welgus, H. G. (1994). Contribution of the C-terminal domain of metalloproteinases to binding by tissue inhibitor of metalloproteinases. *Journal of Biological Chemistry*, **269**, 12692–7.

Baricos, W. H., Cortez, S. L., el Dahr, S. S. & Schnaper, H. W. (1995). ECM degradation by cultured human mesangial cells is mediated by a PA/plasmin/MMP-2 cascade. *Kidney International*, **47**, 1039–47.

Birkedal-Hansen, H., Moore, W. G. I., Bodden, M. K., Windsor, L. J., Birkedal-Hansen, B., DeCarlo, A. & Engler, J. A. (1993). Matrix Metalloproteinases: a review. *Critical Reviews in Oral Biology and Medicine*, **4**, 197–250.

Birkedal-Hansen, H. (1995). Proteolytic remodelling of extracellular matrix. *Current Opinion in Cell Biology*, **7**, 728–35.

Bizot-Foulon, V., Bouchard, B., Hornebeck, W., Dubertret, L. & Bertaux, B. (1995). Uncoordinate of type I and III collagens, collagenase and tissue inhibitor of matrix metalloproteinase 1 along with in vitro proliferative life span of human skin fibroblasts. Regulation by all-trans retinoic acid. *Cell Biology International*, **19**, 129–35.

Bodden, M. K., Windsor, L. J., Caterina, N. C., Yermovsky, A., Birkedal-Hansen, B., Galazka, G., Engler, J. A. & Birkedal-Hansen, H. (1994). Analysis of the TIMP-1/FIB-CL complex. *Annals of the New York Academy of Sciences*, **732**, 84–95.

Bonnin, C. M., Sparrow, M. P. & Taylor, R. R. (1981). Collagen synthesis and content in right ventricular hypertrophy in the dog. *American Journal of Physiology*, **10**, H703.

Bou-Gharios, G., Osman, J., Black, C. & Olsen, I. (1994). Excess matrix accumulation in scleroderma is caused partly by differential regulation of stromelysin and TIMP-1 synthesis. *Clinica Chimica Acta*, **231**, 69–78.

Brown, D. L., Hibbs, M. S., Kearney, M., Loushin, C. & Isner, J. M. (1995). Identification of 92-kD gelatinase in human coronary atherosclerotic lesions. Association of active enzyme synthesis with unstable angina. *Circulation*, **91**, 2125–31.

Burleigh, M. C., Briggs, A. D., Lendon, C. L., Davies, M. J., Born, G. V. R. & Richardson, P. D. (1992). Collagen types I and III, collagen content, GAGs and mechanical strength of human atherosclerotic plaque caps: span-wise variations. *Atherosclerosis*, **96**, 71–81.

Camejo, G., Fager, G., Rosengren, B., Hurt-Camejo, E. & Bondjers, G. (1993). Binding of low density lipoproteins by proteoglycans synthesized by proliferating and quiescent human arterial smooth muscle cells. *Journal of Biological Chemistry*, **268**, 14131–7.

Camejo, G., Hurt-Camejo, E., Olsson, U., Rosengren, B. & Bondjers, G. (1995). Interaction of low density lipoprotein with proteoglycans: molecular basis and consequences. In *Atherosclerosis*, vol. X, ed. F. P. Woodford, J. Davignon & A. Sniderman, pp. 365–8. Amsterdam: Elsevier Science BV.

Cao, J., Sato, H., Takino, T. & Seiki, M. (1995). The C-terminal region of membrane type matrix metalloproteinase is a functional transmembrane domain required for pro-gelatinase A activation. *Journal of Biological Chemistry*, **270**, 801–5.

Castellot, J. J. Jr, Addonizio, M. L., Rosenberg, R. & Karnovsky, M. J. (1981). Cultured endothelial cells produce a heparinlike inhibitor of smooth muscle cell growth. *Journal of Cell Biology*, **90**, 372–9.

Clausell, N., Molossi, S. & Rabinovitch, M. (1993). Increased interleukin-1b and fibronectin expression are early features of the development of the postcardiac transplant coronary arteriopathy in piglets. *American Journal of Pathology*, **142**, 1772–86.

Clausell, N., Molossi, S., Sett, S. & Rabinovitch, M. (1994). In vivo blockade of tumor necrosis factor-α in cholesterol rabbits after cardiac transplant inhibits acute coronary artery neointimal formation. *Circulation*, **89**, 2768–79.

Clark, S. D., Kobayash, D. K. & Welgus, H. G. (1987). Regulation of the expression of tissue inhibitor of metalloproteinases and collagenase by retinoids and glucocorticoids in human fibroblasts. *Journal of Clinical Investigation*, **80**, 1280–8.

Clowes, A. & Schwartz, S. M. (1985). Significance of quiescent smooth muscle migration in the injured rat carotid artery. *Circulation Research*, **56**, 139–45.

Colige, A. C., Lambert, C. A., Nusgens, B. V. & Lapiere, C. M. (1992). Effect of cell–cell and cell–matrix interaction on the response of fibroblasts to epidermal growth factor in vitro. Expression of collagen type I, collagenase, stromelysin and tissue inhibitor of metalloproteinases. *Biochemical Journal*, **285**(part 1), 215–21.

Collier, I. E., Smith, J., Kronberger, A., Bauer, E. A., Wilhelm, S. M., Eisen, A. Z. & Goldberg, G. I. (1988). The structure of the human skin fibroblast collagenase gene. *Journal of*

Biological Chemistry, **263**, 10711–13.

Crabbe, T., Smith, B., O'Connell, J. & Docherty, A. (1994). Human progelatinase A can be activated by matrilysin. *FEBS Letters*, **345**, 14–16.

Darlak, K., Miller, R. B., Stack, M. S., Spatola, A. & Gray, R. D. (1990). Thiol-based inhibitors of mammalian collagenase. *Journal of Biological Chemistry*, **265**, 5199–205.

Davies, M. J., Richardson, P. D., Woolf, N., Katz, D. R. & Mann, J. (1993). Risk of thrombosis in human atherosclerotic plaques: role of extracellular lipid, macrophage, and smooth muscle cell content. *British Heart Journal*, **69**, 377–81.

DeClerck, Y. A., Szpirer, C., Aly, M., Cassiman, J., Eeckhout, Y. & Rousseau, G. G. (1992). The gene for tissue inhibitor of metalloproteinases-2 is localized on human chromosome 17q25. *Genomics*, **14**, 782–4.

Dollery, C. M., McEwan, J. R. & Henney, A. M. (1995). Matrix metalloproteinases and cardiovascular disease. *Circulation Research*, **77**, 863–8.

Edwards, D. R., Murphy, G., Reynolds, J. J., Whitham, S. E., Docherty, A. J., Angel, P. & Health, J. K. (1987). Transforming growth factor-β modulates the expression of collagenase and metalloprotcinase inhibitor. *EMBO Journal*, **6**, 1899–904.

Fritze, L. M., Reilly, C. F. & Rosenberg, R. D. (1985). An antiproliferative heparan sulfate species produced by postconfluent smooth muscle cells. *Journal of Cell Biology*, **100**, 1041–9.

Fuster, V., Badimon, L., Badimon, J. J. & Ghesebro, J. H. (1992). The pathogenesis of coronary artery disease and the acute coronary syndromes (first of two parts). *New England Journal of Medicine*, **326**, 242–50.

Gaire, M., Magbanua, Z., McDonnell, S., McNeil, L., Lovett, D. H. & Matrisian, L. M. (1994). Structure and expression of the human gene for the matrix metalloproteinase matrilysin. *Journal of Biological Chemistry*, **269**, 2032–40.

Galis, Z. S., Muszynski, M., Sukhova, G. K., Simon-Morrissey, E. & Libby, P. (1995a). Enhanced expression of vascular matrix metalloproteinases induced in vitro by cytokines and in regions of human atherosclerotic lesions. *Annals of the New York Academy of Sciences*, **748**, 501–7.

Galis, Z. S., Sukhova, G. K., Kranzhofer, R., Clark, S. & Libby, P. (1995b). Macrophage foam cells from experimental atheroma constitutively produce matrix-degrading proteinase. *Proceedings of the National Academy of Sciences USA*, **92**, 402–6.

Galis, Z. S., Sukhova, G. K., Lark, M. W. & Libby, P. (1994). Increased expression of matrix metalloproteinases and matrix degrading activity in vulnerable regions of human atherosclerotic plaques. *Journal of Clinical Investigation*, **94**, 2493–503.

Goldberg, G. I., Frisch, S. M., He, C., Wilhelm, S. M., Reich, R. & Collier, I. E. (1990). Secreted proteases. Regulation of their activity and their possible role in metastasis. *Annals of the New York Academy of Sciences*, **580**, 375–84.

Guantieri, V., Tamburro, A. M. & Gordini, D. D. (1983). Interactions of human and bovine elastins with lipids: their proteolysis by elastase. *Connective Tissue Research*, **12**, 79–83.

Guyton, J. R. & Klemp, K. F. (1995). Specific features of lipid deposits associated with arterial collagen and elastin. In *Atherosclerosis* vol. X, ed. F. P. Woodford, J. Davignon & A. Sniderman, pp. 360–4. Amsterdam: Elsevier Science BV.

Hassler, O. (1970). The origin of the cells constituting arterial intima thickening. An experimental autoradiographic study with the use of H^3-thymidine. *Laboratory Investigation*, **22**, 286–93.

Henney, A. M., Wakeley, P. R., Davies, M. J., Foster, K., Hembry, R., Murphy, G. & Humphries, S. (1991). Localization of stromelysin gene expression in atherosclerotic plaques by *in situ* hybridization. *Proceedings of the National Academy of Sciences USA*, **88**, 8154–8.

Hoff, H. F. & Wagner, W. D. (1986). Plasma low density lipoprotein accumulation in aortas of hypercholesterolemic swine correlates with modifications in aortic glycosaminoglycan composition. *Atherosclerosis*, **61**, 231–6.

Hosoda, Y., Kawano, K., Yamasawa, F., Ishii, T., Shibata, T. & Inayama, S. (1984). Age-dependent changes of collagen and elastin content in human aorta and pulmonary artery. *Angiology*, **35**, 615–21.

Huhtala, P., Chow, L. T. & Tryggvason, K.(1990). Structure of the human type IV collagenase gene. *Journal of Biological Chemistry*, **265**, 11077–82.

Huhtala, P., Tuuttila, A., Chow, T., Lohi, J., Keski-Oja, J. & Tryggvason, K. (1991). Complete structure of the human gene for 92-kDa type IV collagenase. Divergent regulation of expression for the 92- and 72-kilodalton enzyme genes in HT-1080 cells. *Journal of Biological Chemistry*, **266**, 16485–90.

Imai, K., Yokohama, K., Nakanishi, I., Ohuchi, E., Fujii, Y., Nakai, N. & Okada, Y. (1995). Matrix metalloproteinase 7 (matrilysin) from human rectal carcinoma cells. Activation of the precursor, interaction with other matrix metalloproteinases and enzymic properties. *Journal of Biological Chemistry*, **270**, 6691–7.

Jaeger, E., Rust, S., Scharffetter, K., Roessner, A., Winter, J., Buchholz, B., Althaus, M. & Rauterberg, J. (1990). Localisation of cytoplasmic collagen mRNA in human aortic coarctation: mRNA enhancement in high blood pressure-induced intimal and medial thickening. *Journal of Histochemistry and Cytochemistry*, **38**, 1365.

Knauper, V., Murphy, G. & Tschesche, H. (1994). Neutrophil procollagenase can be activated by stromelysin-2. *Annals of the New York Academy of Sciences*, **732**, 367–8.

Knauper, V., Wilhelm, S. M., Seperack, P. K., DeClerck, Y. A., Langley, K. E., Osthues, A. & Tschesche, H. (1993). Direct activation of human neutrophil procollagenase by recombinant stromelysin. *Biochemical Journal*, **295**, 581–6.

Lendon, C. L., Davies, M. J., Born, G. V. R. & Richardson, P. D. (1991). Atherosclerotic plaque caps are locally weakened when macrophage density is increased. *Atherosclerosis*, **87**, 87–90.

Libby, P. (1995). Molecular bases of the acute coronary syndromes. *Circulation*, **91**, 2844–50.

Mackay, A. R., Ballin, M., Pelina, M. D., Farina, A. R., Nason, A. M., Hartzler, J. L. & Thorgeirsson, U. P. (1992). Effect of phorbol ester and cytokines on matrix metalloproteinase and tissue inhibitor of metalloproteinase expression in tumour and normal cell lines. *Invasion and Metastasis*, **12**, 168–84.

Matrisian, L. M. & Hogan, B. L. M. (1990). Growth factor-regulated proteases and extracellular matrix remodelling during mammalian development. *Current Topics in Developmental Biology*, **24**, 219–59.

Miyazaki, K., Umenishi, F., Funahashi, K., Koshikawa, N., Yasumitsu, H. & Umeda, M. (1992). Activation of TIMP-2/progelatinase A complex by stromelysin. *Biochemical and Biophysical Research Communications*, **185**, 852–9.

Molossi, S., Clausell, N. & Rabinovitch, M. (1995). Reciprocal induction of tumor necrosis factor-α and interleukin-β activity mediates fibronectin synthesis in coronary artery smooth muscle cells. *Journal of Cellular Physiology*, **163**, 19–29.

Morton, L. F. & Barnes, M. J. (1982). Collagen polymorphism in the normal and diseased blood vessel wall: Investigation of collagen types I, III and V. *Atherosclerosis*, **42**, 41–51.

Muller, D., Quantin, B., Gesnel, M.C., Millon-Collard, R., Abecassis, J. & Breathnach, R. (1988). The collagenase gene family in humans consists of at least four members. *Biochemical Journal*, **253**, 187–92.

Murphy, G. & Reynolds, J. (1993). Extracellular matrix degradation. In *Connective Tissue and its Heritable Disorders*, ed. P. M. Royce & B. Steinman, pp. 287–316. New York: Wiley-Liss.

Murphy, G., Cockett, M. I., Stephens, P. E., Smith, B. J. & Docherty, A. J. P. (1987). Stromelysin is an activator of procollagenase. A study with natural and recombinant enzymes. *Biochemical Journal*, **248**, 265–8.

Murphy, G., Reynolds, J. J. & Werb, Z. (1985). Biosynthesis of tissue inhibitor of metalloproteinases by human fibroblasts in culture. Stimulation by 12-*O*-tetradecanoylphorbol-13-acetate and interleukin 1 in parallel with collagenase. *Journal of Biological Chemistry*, **260**, 3079–83.

Newby, A. C., Southgate, K. M. & Davies, M. (1994). Extracellular matrix degrading metalloproteinases in the pathogenesis of arteriosclerosis. *Basic Research in Cardiology*, **89**(Suppl. 1), 59–70.

Nikkari, S. T., O'Brien, K. D., Furguson, M., Hatsukami, T., Welgus, H. G., Aplers, C. E. & Clowes, A. W. (1995). Interstitial collagenase (MMP-1) expression in human carotid atherosclerosis. *Circulation*, **92**, 1393–8.

Ogata, Y., Enghild, J. J. & Nagase, H. (1992). Matrix metalloproteinase 3 (stromslysin) activates the precursor for the human matrix metalloproteinase 9. *Journal of Biological Chemistry*, **267**, 3581–4.

Olsen, B. R. (1995). New insights into the function of collagens from genetic analysis. *Current Opinion in Cell Biology*, **7**, 720–7.

Pauly, R. R., Passaniti, A., Crow, M., Kinsella, J. L., Rapadopoulos, N., Monticone, R,. Lakatta, E. G. & Martin, G. R. (1992). Experimental models that mimic the differentiation and dedifferentiation of vascular cells. *Circulation*, **86**(Suppl. III), III-68–III-73.

Pauly, R. R., Passaniti, A., Bilato, C., Monticone, R., Cheng, L., Papadopoulos, N., Gluzband, Y. A., Smith, L., Weinstein, C., Lakatta, E. G. & Crow, M. T. (1994). Migration of cultured vascular smooth muscle cells through a basement membrane barrier requires type IV collagenase activity and is inhibited by cellular differentiation. *Circulation Research*, **75**, 41–54.

Rabinovitch, M. (1995). Elastase and cell extracellular matrix interactions in pathogenesis of intimal proliferation. In *Atherosclerosis*, vol. X, ed. F. P. Woodford, J. Davignon & A. Sniderman, pp. 338–49. Amsterdam: Elsevier Science BV.

Richardson, P. D., Davies, M. J. & Born, G. V. R. (1989). Influence of plaque configuration and stress distribution of fissuring of coronary atherosclerotic plaques. *Lancet*, **ii**, 941–4.

Ross, R. (1993). The pathogenesis of atherosclerosis: a perspective for the 1990s. *Nature*, **362**, 801–9.

Sage, H., Crouch, E. & Bornstein, P. (1979). Collagen synthesis by bovine aortic endothelial cells in culture. *Biochemistry*, **18**, 5433–42.

Sang, Q. X., Birkedal-Hansen, H. & Van Wart, H. E. (1995). Proteolytic and non-proteolytic activation of human neutrophil progelatinase B. *Biochimca et Biophysica Acta*, **1251**, 99–108.

Sato, H., Takino, T., Okada, Y., Cao, J., Shinagawa, A., Yamamoto, E. & Seiki, M. (1994). A matrix metalloproteinase expressed on the surface of invasive tumour cells. *Nature*, **370**, 61–5.

Shapiro, S. D., Fliszar, C. J., Broekelmann, T. J., Mecham, R. P., Senior, R. M. & Welgus, H. G. (1995). Activation of the 92-kDa gelatinase by stromelysin and 4-aminophenylmercuric acetate. *Journal of Biological Chemistry*, **270**, 6351–6.

Stary, H. C., Blankenhorn, D. H., Chandler, B., Glagov, S., Insull, Jr, W., Richardson, M., Rosenfeld, M. E., Schaffer, S. A., Schwartz, C. J., Wagner, W. D. & Wissler, R. W. (1992). A definition of the intima of human arteries and of its atherosclerosis-prone regions. *Arteriosclerosis and Thrombosis*, **12**, 120–34.

Stary, H. C., Chandler, A. B., Glagov, S., Guyton, J. R., Insull, W., Resenfeld, M. E., Schaffer,

S. A., Schwartz, C. J., Wagner, W. D. & Wissler, R. W. (1994). A definition of initial, fatty streak, and intermediate lesions of atherosclerosis. *Arteriosclerosis and Thrombosis*, **14**, 840–56.

Stary, H. C., Chandler, A. B., Dinsmore, R. E., Fuster, V., Glagov, S., Insull, Jr, W., Rosenfeld, M. E., Schwartz, C. J., Wagner, W. D. & Wissler, R. W. (1995). A definition of advanced types of atherosclerotic lesions and a histological classification of atherosclerosis. *Arteriosclerosis, Thrombosis and Vascular Biology*, **15**, 15512–31.

Stetler-Stevenson, W. G., Brown, P. D., Onisto, M., Levy, A. T. & Liotta, L. A. (1990). Tissue inhibitor of metalloproteinase-2 (TIMP-2) mRNA expression in tumor cell lines and human tumor tissues. *Journal of Biological Chemistry*, **265**, 13933–8.

Stetler-Stevenson, W. G., Krutzsch, H. C. & Liotta, L. A. (1992). TIMP-2: identification and characterization of a new member of the metalloproteinase inhibitor family. *Matrix*, **1**(Suppl.), 299–306.

Strongin, A. Y., Collier, I., Bannikov, G., Marmer, B. L., Grant, G. A. & Goldberg, G. I. (1995). Mechanism of cell surface activation of 72-kDa type IV collagenase. *Journal of Biological Chemistry*, **270**, 5331–8.

Suzuki, K., Enghild, J. J., Morodomi, T., Salvesen, G. & Nagase, H. (1990). Mechanisms of activation of tissue procollagenase by matrix metalloproteinase 3 (stromelysin). *Biochemistry*, **29**, 10261–70.

Tyagi, S. C., Meyer, L., Schmaltz, R. A., Reddy, H. K. & Voelker, D. J. (1995). Proteinases and restenosis in the human coronary artery: extracellular matrix production exceeds the expression of proteolytic activity. *Atherosclerosis*, **116**, 43–57.

Wight, T. N., Schonherr, E., Jarvelainen, H., Kinsella, M., Evanko, S. & Lemire, J. (1995). Regulation of proteoglycan synthesis by vascular cells. In *Atherosclerosis*, vol. X, ed. F. P. Woodford, J. Davignon & A. Sniderman, pp. 350–4. Amsterdam: Elsevier Science BV.

Weber, B. H., Vogt, G., Pruett, R. C., Stöhr, H. & Felbor, U. (1994). Mutation in the tissue inhibitor of metalloproteinases-3 (TIMP3) in patients with Sorsby's fundus dystrophy. *Nature Genetics*, **8**, 352–6.

Willard, H. F., Durfy, S. J., Mahtan, M. M., Dorkins, H., Davized, K. E. & Williams, B. R. G. (1989). Regional localization of the TIMP gene on the human X chromosome. *Human Genetics*, **81**, 234–8.

Woessner, J. F. Jr (1991). Matrix metalloproteinases and their inhibitors in connective tissue remodelling. *FASEB Journal*, **5**, 2145–54.

Van Wart, H. E. & Birkedal-Hansen, H. (1990). The cysteine switch: a principle of regulation of metalloproteinase activity with potential applicability to the entire matrix metalloproteinase gene family. *Proceedings of the National Academy of Sciences of the USA*, **87**, 5578–82.

Ye, S., Eriksson, P., Hamsten, A., Kurkinen, M., Humphries, S. E. & Henney, A. M. (1996). Progression of coronary atherosclerosis is associated with a common genetic variant of the human stromelysin 1 promoter which results in reduced gene expression. *Journal of Biological Chemistry*, **271**, 13055–60.

Ye, S., Watts, G. F., Mandalia, S., Humphries, S. E. & Henney, A. M. (1995). Genetic variation in the human stromelysin promoter is associated with progression of coronary atherosclerosis. *British Heart Journal*, **73**, 209–15.

Ylä-Herttuala, A., Solakivi, T., Hirvonen, J., Laaksonen, H., Möttönen, M., Pesonen, E., Raekallio, J., Akerblom, H. K. & Nikkari, T. (1987). Glycosaminoglycans and apolipoproteins B and A-I in human aortas: chemical and immunological analysis of lesion-free aortas from children and adults. *Arteriosclerosis*, **7**, 333–40.

10

Restenosis

P. CHAN and S. HEPPLE

Introduction

Restenosis is a common and serious problem after arterial bypass or angioplasty. The pathophysiological processes contributing to restenosis may be considered as a model of the vessel wall response to injury, and of early atherosclerosis (Ross, 1993).

Pathology

Restenosis causes a mechanical obstruction to flow, after an initially successful vascular procedure. It can be considered to have three components:

1. elastic recoil after vessel stretching
2. vessel wall thickening
3. circumferential constriction

Studies of restenotic lesions obtained at operation or post-mortem have revealed substantial thickening of the intimal layer of the vessel wall (number 2, above), the major component of restenosis. The thickened intima is composed of fibrocellular connective tissue of variable cellularity, surrounded by extracellular matrix of collagen and ground substance. The cells are vascular smooth muscle, which proliferate in the intima and secrete matrix protein, probably after initial migration from the vessel media. In the early stages, the cellular component is prominent; later more extracellular matrix is observed.

This process is seen after all vascular injury, whether it proceeds to restenosis or not, and represents vascular healing. Restenosis lesions contain more intimal material, compromising the vessel lumen.

These structural changes have been recognized since the early days of vascular surgery (Carrel & Guthrie, 1986). It has been described as 'fibrosis' of artery or graft, and called intimal, neointimal or fibrous hyperplasia, early or accelerated atherosclerosis (Imparato et al, 1972; DeWeese & Robb, 1977). In this chapter it is referred to as myointimal hyperplasia (MIH), reflecting the smooth muscle origin of the cellular proliferation. This term however underestimates the importance of extracellular matrix secretion, which may constitute up to 70% of the volume of the restenotic lesion. *MIH represents physiological vascular healing; restenosis is pathological and might involve different mechanisms.*

Ultrastructural studies of MIH have clarified its cytopathology. The predominant cell type is the smooth muscle cell (SMC). Cells similar to fibroblasts and cells of intermediate appearance are also seen. The uninjured artery has no fibroblasts in the intima and media, and vascular (SMCs) are the major component of the media, and occasionally present in the intima.

Proliferating SMCs probably originates from the media, but they may come from underlying adventitia. After grafting of uninjured vein into the arterial circulation, the media changes, SMCs hypertrophy, adopt the synthetic phenotype, and elaborate extracellular matrix and collagen. These medial SMCs may migrate into the intima, and proliferate (Dilley et al, 1988). Similar changes in adventitial fibroblasts, with additional myofibroblast differentiation, have been observed in a pig coronary artery model of balloon overstretch injury (Scott et al, 1996). There is still no direct proof that cells migrate through an intact medial layer to proliferate in the intima, but in a pig coronary balloon injury model there is myointimal hyperplasia, apparently continuous with adventitial hyperplasia of SMCs. This is only found in the artery where the media has split and the intima is in contact with the external elastic lamina (J. Gunn, personal communication).

SMCs and fibroblasts may not be distinct cell types, but can differentiate in both directions from a common mesenchymal origin (Sottiurai 1983). In cell culture studies, cells of vascular smooth muscle origin can be induced to differentiate into contractile (smooth muscle-like) and synthetic (fibroblast-like) phenotypes (Chamley-Campbell et al, 1979).

These appearances cause confusion between vascular 'fibrosis' and the cellular appearance of MIH. Proliferating SMCs can adopt a phenotype similar to a fibroblast, secrete collagen and ground substance, producing a copious extracellular matrix. Thus arterial and venous 'fibrosis' represents the mature lesion of MIH.

Are MIH and restenosis different in different parts of the circulation? Although risk factors for restenosis vary, the incidence of restenosis is remarkably similar (25–40%) after procedures in all arterial beds. Histological appearances of restenosis are similar in coronary angioplasty, prosthetic surgical bypass, venous reconstruction and arteriovenous fistula. If surrounding tissue were excluded, it would not be possible to distinguish between a histological section of coronary restenosis and any other restenosis.

We have shown that a cellular trait in human vascular smooth muscle associated with restenosis is found throughout the circulation (arterial and venous, of a single individual (Munro et al, 1994). In spite of differences in physiology within the circulation, it is possible that the response to injury, and the pathological response of restenosis is similar. Restenosis does not appear to vary from site to site.

The stimulus to MIH is vessel wall trauma. Cellular proliferation is mediated by peptide growth factors. Following endothelial denudation and platelet accumulation, platelet activation and degranulation release a factors which stimulate medial SMCs, (platelet-derived growth factor (PDGF), and also TGF-β, serotonin and platelet factor 4). Damaged vascular wall cells release basic fibroblast growth factor (bFGF). These factors are mitogenic for smooth muscle (Ross & Glomset, 1973) and chemotactic for SMCs (Bell & Madri, 1989), stimulating their proliferation and migration into the intima.

Growth factors from proliferating SMCs may allow the process to continue after the resolution of the original platelet stimulation (Sjolund et al, 1988; Golden et al, 1990). This paracrine stimulation may be important in determining which lesions will progress and which remain self-limiting.

The relative importance of different growth factors in the aetiology of MIH in humans is not known. Platelet-derived growth factor (PDGF) transcripts have been found by in situ hybridization in atherosclerotic plaques (Wilcox et al, 1988), and a PDGF-like mitogen is secreted by cultured vascular SMCs from anastomotic hyperplastic lesions (Birinyi et al, 1989). PDGF is expressed by cultured human venous endothelium and by intimal cells in healing PTFE grafts. (Limmani et al, 1988; Golden et al, 1990) TGF-β transcripts are more frequently expressed in human coronary artery restenosis tissue than in atherosclerotic plaques (Nikol et al, 1992). Antibodies to single growth factors diminish but do not abolish the rat carotid model hyperplastic response to injury.

Intimal hyperplasia may be important in development of atherosclerosis. Following vessel wall injury and vascular SMC proliferation (Ross & Glomset, 1973), development of the atherosclerotic lesion depends on 'progression factors' which include vascular SMC proliferative capacity, lipid uptake and the inflammatory response. Vascular injury may be physical, with endothelial denudation and platelet activation as described above; or biochemical, perhaps associated with lipid peroxidation. This 'response to injury' hypothesis is now the dominant theory, focusing interest on the vascular SMC and its growth characteristics.

Is MIH the main cause of restenosis ? Structural studies of post-mortem coronary arteries or reoperative peripheral bypass graft material support this theory (Whittemore et al, 1981; Sottiurai et al, 1983; Nobuyoshi et al, 1991; Waller et al, 1991). Recent in vivo coronary artery studies using intravascular ultrasound have shown that a decrease in the cross-sectional area of the whole artery might be more important (Mintz et al, 1996). Mechanisms for this phenomenon are not known but experimental studies suggest that adventitial constrictive scarring, vessel wall cellular apoptosis, and extracellular matrix remodelling, termed vascular remodelling, may play a part (Isner, 1994; Glagov, 1994). Vascular remodelling has not yet been shown to play a major role in human restenosis. At least in histopathological studies.

Vascular remodelling certainly occurs after angioplasty and may contribute to restenosis, particularly in small arteries injured by overstretch or atherectomy. More than 20% of subjects in the Mintz study with increases in arterial cross-sectional area still developed luminal stenoses. It is less likely to cause vein conduit restenoses after surgical bypass.

Elastic recoil of the vessel after balloon angioplasty may be a less important factor in human restenosis, and is mentioned later.

Technical aspects

The clinical symptoms and signs of restenosis, usually obvious, include recurrence of the ischaemia which preceded the intervention; however, many restenoses occlude before clinically apparent events recur (Taylor et al, 1990). An objective definition of restenosis is desirable and usuallyinvolves imaging of the intervention site.

Angiography may not show restenosis because vascular remodelling may enlarge the vessel eccentrically (Glagov et al, 1987). The definition of restenosis as a haemodynamically significant stenosis is probably adequate for a procedure like vein grafting, where there was no major pre-exisiting stenosis (Fig. 10.1), but the definition is confused when considering partially successful primary angioplasty procedures which do not fully restore the lumen.

Restenosis can be defined as a measured change from the primary post procedure image greater than two standard deviations from observer and repeat imaging error, which is functionally important. In coronary angioplasty studies, 50% loss of initial luminal gain is often regarded as restenosis; but this is dependent on whether that initial gain was large or small.

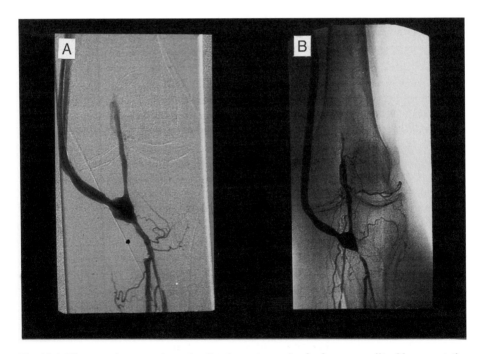

Fig. 10.1. These angiograms show the distal anastomosis of a femoropopliteal bypass at the time of surgery (A) and 6 months after operation when the patient was detected to have an asymptomatic stenosis affecting the popliteal artery just distal to the anastomosis. (B) The graft is constructed from prosthetic material (PTFE) with an interposed cuff of saphenous vein.

Restenosis rates may, therefore, be reported differently. When Beatt and colleagues applied the the first two definitions (any haemodynamic stenosis and any change from post procedure image) to a single set of pre- and post-coronary angioplasty images, (restenosis rates of 24% and 33%) less than 50% of patients from the first definition were included in the second definition (Beatt et al, 1990).

The literature on restenosis is therefore difficult to interpret. Measurement error is significant, particularly in the coronary circulation. For example, the within-subject standard deviation in coronary arterial images was found to be 0.36 mm, (Beatt et al, 1990) but in a recent angioplasty stent restenosis study, mean luminal diameter in the stented compared with the non-stented group was 0.11 mm (± 0.62 mm), well within the defined measurement error of this image-analysis method (Fischman et al, 1994).

Models of restenosis

Clowes has studied cellular events following balloon catheter arterial injury in the rat carotid. Maximal SMC proliferation occurred 2–4 days after arterial wall injury (measured by labelled thymidine incorporation) but continued SMC proliferation depended on endothelial coverage. The thymidine index returns to baseline values 4–8 weeks after injury in arterial segments covered by endothelium, but remained high in chronically denuded arterial segments.

Vasoconstriction caused by SMC contraction and producing 75% luminal stenosis occurred around 2 weeks after injury. From the first week, intimal thickening was measureable and became prominent by 4–12 weeks after injury. From 2–12 weeks the intimal vascular SMC numbers hardly change, the arterial wall thickens as cells synthesise and accumulate connective tissue (Clowes et al, 1983).

This rat model is the most frequently studied model of vascular healing. Many others exist, using other types and sites of vascular injury in most species of common laboratory animals. A variety of surgical approaches with autogenous and prosthetic bypasses has also been used to study haemodynamic influences on MIH in conditions of varying blood flow.

MIH may not be similar in humans and animals as restenosis is relatively common in humans and rare in animal models. Unfortunately, animal models have had to be used to validate treatments for MIH, and to study the mechanical factors that may be involved in stimulating MIH. Considerable differences appear to exist between the responses of vascular SMC to growth factor stimuli and inhibition in different species (Castellot et al, 1989).

Mechanical factors and restenosis

Haemodynamic factors such as blood flow have been shown to correlate with development of MIH. Normal laminar flow pattern in arteries includes a relatively slower moving layer next to the artery wall known as the boundary layer. In conditions of slow flow or turbulence, flow in the boundary layer may be static or even reversed; this is known as boundary layer separation. It has been suggested that the prolonged contact with platelets and other blood constituents in a boundary layer separation may contribute to arterial wall pathology. Slow flow or turbulence may produce low tangential, or shear stress on the neighbouring arterial wall.

In a dog femoro–femoral crossover bypass model there is a rather weak correlation between these areas of low shear stress and subsequent intimal hyperplasia (Rittgers, 1978). Using a plexiglass model of an end-to-side 45° anastomosis, a complex helicospiral flow pattern was produced at normal arterial pressure and pulsation. Areas of localized low shear stress corresponded with two common sites of intimal hyperplasia: the toe of the anastomosis and the floor of the recipient artery opposite the aperture (Bassiouny et al, 1992; Ojha et al, 1990).

High shear stress may also be a factor in intimal hyperplasia. Inserting a vein graft into the arterial circulation causes a high wall shear stress, and subsequent vein wall thickening then returns the wall shear stress towards normal. Rigid external support of the vein graft will reduce the high shear stress, and tends to reduce intimal hyperplasia (Kohler et al, 1989). In human studies of femoropopliteal bypass and arteriovenous fistulas (constructed for dialysis access) using vessel wall Doppler tracking, high shear stress is indeed associated with restenosis (Hofstra et al, 1995).

In a canine arterivenous femoral PTFE loop model, Fillinger found that turbulence correlated with the development of intimal hyperplasia (Fillinger et al, 1989, 1990). At an anastomosis, where the stiff artificial graft meets the compliant artery, there is a postulated 'compliance mismatch', responsible for setting up deleterious patterns of blood flow, with areas of low/high shear stress, boundary layer separation, etc. which may ultimately lead to intimal hyperplasia. This is unlikely to occur in autogenous vein grafts, or in MIH occurring after angioplasty. Direct evidence for this 'mismatch' theory is based on an experiment with 14 dogs, with paired glutaraldehyde-treated autografts differing only in compliance being inserted into femoral arteries; eight stiff and two compliant grafts thrombosed within 3 months (Abbott et al, 1987). In contrast, Hofstra's studies of human prosthetic grafts do not show any relation between compliance mismatch and restenosis (Hofstra et al, 1995b).

In summary, many mechanical factors have been postulated as important determinants of intimal hyperplasia. Some are interrelated; all may correlate with sites of excessive endothelial and intimal injury and lead up to restenosis. In a diseased circulation, these may not be treatable and there might also be limits to improving haemodynamic results by altering anastomotic and angioplasty techniques.

Treatment for restenosis

Treatment of an established restenosis is similar to primary stenosis. The incidence of further stenosis after re-angioplasty or surgical correction is 50–60%, compared with 30–40% for first time coronary angioplasty. This applies even if the first restenosis occurred remote from the second operative site (Bresee et al, 1991; Berger et al, 1992). In a register of all early coronary angioplasties, the most powerful risk factor was having suffered a previous restenosis (Holmes et al, 1984). This implies individual predilection to restenosis. Although correction of restenosis is worthwhile, some patients will restenose many times.

There may not be an individual predilection to restenosis if the risk of restenosis is linked to morphological characteristics of the stenosing lesion or of the procedure, or if restenosis is a continuous variable with an arbitrary division between normal vascular healing and pathological restenosis.

Various anatomical and procedure-related variables which may predispose to restenosis in coronary angioplasty are outlined in Table 10.1. Most of the data in Table 10.1 is derived from large series by retrospective review and posthoc subgroup analysis, a method which tends to produce false positive correlations. Gibson et al (1993) produced a mathematical model which was applied to restenoses in patients having either multiple procedures or single lesion procedures. They wished to determine whether there was a correlation in behaviour of multiple lesions within single patients. The model revealed that restenosis in patients with multiple lesions could be accurately predicted by assuming independent restenosis risks for each lesion. This model therefore favoured lesion-specific risk factors over patient-related risk factors. This study is flawed by the high incidence of restenosis lesions in both groups, especially in the single-lesion compared with the multi-lesion group. Weintraub et al (1993) tried to apply correlates derived from multivariate analysis of 2500 patients to predict restenosis in a subsequent cohort of 1506 patients. Although the observed incidence of restenosis fitted well with the predicted incidence, restenosis in the subsequent cohort was poorly predicted, with a power of nearly zero.

Does restenosis represent a continuous variable? Studies analysing follow-up coronary angiograms showed that late loss of luminal diameter followed a normal distribution (Rensing et al, 1992). A recent, statistically precise study has shown how this finding could have resulted from the known measurement error of quantitiative coronary angiography. Lehmann et al (1996) then described a bimodal distribution of lesions on follow-up angiography; one shows considerable restenosis and a second shows very little, with few intermediates. These data applied to lesions rather than patients, although in most patients only a single lesion was studied, and a bimodal grouping of lesions would roughly translate into a bimodal grouping of patients, providing some support for the concept that there is an individual risk for restenosis. These data do suggest that restenosis is not likely to be a continuous variable.

The aim of most restenosis research is to define a strategy to prevent restenosis after intervention. There have been two main lines of research: to develop procedures that might reduce restenosis and to discover drugs that reduce the severity of restenosis after standard procedures.

Most devices developed to reduce restenosis have not been subjected to properly conducted trials and published preliminary results have usually appeared more promising than subsequent clinical experience. Laser angioplasty may produce more restenosis than conventional angioplasty (Lammer et al, 1993). Atherectomy in coronary arteries or the femoropopliteal segment is no more successful than angioplasty (Vroegindeweij et

Table 10.1. *Proposed clinical correlates of coronary restenosis post angioplasty*

Patient-related factors	
Unstable angina	Leimgruber et al, Weintraubet al (1993)
Young age	Glazier et al (1987)
Old age	Weintraub et al (1993)
Diabetes,	Lambert et al (1988), Weintraub et al (1993)
Hypertension	Weintraub et al (1993)
Lesion related factors	
Proximal LAD site	Ellis, Ardissino et al (1991), Leimgruber et al (1994), Foley et al (1994), Hirshfeld et al (1994), not Herrmans
Bend point site	Ellis,
High grade stenosis preangioplasty	Lambert, Weintraub et al (1993), Hirshfeld et al (1991)
Eccentric lesion	Weintraub et al (1993), Hirshfeld et al (1991)
Long lesion	Bourassa et al (1991), Ardissino et al (1992), Hirshfeld et al (1991), Rensing et al (1991)
Procedure-related factors	
Absence of fracture/tear/dissection	Jain et al (1994), Leimgruber et al (1986), Weintraub et al (1993), Tenaglia et al (1992)
Existence of major dissection	Jain et al (1994), not Hermans
Greater number of balloon inflations	Glazier et al (1989)
Hyperventilation-induced vasospasm	Ardissino et al (1991)
Number of lesions dilated	LeFeuvre et al (1994)
Residual stenosis after angioplasty	Bourassa et al (1994), Ellis et al (1988), Lambert et al (1988), LeFeuvre et al (1994), Leimgruber et al (1989b)
Relatively high gain after stent/angioplasty	DeJaegere et al (1996), Rensing et al (1992a,b)
Relatively small gain after stent	STRESS

al, 1995; Holmes et al, 1994) and might actually cause more restenosis. Stenting coronary arteries in two large multicenter trials produced a modest reduction in restenosis rates from around 35% to around 25% (Serruys et al, 1994; Fischman et al, 1994). Stenting of peripheral arteries has not been well studied, and conclusions cannot be inferred from the coronary artery results.

Can the restenosis be lowered by improvements in existing techniques? Does leaving a smoother intimal outline, or dilating an angioplasty site more widely, or handling a vein bypass more gently to less restenosis? Improvements in general technique will usually produce better results but this is not due to effects on restenosis. In humans neither depth of angioplasty nor deeper atherectomy have a therapeutic effect on restenosis (Hermans et al, 1992a; Kuntz et al, 1992). It has been suggested that a smoother arterial wall or angiographically 'better' result after angioplasty avoids restenosis, but there is very little controlled data to support this concept.

A study of patients with bilateral carotid disease who had endarterectomy on one side and vein interposition bypass on the other revealed no differences in the (very low) restenosis rate (Fabiani, 1994). Changes in angle of anastomosis or in vein bypass techniques have hardly influenced the development of MIH (Storm et al, 1975; Bond et al, 1976; Breyer et al, 1976; Quigley et al, 1986).

The range and number of candidate drugs for prevention of restenosis is truly impressive. Over 50 agents have completed the course from promising in vitro and animal experiments through to randomized trials, usually in coronary angioplasty restenosis.

None of these large number of agents, which all reduce MIH in animal vascular injury, have inhibited restenosis in humans (Table 10.2).

Why the disparity between animal and human results? It is possible that in human trials the agent did affect restenosis, but may have been administered in too low dosage (heparin, Ellis et al, 1989), in too high dosage (angiopeptin, Emmanuelsson et al, 1995), at incorrect frequency (cilazipril, Faxon et al, 1995) or the methodology of quantitative angiography may be too demanding a criterion. It is quite possible that existing animal methods do not correctly model human restenosis, because those methods study physiological MIH rather than pathological restenosis. Restenosis may not just be 'too much MIH', but might involve different or additional mechanisms.

Human restenosis

Future strategies to reduce restenosis will involve more research into the processes of human restenosis. Human restenosis can be considered as the sum of three vascular responses: (1) myointimal hyperplasia, (2) elastic recoil of the vessel wall, (3) constrictive remodelling of the vessel wall.

There may be differences between myointimal hyperplasia in humans and in animal models. In balloon angioplasty, there is a preexisting human atherosclerotic lesion, but this is not present in most animal models. There may also be differences in human SMC responses. We found that resistance to heparin inhibition, detectable in vascular SMC culture, was a risk factor in both retrospective and prospective human restenosis cohorts (Chan et al, 1993; Refson et al, 1996). This heparin resistance appears to define a subtype of vascular SMC present in most human vessels, but only rarely found in animals (Chan, 1994; Barzu et al, 1994; SanAntonio et al, 1993).

Elastic recoil is important in angioplasty restenosis, but not in bypass graft stenosis. It is apparent in animal models of balloon injury to arteries (Clowes et al, 1983) and is unlikely to account for unique features in human restenosis.

Vascular remodelling probably involves many processes, as an adaptive response to vessel injury. Glagov noted that arteries with atherosclerotic plaque often displayed compensatory enlargement (Glagov et al, 1987). Subsequently, studies using intra-vascular ultrasound have shown that constrictive remodelling in angioplastied segments, worsens restenosis; and may be more significant than myointimal hyperplasia (Mintz et al, 1996).

Table 10.2. *Human restenosis trials*

Class of agent	Agent	Trial acronym (if any)	Numbers in trial
Heparin	unfractionated		419
	enoxaparin LMW	ERA	458
Antiplatelet agents	aspirin/dipyridamole		203,453,79,40,249,207, 549
	ticlopidine		236, 179
	ketanserin		43, 658
	thromboxane A2 synthase inhibitors		707,33, 755,1089
	prostacyclin	CARPORT, M-HEART, GRASP	311, 286
Anticoagulant	warfarin		110, 119
	coumadin		248
Fish oils	EPA preparations	FORT	82,108,204, 194, 108, 119, 107, 204
ACE inhibitors/ A2 antagonist	cilazipril	MERCATOR, MARCATOR	595, 1436
	enalapril		95
	quinapril		ongoing
Calcium channel blockers	diltiazem		94, 201
	nifedipine	QUIET	241
Steroids	methylprednisolone	M-HEART	66,722, 102,
Lipid-lowering agents	lovastatin	L-ART	157, 404
	LDL-apheresis		66
Growth factor antagonist	angiopeptin		553
	trapidil	STARC	72, 254
Antiproliferative agents	colchicine	CART	197,253

Note: This is not a complete list of restenosis trials. All trials cited are randomized, usually placebo controlled or aspirin controlled trials of restenosis, mostly after coronary angioplasty, generally defined by repeat angiography. Most trials have shown no effect on postprocedure restenosis. Often a small study indicates a promising significant effect of an agent, only to be disproved by a multicentre, randomized, controlled, larger trial at a later date (e.g. lovastatin).

Similar changes of arterial remodelling have been described after angioplasty in the pig coronary, normal rabbit iliac and femoral , and hypercholesterolemic rabbit iliac arteries (Post et al, 1994; Kakuta et al, 1994). The proportional contribution of remodelling and MIH to restenosis remains controversial. Post attributes between 52 and 89% of late luminal loss to constrictive remodelling. Kakuta showed little difference in MIH between restenotic and non-restenotic groups. Gertz et al, working with hypercholesterolaemic rabbits, showed no geometric remodelling and implicated preexisting lesion morphology (Gertz et al, 1994). Lafont showed a poor correlation between late lumen loss and both constriction and MIH, but favoured remodelling as the main determinant of narrowing after balloon injury in hypercholesterolemic rabbits (Lafont et al, 1995). These models may not resemble humans; it is also possible that the relative roles of remodelling and MIH may vary considerably between individuals (this is seen in the above experiments) and from site to site within individuals.

Although the processes of human restenosis are not yet adequately defined therapeutic research continues. There is much current interest in systems of local delivery and in gene therapy. Local delivery systems, for example through angiographic catheters may be used to target high dose drugs (Lambert et al, 1994) or other agents, such as beta irradiation (Verin et al, 1995), or intact endothelial seeding (Thompson et al, 1994) to the site of arterial injury after angioplasty. These approaches may allow higher doses of agents to be targetted more selectively.

Gene therapy relies on local delivery of nucleotide material into the vascular wall at the site of injury. This approach targets the control mechanism for cellular events leading to restenosis (Ohno et al, 1994). There is, however, a major problem with targetting. Current animal experience with antisense nucleotides is directed at oncogenes which are equivalent to non-specific cytostatic therapy; to be effective in vascular restenosis they must be delivered using a balloon catheter to the angioplasty site. Possibly, other cytostatic agents would also be effective when given by the same route. This might include therefore some agents which failed to reduce restenosis when given systemically. Local intravascular radiotherapy has also been attempted taking the concept of local cytostasis to a 'logical' extreme.

Conclusions

Restenosis is a continuing problem. More than 100 randomized trials and 50 agents have been tested without success. The only consistently successful treatment is endovascular stenting, and even these improvements are modest. Population studies of restenosis suggest that there is probably an at-risk population. The nature of this risk has not been identified and the molecular basis of restenosis is proving similarly elusive.

References

Abbott, W. M., Megerman, J. M., Hasson, J. E., L'Italien, G. & Warnock D. (1987). Effect of compliance mismatch upon vascular graft patency. *Journal of Vascular Surgery*, **5**, 376–82.

Ardissino, D., Barberis, P., deServi, S., Merlini, P. A., Bramucci, E., Falcone, C. & Specchia, G. (1991). Abnormal coronary vasoconstriction as a predictor of restenosis after successful coronary angioplasty in patients with unstable angina pectoris. *New Engand Journal of Medicine*, **325**, 1053–7.

Barzu, T., Hebert, J. M., Desmouliere, A., Carayon, P. & Pascal, M. (1994). Characterisation of rat aortic smooth muscle cells resistant to the antiproliferative effect of heparin after long term heparin treatment. *Journal of Cellular Physiology*, **160**, 239–48.

Bassiouny, H. S., White, S., Glagov, S., Choi, E., Giddens, D. P. & Zarins, C. K. (1992). Anastomotic intimal hyperplasia: mechanical injury or flow induced. *Journal of Vasular Surgery*, **15**, 708–17.

Beatt, K. J., Serruys, P. W. & Hugenholtz, P. G. (1990). Restenosis after coronary angioplasty: new standards for clinical studies. *Journal of the American College of Cardiology*, **15**, 491–8.

Bell, L. & Madri, J. A. (1989). Effect of platelet factors on migration of cultured bovine endothelial and smooth muscle cells. *Circulation Research*, **65**, 1057–65.

Berger, P. B., Bell, M. R., Holmes, D. R., Hammes, L., Kosanke, J. L. & Bresee, S. J. (1992). Effect of restenosis after an earlier angioplasty at another coronary site on the frequency of restenosis after a subsequent coronary angioplasty. *American Journal of Cardiology*, **69**, 1086–9.

Birinyi, L. K., Warner, S. J. C., Salomon, R. N., Callow, A. D. & Libby, P. (1989). Observations on human SMCs from hyperplastic lesions of prosthetic bypass grafts: production of a PDGF-like mitogen and expression of a gene for PDGF receptor – a preliminary study. *Journal of Vascular Surgery*, **10**, 157–65.

Bond, M. G., Hostetler, J. R., Karayannacos, P. E., Geer, J. C. & Vasko, J. S. (1976). Intimal changes in arteriovenous bypass grafts. *Journal of Thoracic and Cardiovascular Surgery*, **71**, 907–16.

Bourassa, M. G., Lesperance, J., Eastwood, C., Schwartz, L., Cote, G., Kazim, F. & Hudon G. (1991). Clinical, physiologic, anatomic and procedural factors predictive of restenosis after PTCA. *Journal of the American College of Cardiology*, **18**, 368–76.

Bresee, S. J., Jacobs, A. K., Garber, G. R., Ruocco, N. A., Mills, R. M., Bergelson, B. A., Ryan, T. J. & Faxon, D. P. (1991). Prior restenosis predicts restenosis after coronary angioplasty of a new significant narrowing. *American Journal of Cardiollogy*, **68**, 1158–62.

Breyer, R. H., Spray, T. L., Kastl, D. G. & Roberts, W. C. (1976). Histologic changes in saphenous vein aortocoronary bypass grafts. *Journal of Thoracic and Cardiovascular Surgery*, **72**, 916–24.

Carrel, A. & Guthrie, C. C. (1986). Uniterminal and biterminal venous transplantation. *Surgical and Gynecological Obstetrics*, **2**, 266–86.

Castellot, J. J., Pukac, L. A., Caleb, B. J., Wright, T. C. & Karnovsky, M. J. (1989). Heparin selectively inhibits a protein kinase C dependent mechanism of cell cycle progression in claf aortic smooth muscle cells. *Journal of Cellular Biology*, **109**, 3147–55.

Chamley-Campbell, J. H., Campbell, G. R. & Ross, R. (1979). The smooth muscle cell in culture. *Physiology Reviews*, **59**, 1–61.

Chan, P. (1994). Cell biology of human vascular smooth muscle. *Annals of the Royal College of Surgery*, **76**, 298–303.

Chan, P., Patel, M., Betteridge, L., Munro, E., Schachter, M., Wolfe, J. & Sever, P. (1993). Abnormal growth regulation of vascular smooth muscle cells by heparin in patients with restenosis. *Lancet* **341**, 341–2.

Clowes, A. W., Reidy, M.A. & Clowes, M. M. (1983). Mechanisms of stenosis after arterial injury. *Laboratory Investigation*, **49**, 208–15.

DeJaegere, P., Serruys, P. W., Bertrand, M., Wiegand, V., Marquis, J. F., Vrolicx, M.,

Piessens, J., Valeix, B., Kober, G., Bonnier, H., Rutsch, W. & Uebis, R. (1993). Angiographic predictors of restenosis after Wiktor stent implantation in native coronary arteries. *American Journal of Cardiology*, **72**, 165–70.

DeWeese, J. A. & Rob, C. G. (1977). Autogenous vein grafts: ten years later. *Surgery*, **82**, 755–84.

Dilley, R. J., McGeachie, J. K. & Prendergast, F. J. (1988). A review of the histologic changes in vein-to-artery grafts, with particular reference to intimal hyperplasia. *Archives of Surgery*, **123**, 691–6.

Ellis, S. G., Roubin, G. S., Wilentz, J., Douglas, J. S. & King, S. B. (1989a). Effect of 18- to 24-hour heparin administration for prevention of restenosis after uncomplicated coronary angioplasty. *American Heart Journal*, **117**, 777–82.

Ellis, S. G., Roubin, G. S., King, S. B., Douglas, J. S. & Cox W. R. (1989b). Importance of stenosis morphology in the estimation of restenosis risk after elective PTCA. *American Journal of Cardiology*, **63**, 30–4.

Ellis, S. G., Shaw, R. E., Gershony, G., Thomas, R., Roubin, G. S., Douglas, J. S., Topol, E. J., Startzer, S. H., Myler, R. K. & King, S. B. (1989c). Risk factors, time course and treatment effect for restenosis after sucessful PTCA of chronic total occlusion. *American Journal of Cardiology*, **63**, 897–901.

Emmanuelsson, H., Beatt, K. J., Bagger, J. P., Balcon, R., Heikkila, J., Piessens, J., Schaffer, M., Suryapranta, H. & Foegh, M. (1995). Long-term effects of angiopeptin in coronary angioplasty. Reduction in clinical events but not angiographic restenosis. *Circulation* **91**, 1689–96.

Fabiani, J. N., Julia, P., Chemla, E., Birmbaum, P. L., Chardigny, C., D'Attelis, N. & Renaundin, J. M. (1994). Is the incidence of recurrent carotid stenosis influenced by the choice of surgical technique? Carotid endoterectomy versus saphenous vein bypass. *Journal of Vascular Surgery*, **20**, 821–5.

Faxon, D. P. & MARCATOR study group. (1995). Effect of high dose angiotensin converting enzyme inhibition on restenosis: final results of the MARCATOR study, a double blind, placebo controlled trial of clilazapril. *Journal of the American College of Cardiology*, **2**, 362–9.

Fillinger, M. F., Reinitz, E. R., Schwartz, R. A., Resetarits, D. E., Paskanik, A. M. & Bredenberg, C. E. (1989). Beneficial effect of banding on venous intimal-medial hyperplasia in arteriovenous loop grafts. *American Journal of Surgery*, **158**, 87–94.

Fillinger, M. F., Reinitz, E. R., Schwartz, R. A., Resetarits, D. E., Paskanik, A. M., Bruch, D. & Bredenberg, C. E. (1990). Graft geometry and venous intimal-medial hyperplasia in arteriovenous loop grafts. *Journal of Vascular Surgery*, **11**, 556–66.

Fischman, D. L., Leon, M. B., Baim, D. S., Schatz, R. A., Savage, M. P., Penn, I., Detre, K., Veltri, L., Ricci, D., Nobuyoshi, M. & Stent Restenosis Study Investigators. (1994). A randomised comparison of coronary stent placement and balloon angioplasty in the treatment of coronary artery disease. *New England Journal of Medicine*, **331**, 496–501.

Foley, D. P., Melkert, R. & Serruys, P. W. (1994). Influence of coronary vessel size on the renarrowing process and late angiographic outcome afer successful balloon angioplasty. *Circulation*, **90**, 1239–51.

Gertz, S. D., Gimple, L. W., Banai, S., Ragosta, M., Powers, E. R., Roberts, W. C., Perez, L. S. & Sarembock, I. J. (1994). Geometric remodelling is not the principal pathogenic process in restenosis after balloon angioplasty; evidence from correlative angiographic histomorphometric studies of atherosclerotic arteries in rabbits. *Circulation*, **90**, 3001–8.

Gibson, C. M., Kuntz, R. E., Nobuyoshi, M., Rosner, B. & Baim, D. S. (1993). Lesion to lesion independence of restenosis after treatment by conventional angioplasty, stenting or directional atherectomy. *Circulation*, **87**, 1123–9.

Glagov, S., Weisenberg, E., Zarins, C. K., Stankunavicius, R. & Kolettis, G. J. (1987). Compensatory enlargement of human atherosclerotic coronary arteries. *New England Journal of Medicine*, **316**, 1371–5.

Glagov, S. (1994). Intimal hyperplasia, vascular modeling and the restenosis problem. *Circulation*, **84**, 2888–91.

Glazier, J. J., Varricchione, T. R., Ryan, T. J., Ruocco, N. A., Jacobs, A. K. & Faxon, D. P. (1989). Factors predicting recurrent restenosis after PTCA. *American Journal of Cardiology*, **63**, 902–5.

Golden, M. A., Au, Y. P. T., Kenagy, R. D. & Clowes, A. W. (1990). Growth factor gene expression by intimal cells in healing PTFE grafts. *Journal of Vascular Survery*, **11**, 580–5.

Hermans, W., Rensing, B., Foley, D., Deckers, J., Rutsch, W., Emanuelsson, H., Danchin, N., Wijns, W., Chappuis, F. & Serruys, P. (1992a). Therapeutic dissection after successful coronary balloon angioplasty; no influence on restenosis or clinical outcome in 693 patients. *Journal of the American College of Cardiology*, **20**, 767–80.

Hermans, W., Rensing, B., Kelder, J. C., de Feyter, P. J. & Serruys, P. (1992b). Postangioplasty restenosis rate between segments of the major coronary arteries. *American Journal of Cardiology*, **69**, 194–200.

Hirschfeld, J. W., Schwartz, J. S., Jugo, R., Macdonald, R. G., Goldberg, S., Savage, M. P., Bass, T. A., Vetrovec, G., Cowley, M., Taussig, A. S., Whitworth, H. A., Margolis, J. R., Hill, J. A & Pepine, C. J. (1991). Restenosis after coronary angioplasty: a multivariate statistical model to relate lesion and procedure variables to restenosis. *Journal of the American College of Cardiology*, **18**, 647–56.

Hofstra, L., Bergmans, D., Leunissen, K., Hoeks, A., Kitslaar, P., Daemen, M. & Tordior, J. (1995a). *Anastomotic intimal hyperplasia in prosthetic arteriovenous fistulas for hemodialysis is associated wwith intial high shear rate and not with mismatch in elastic properties*. PhD Thesis, University of Limburg, Maastricht.

Hofstra, L., Hoeks, A., Tordior, J., Bergmans, D., Daemen, M. & Kitslaar, P. (1995b). *Mechanical factors predisposing to intimal hyperplasia in peripheral bypass grafts constructed with the use of autologous vein; a prospective analysis*. PhD Thesis, University of Limburg, Maastricht.

Holmes, D. R., Topol, E. J., Adelman, A. G., Cohen, E. A. & Califf, R. M. (1994). Randomised trials of directional coronary atherectomy: implications for clinical practice and future investigation. *Journal of the American College of Cardiology*, **24**, 431–9.

Holmes, D. R., Vlietstra, R. E., Smith, H. C., Vetrovec, G. W., Kent, K. M., Cowley, M. J., Faxon, D. P., Gruentzig, A. R., Kelsey, S. F., Detre, K. M., Vanraden, M. J. & Mock, M. B. (1984). Restenosis after percutaneous transluminal coronary angioplasty: a report from the PTCA registry of the National Heart Lung and Blood Institute. *American Journal of Cardiology*, **53**, 77C–81C.

Imparato, A. M., Bracco, A., Kim, G. E. & Zeff, R. (1972). Intimal and neointimal fibrous proliferation causing failure of arterial reconstructions. *Surgery*, **72**, 1007–17.

Isner, J. M. (1994). Vascular remodeling; honey, I think I shrunk the artery. *Circulation*, **89**, 2937–42.

Jain, S. P., Jain, A., Collins, T. J., Ramee, S. R. & White, C. J. (1994). Predictors of restenosis: a morphometric and quantitative evaluation by intravascular ultrasound. *American Heart Journal*, **128**, 664–73.

Kakuta, T., Currier, J. W., Haudenschild, C. C., Ryan, T. J., Faxon, D. P. (1994). Differences in compensatory vessel enlargement, not intimal formation, account for restenosis after angioplasty in the hypercholesterolemic rabbit model. *Circulation*, **89**, 2809–15.

Kohler, T. R., Kirkman, T. & Clowes, A. W. (1989). The effect of rigid external support on vein graft adaptation to the arterial circulation. *Journal of Vascular Surgery*, **9**, 277–85.

Kuntz, R. E., Hinohara, T., Safian, R. D., Selmon, M. R., Simpson, J. B. & Baim, D. S. (1992). Restenosis after directional coronary atherectomy; effect of luminal diameter and deep wall excision. *Circulation*, **86**, 1394–9.

Lafont, A., Guzman, L. A., Whitlow, P. L., Goormastic, M., Cornhill, J. F. & Chisholm, G. M. (1995). Restenosis after experimental angioplasty. Intimal medial and adventitial changes associated with constrictive remodelling. *Circulation Research*, **76**, 996–1002.

Lambert, M., Bonan, R., Cote, G., Crepeau, J., deGuise, P., Lesperance, J., David, P. R. & Waters D. D. (1988). Multiple coronary angioplasty: a model to discriminate systemic and procedural factors related to restenosis. *Journal of the American College of Cardiology*, **12**, 310–14.

Lambert, T. L., Dev, V., Rechavia, E., Forrester, J. S., Litvack, F. & Eigler, N. L. (1994). Localised arterial wall drug delivery from a polymer coated removable metallic stent. *Circulation*, **90**, 1003–11.

Lammer, J., Pilger, E., Ddecrinirs, M., Quehenberger, F., Klein, G. E. & Stark, G. (1993). Pulsed excimer laser versus continuous wave laser versus conventional angioplasty of peripheral arterial occlusions: prospective controlled randomised trial. *Lancet*, **340**, 1183–8.

LeFeuvre, C., Bonan, R., Lesperance, J., Gosselin, G., Joyal, M. & Crepeau, J. (1994). Predictive factors for restenosis after multivessel PTCA. *American Journal of Cardiology*, **73**, 840–4.

Lehmann, K. G., Melkert, R. & Serruys, P. W. (1996). Contributions of frequency distribution analysis to the understanding of coronary restenosis. *Circulation*, **93**, 1123–32.

Leimgruber, P. P., Roubin, G. S., Hollman, J., Cotsonis, G. A., Meier, B., Douglas, J. S., King, S. B. & Gruentzig, A. R. (1986). Restenosis after successful coronary angioplasty in patients with single vessel disease. *Circulation*, **73**, 710–17.

Limmani, A., Fleming, T., Molina, R., Hufnagel, H., Cunningham, R. E., Cruess, D. F. & Sharefkin, J. B. (1988). Expression of genes for PDGF in adult human venous endothelium. *Journal of Vascular Surgery*, **7**, 10–19.

Mintz, G. S., Popma, J. J., Pichard, A. D., Kent, K. M., Satler, L. F., Wong, C., Hong, M. K., Kovach, J. A. & Leon, M. B. (1996). Arterial remodelling after coronary angioplasty, a serial intravascular ultrasound study. *Circulation*, **94**, 35–43.

Munro, E., Chan, P., Patel, M., Betteridge, L., Gallagher, K., Schachter, M., Sever, P. & Wolfe, J. (1994). Consistent responses of the human vascular smooth muscle cell in culture: implications for restenosis. *Journal of Vascular Surgery*, **20**, 482–7.

Nikol, S., Isner, J. M., Pickering, J. G., Kearney, M., Leclerc, G. & Weir, L. (1992). Expression of transforming growth factor beta 1 is increased in human vascular restenotic lesions. *Journal of Clinical Investigation*, **90**, 1582–92.

Nobuyoshi, M., Kimura, T., Ohnishi, H., Horiuchi, H., Nosaka, H., Hamasaki, N., Yokoi, H. & Kim, K. (1991). Restenosis after PTCA; pathologic observations on 20 patients. *Journal of the American College of Cardiology*, **17**, 433–9.

Ohno, T., Gordon, D., San, H., Pompili, V. J., Imperiale, M. J., Nable, G. J. & Nabel, E. G. (1994). Gene therapy for vascular smooth muscle cell proliferation after arterial injury. *Science*. **265**, 781–4.

Ojha, M., Ethier, C. R., Johnston, K. W. & Cobbold, R. S. (1990). Steady and pulsatile flow fields in an end-to-side anastomosis model. *Journal of Vascular Surgery*, **12**, 747–53.

Post, M. J., Borst, C. & Kuntz, R. E. (1994). The relative importance of arterial remodelling compared with intimal hyperplasia in lumen renarrowing after balloon angioplasty. *Circulation*, **89**, 2816–21.

Quigley, M. R., Bailes, J. R., Kwaan, H. C., Cerullo, L. J. & Block, S. (1986). Comparison of myointimal hyperplasia in laser-assisted and sutured anastomosed arteries, a preliminary study. *Journal of Vascular Surgery*, **4**, 217–19.

Refson, J., Schachter, M., Patel, M., Hughese, A., Munro, E., Chan, P., Wolfe, J. & Sever, P. (1995). Correlation of heparin binding with responsiveness in human vascular smooth muscle. *Biochemical Society Transactions*, **23**, 172S.

Rensing, B. J., Hermans, W. R., Vos, J., Beatt, K. J., Bossuyt, P., Rutsch, W. & Serruys, P. W. (1992a). Angiographic risk factors of luminal narrowing after coronary balloon angioplasty using balloon measurements to reflect stretch and elastic recoil at the dilatation site. *American Journal of Cardiology*, **69**, 584–91.

Rensing, B. J., Hermans, W. R., Deckers, J. W., deFeyters, P. J., Tijseen, J. G. & Serruys, P. W. (1992b). Lumen narrowing after PTCA follows a near Gaussian distribution: a quantitative angiographic study in 1445 successfully dilated lesions. *Journal of the American College of Cardiology*, **19**, 939–45.

Rittgers, S. E., Karayiannicos, P. E., Guy, J. F. (1978). Velocity distribution and intimal proliferation in autogenous vein grafts in dogs. *Circulation Research*, **42**, 792–801.

Ross, R. (1993). The pathogenesis of atherosclerosis; a perspective for the 1990s. *Nature*, **362**, 801–9.

Ross, R. & Glomset, J. A. (1973). Atherosclerosis and the arterial smooth muscle cell. *Science*, **180**, 1332–9.

Sanantonio, J. D., Karnovsky, M. J., Ottlinger, M. E., Schillig, R. & Pukac, L. A. (1993). Isolation of heparin insensitive aortic smooth muscle cells. *Arteriosclerosis and Thrombosis*, **13**, 748–57.

Scott, N. A., Cipolla, G. A., Ross, C. E., Dunn, B., Martin, F. H., Simonet, L. & Wilcox, J. N. (1996). Identification of a potential role for the adventitia in vascular lesion formation after balloon overstretch of porcine coronary arteries. *Circulation*, **93**, 2178–87.

Serruys, P. W., deJaegers, P., Kiememeij, F., Macaya, C., Rutsch, W., Heyndrickx, G., Emanuelsson, H., Marco, J., Legrand, V. & Materne, P. (1994). A comparison of balloon-expandable stent implantation with balloon angioplasty in patients with coronary artery disease. *New England Journal of Medicine*, **331**, 489–95.

Sjolund, M., Hedin, U., Sejersen, T., Heldin, C. H. & Thyberg, J. (1988). Arterial smooth muscle cells express PDGF a chain mRNA, secrete a PDGF-like protein, and bind exogenous PDGF in a phenotype and growth state dependent manner. *Journal of Cell Biology*, **106**, 403–13.

Sottiurai, V. S., Yao, J. S. T., Flinn, W. R. & Batson, R. C. (1983). Intimal hyperplasia and neointima: an ultrastructural analysis of thrombosed grafts in humans. *Surgery*, **93**, 809–17.

Storm, F. K., Gierson, E. D., Sparks, F. C. & Barker, W. F. (1975). Autogenous vein bypass grafts: biological effects of mechanical dilatation and adventitial stripping in dogs. *Surgery*, **77**, 261–7.

Taylor, P. R., Wolfe, J. H., Tyrrell, M. R., Mansfield, A. O., Nicolaides, A. N. & Houston, R. E. (1990). Graft stenosis: justification for one year surveillance. *British Journal of Surgery*, **77**, 1125–8.

Tenaglia, A. N., Buller, C. E., Kisslo, K. B., Phillips, H. R., Stack, R. S. & Davidson, C. J. (1992). Intracoronary ultrasound predictors of adverse outcomes after coronary artery interventions. *Journal of the American College of Cardiology*, **20**, 1385–90.

Thompson, M. M., Budd, J. S., Eady, S. L., Underwood, M. J., James, R. F. & Bell, P. R. (1994). The effect of transluminal endothelial seeding on myointimal hyperplasia following angioplasty. *European Journal of Vascular Surgery*, **8**, 423–34.

Verin, V., Popowski, Y., Urban, P., Belenger, J., Redard, M., Costa, M., Widmer, M. C., Rouzaud, M., Nouet, P., Grob, E., Schwager, M., Kurtz, J. M. & Rutishauer, W. (1995). Intra-arterial beta irradiation prevents neointimal hyperplasia in a hypercholesterolemic rabbit restenosis model. *Circulation*, **92**, 2284–90.

Vroegindeweij, D., Tielbeek, A. V., Buth, J., Schol, F., Hop, W. & Landman, G. (1995).

Directional atherectomy versus balloon angioplasty in segmental femoropopliteal artery disease: two year follow-up with color-flow duplex scanning. *Journal of Vascular Surgery*, **21**, 255–69.

Waller, B. F., Pinkerton, C. A., Orr, C. M., Slack, J. D., VanTassel, J. W. & Peters, T. (1991). Morphological observations late after clinically successful coronary balloon angioplasty. *Circulation*, **83**, 128–41.

Weintraub, W. S., Kosinski, A. S., Brown, C. L. & King, S. B. (1993). Can restenosis after coronary angioplasty be predicted from clinical variables? *Journal of the American College of Cardiology*, **21**, 6–14.

Whittemore, A. D., Clowes, A. W., Couch, N. P. & Mannick, J. A. (1981). Secondary femoropopliteal reconstruction. *Annals of Surgery*, **193**, 35–42.

Wilcox, J. N., Smith, K. M., Williams, L. T., Schwartz, S. M. & Gordon, D. (1988). PDGF mRNA detection in human atherosclerotic plaques by in situ hybridisation. *Journal of Clinical Investigation*, **82**, 1134–43.

11

Abdominal aortic aneurysm

J. T. POWELL

Introduction

The aorta has to withstand the load imposed by arterial blood pressure for a lifetime. The microanatomy of the aorta reflects this burden and the media is thick, composed of numerous concentric lamellae of elastic connective tissue and smooth muscle cells. In youth and health elastin is the principal load bearing component of the aorta with collagen fibres only being recruited at the highest loads (Burton, 1954). Other microfibrils, including fibrillin rich fibrils, also contribute to load bearing. The abdominal aorta, distal to the renal arteries, is the aortic segment with least elastin and least nutrient vasa vasorum in the adventitia. With ageing this segment of the aorta is vulnerable to weakening and fusiform aneurysmal dilatation, abdominal aortic aneurysms being present in approximately 5% of men aged 65 years or older.

Definition of an abdominal aortic aneurysm

The normal diameter of the infrarenal aorta is 1.5–2.2 cm, with taller patients tending to have wider aortas. The infrarenal aorta is conveniently assessed by ultrasonography. A localized fusiform dilatation clearly is evidenced when the proximal and distal aortic diameters are much smaller than the maximum diameter. One suggested definition of an abdominal aortic aneurysm (AAA) is when the ratio of maximum diameter to infrarenal diameter exceeds 1.5 cm. However, the resolution and visualization of the suprarenal aorta by ultrasonography is poor (Ellis et al, 1991). A more convenient and widely accepted definition of an aneurysm is when the maximum anterior-posterior diameter exceeds 3 cm.

Clinical examination often fails to detect the smallest aneurysms (3–5 cm) but larger aneurysms are readily detected by clinical examination. The largest aneurysms may reach from 10 to 15 cm in diameter, but the larger the aneurysm the higher the risk of catastrophic rupture.

Disease burden and epidemiology

Studies in three continents have indicated that the incidence of AAA is increasing (Fowkes et al, 1989). AAA was one of the outcomes documented in the Framingham Study and has been associated strongly with smoking. Two other epidemiological studies have identified hypertension as a risk factor for AAA (Strachan, 1991; Reed et al, 1992). In Strachan's study diastolic blood pressure and the smoking of hand rolled cigarettes were associated with a greatly increased risk of death from ruptured AAA. It also is the authors prejudice that AAA is usually a smoking related disorder and the increasing incidence of AAA lags 30–40 years behind the rise of cigarette consumption (Henney et al, 1993). The recommended treatment option for all larger aneurysms (>5.5 cm) is elective aortic graft replacement surgery or endovascular repair. Aortic biopsy is readily available at the time of open surgery. Even though the number of elective aneurysm repairs performed each year grows rapidly, so too do the number of emergency operations for ruptured AAA. With the population of 65 + years expected to almost double by 2025 the burden of AAA on health resources is enormous.

Screening studies and clues to the aetiology of abdominal aortic aneurysm

Ultrasonographic screening studies of the general population >65 years of age have demonstrated the presence of AAA in approximately 5% of men. The prevalence of AAA in women is much lower. The screening of particular groups have indicated predisposing risk factors (Table 11.1) (Henney et al, 1993).

Screening hypertensive patients has provided a low yield of AAA but about 10% of patients with intermittent claudication have an AAA and approximately 25% of the brothers of patients with AAA also have an AAA detected on screening. Such studies indicate a strong familial tendency to AAA, although this maybe environmental rather than genetic. These studies also indicate a common risk factor for peripheral atherosclerosis and AAA: smoking, dyslipidaemia and hypertension are possible common risk factors. Interestingly AAA is rare amongst patients with type II diabetes.

Histopathology

The aneurysm wall as observed at surgery is lined with laminated thrombus, which must act to deny luminal nutrition to the aortic wall. Underneath this extensive intimal atherosclerosis is the rule (Figure 11.1). Beneath this the media is very thin and atrophic, there is fibrous replacement with few smooth muscle cells being observed. The medial connective tissue has become collagen rich and the elastic fibres are very disrupted, with the elastin content being very reduced. The adventitia has undergone compensatory thickening and neovascularization. In larger aneurysms an extensive inflammatory infiltrate (mainly B cells and macrophages) in the adventitia is an important finding (Koch et al, 1990). Although the media thins and the elastin content is very low, there is compensatory increase in both adventitial collagen and thickness.

Table 11.1. *Screening for abdominal aortic aneurysm*

	Prevalence of AAA (%)
Population (> 65 years general practice)	2–6
Patients with hypertension	1
Patients with peripheral arterial disease	10–12
Brothers of patients with AAA	20–30

AAA: abdominal aortic aneurysm.

Biomechanical properties of the abdominal aorta

With ageing the elastic resilience of the aorta is lost gradually and this accords with a declining elastin content and increasing content of polar glycoproteins in the media. In youth the dry weight elastin content of the aortic wall is approximately 35% compared with about 25% at the age of 70 years and only 8–10% or less in an AAA wall. The aneurysmal wall also is very inelastic and stiff and the stiffness or loss of elasticity appears to depend upon both the elastin content and genetic variation in the type III collagen and fibrillin genes (MacSweeney et al, 1992; Powell et al, 1993).

Cell biology and biochemical perspectives

It is very difficult to propagate in culture smooth muscle cells isolated from the adult abdominal aorta (Powell & Greenhalgh, 1989). In contrast, cell isolated from the adult thoracic aorta can be passaged readily. It is these cells that, as the aorta develops, synthesize the load-bearing connective tissue components of the aortic media: elastin, types I, III, V collagen, microfibril associated glycoproteins and fibrillin. Smooth muscle cells isolated from adult abdominal aortic media synthesize collagens type I and III but not elastin in culture.

The instillation of elastase into canine aorta in vivo or human vessels in vitro is sufficient to cause aneurysmal dilatation and has been used to provide an animal model of AAA (Dobrin et al, 1984; Anidjar et al, 1990). Such aneurysms do not rupture unless collagenase also is installed. These experiments have given rise to a widely held hypothesis for aneurysmal dilatation in the aorta:

elastinolysis → aortic dilatation
collagenolysis → aneurysm rupture

Not surprisingly many workers have identified increased elastase activity in both the blood and aortic wall of patients with AAA (Powell & Greenhalgh, 1989). Elastin is very resistant to both chemical and enzymic degradation and only a few enzymes are known to degrade elastin: these include leukocyte elastase (a serine protease) and

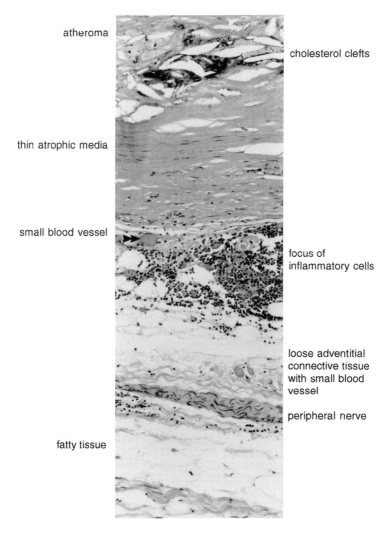

atheroma

cholesterol clefts

thin atrophic media

small blood vessel

focus of
inflammatory cells

loose adventitial
connective tissue
with small blood
vessel

peripheral nerve

fatty tissue

Fig. 11.1. Histopathology of the aneurysm.

matrix metalloproteinases (MMPs), including gelatinases A and B (MMP-2 and MMP-9, respectively), and a metalloelastase (MMP-12). All these enzymes degrade insoluble elastin. Elastinolytic activities reported on the basis of the hydrolysis of soluble substrates must be viewed with suspicion. Recently two of the enzymes with known elastinolytic activity have been described in AAA wall: gelatinase A (MMP-2) and gelatinase B (MMP-9). These enzymes are likely to contribute to the vascular

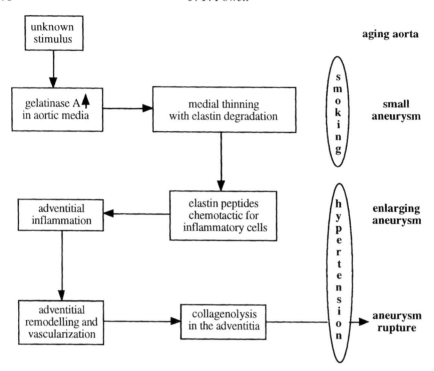

Fig. 11.2. Pathogenesis of the abdominal aortic aneurysm.

remodelling in the AAA wall. As elastin peptides are known to be chemotactic for inflammatory cells Scheme 1 below accords with our current knowledge about aneurysmal dilatation. Smaller aneurysms have most gelatinase A and least adventitial inflammation and gelatinase B has been localized in the adventitial macrophages of larger aneurysms.

Inflammation is an important feature of the aneurysm biopsy, with a variable infiltrate of chronic inflammatory cells (B cells and macrophages) in the adventitia and T cells commonly are found as a cuff around the neovasculature in the adventitia. There is no evidence that this inflammation is a response to specific antigens, although viral infection with cytomegalovirus has been suggested to have a pathogenic role in inflammatory aneurysms (Yonemitus et al, 1996). These inflammatory aneurysms are defined clinically by the dense periaortic fibrosis, which makes surgical resection more difficult. Such inflammatory aneurysms are not common and in the most common form the chronic inflammation may be a response to hypoxia or a result of a unique stromal environment which favours inflammatory cells residence and proliferation. Irrespective of its origin, this influx of inflammatory cells will play a prominent part in the connective tissue remodelling in the aortic wall.

The genetics of AAA

The strong familial predisposition to AAA raises the question of an inherited disorder manifest late in life. Two well-characterized genetic disorders have been associated with aortic fragility (Ehlers Danlos type IV syndrome) and aortic rupture (Marfan syndrome). These disorders are caused by mutations in the type III collagen gene (chromosome 2) and the fibrillin gene (chromosome 15), respectively. Both direct gene sequencing studies and population molecular genetics has failed to demonstrate that mutations or genetic variation in either the fibrillin or type III collagen genes are a common cause of AAA (Powell et al, 1993). Similarly, variation in the elastin gene is not a common cause of AAA, however, variation in both the fibrillin and type III collagen gene is associated with the biomechanical properties of the aneurysm wall (Figure 11.3).

Apart from the influence of gene variation on the biomechanical properties of the aorta there has been reported an association between genetic variation on chromosome 16 and AAA in both Scandinavian and British populations (Powell et al, 1990). The particular region on the long arm of chromosome 16 encodes for genes involved in lipid transport (CETP) and for gelatinase A. Gelatinase A is another candidate gene to explain the familial tendency to AAA, but no definitive studies have been reported. As metalloproteinases, both gelatinase A and B are inhibited by tissue inhibitors of metalloproteinases (TIMPs); however, genetic variation in TIMP 1 is not a common cause of AAA.

The genetics of AAA remains an unsolved problem and several centres are collecting and pooling families enriched in AAA for a more systematic approach to this problem.

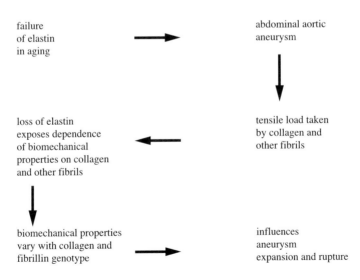

Fig. 11.3. Abdominal aortic aneurysm: a genetic disorder of the elderly?

The cause of abdominal aortic aneurysm

There are champions of two causes of AAA: atherosclerosis and inheritance. My personal viewpoint is that AAA is a multifactorial disorder with complex environmental–genetic interactions, stimulating an adventitial inflammatory response which is critical to the aortic remodelling. In those who develop AAA at a young age (< 60 years) the genetic contribution is stronger while the environmental contribution is greater for those developing AAA in the seventh and eighth decades (Henney et al, 1993). If we all lived to 120 years we might all develop AAA as the elastin in the abdominal aorta wears out and is not replaced. Many more references relating to the pathogenesis of AAA are included in a recent review (MacSweeney et al, 1994).

References

Anidjar, S., Salzmann, J. L., Gentric, D., Lagueau, P., Camilleri, J.-P. & Michel, J.-B. (1990). Elastase induced experimental aneurysms in rats. *Circulation,* 82, 973–81.

Burton, A. C. (1954). Relationship of structure to function of the tissues of the wall of blood vessels. *Physiology Reviews,* 34, 619–42.

Dobrin, P. B., Baker, W. H. & Gley, W. C. (1984). Elastolytic and collagenolytic studies of arteries: Implications for the mechanical properties of arteries. *Archives of Surgery* 119, 405–9.

Ellis, M., Powell, J. T., Greenhalgh, R. M. (1991). The limitations of ultrasound for the surveillance of abdominal aortic aneurysms. *British Journal of Surgery,* 78, 614–16.

Fowkes, F. G. R., MacIntyre, C. C. A. & Ruckley, C. V. (1989). Increasing incidence of aortic aneurysms in England and Wales. *British Medical Journal,* 298, 33–5.

Henney, A. M., Adiseshiah, M., MacSweeney, S. T. R., et al. (1993). Abdominal aortic aneurysm. *Lancet,* 341, 215–20.

Koch, A. E., Haines, G. K., Rizzo, R. J., Radosevich, J. A., Pope, R. M., Robinson, R. G. & Pearce, W. H. (1990). Human abdominal aortic aneurysms. Immunophenotypic analysis suggesting an immune-mediated response. *American Journal of Pathology,* 137, 1199–213.

MacSweeney, S. T. R., Powell, J. T. & Greenhalgh, R. M. (1994). The pathogenesis of abdominal aortic aneurysm: A review. *British Journal of Surgery,* 81, 935–41.

MacSweeney, S. T. R., Young, G., Greenhalgh, R. M. & Powell, J. T. (1992). The mechanical properties of the aneurysmal aorta. *British Journal of Surgery,* 79, 1281–4.

Powell, J. T., Adamson, J., MacSweeney, S. T. R. et al. (1993). The influence of type III collagen genotype on aortic diameter and disease. *British Journal of Surgery,* 80, 1246–8.

Powell, J. T., Bashir, A., Dawson, S., Vine, N., Humphries, S. E., Henney, A. & Greenhalgh, R. M. (1990). Variations on chromosome 16 are associated with abdominal aortic aneurysms. *Clinical Science,* 78, 13–16.

Powell, J. T. & Greenhalgh, R. M. (1989). Cellular, enzymatic and genetic factors in the pathogenesis of abdominal aortic aneurysm. *Journal of Vascular Surgery,* 9, 297–304.

Reed, D., Reed, C., Stemmerman, G. & Hayashi, T. (1992). Are aortic aneurysms caused by atherosclerosis? *Circulation,* 85, 205–11, comment p. 378.

Strachan, D. P. (1991). Predictors of death from aortic aneurysm among middle-aged men: the Whitehall Study. *British Journal of Surgery,* 78, 401–4.

Yonemitus, Y., Nakagawa, K., Tanaka, S., Mori, R., Sugimachi, K. & Sueshi, K. (1996). *In situ* detection of frequent and active infection of human cytomegalovirus in inflammatory abdominal aortic aneurysms: possible pathogenic role in sustained chronic inflammatory reaction. *Laboratory Investigation,* 74, 723–36.

12

Vascular complications of diabetes and the role of advanced glycosylation end products

H. VLASSARA, R. BUCALA and A. STITT

Introduction

With the introduction of insulin in the 1920s, the life expectancy of diabetics was markedly improved; however, this therapy heralded a previously unseen aspect of diabetes which took the form of severe and progressive complications, which even today are not wholly understood and remain largely unpreventable. It has now been established that persistent hyperglycaemia is the principal and underlying cause of diabetic complications (Diabetes Control & Complications Trial Research Group, 1993) and diabetics may suffer one or a number of debilitating complications which may be manifested in several organ systems in the form of retinopathy, nephropathy, neuropathy, hypertension, peripheral vasculopathy and as an increased risk of atherosclerosis. Although somewhat variable in distribution and frequency of vascular complications between insulin-dependent (IDDM) and non-insulin dependent (NIDDM) diabetics (Donahue & Orchard, 1992), both groups are generally equally prone to such vasculopathies, after correcting for disease duration. Diabetic vascular disease has been conveniently divided into two main groups, those involving the capillary beds as microvascular disease and those where the arteries and arterioles are affected (macrovascular disease). In the following review we adopt this distinction to provide a general overview of both classes of vasculopathy with an emphasis on the role of advanced glycation endproducts (AGEs) in the pathogenesis of the diverse complications which characterize this disease.

Etiological mechanisms of diabetic vasculopathy
Advanced glycation endproducts

The non-enzymatic glycation of proteins by aldehyde or keto-groups of reducing sugars, a process known as the Maillard reaction, eventually leads to the formation of advanced glycation endproducts (AGE) (Koenig & Cerami, 1975; Bucala et al, 1992). AGE moieties persist for the lifetime of the protein or lipid to which they are attached, can display distinctive fluorescence and have the ability to crosslink substates. Such irreversible glucose-derived crosslinks have been shown to accumulate with age and

Table 12.1. *Cellular components of the AGE-Receptor system, cell types and biological functions*

Cell types	Components	Functions
Monocyte/macrophages Peritoneal, circulating, U937, J774, HL-60	AGE-R$_1$ (OST-48) AGE-R$_2$ (80 k-H) AGE-R$_3$ (Gal-3 or GBP-35)	Binding, endocytosis, degradation ↑Cytokine production (TNF-α, IL-Iβ, IL-6, IFNγ) ↑Growth factor induction (PDGF, IGF-IA, TGF-β1, EGF, EGF-R)
T lymphocytes (CD4$^+$, CD8$^+$)	R AGE (amphoterin-receptor)	Chemotaxis Upregulation by TNF-α, AGE
Endothelial cells Macrovascular Microvascular		Downregulation by insulin ↑Permeability ↑Tissue factor
Mesangial cells		⇩Thrombomodulin
Renal tubular cells		↑Adhesion molecules (ICAM-1, VCAM-1)
Fibroblasts		↑Matrix proteins (fibronectin, collagen IV, laminin, HSPG)
Smooth muscle cells		↑Oxidant stress
Neuronal cells		↑NF$\kappa\beta$
Glia Astroglia Microglia		

in increased amounts in diabetes (Monnier & Cerami, 1981; Kohn et al, 1984). Significantly, AGEs have been implicated as causal factors in several aspects of vascular complications of diabetes (Makita et al, 1992a; Vlassara et al, 1994; Reiser, 1991) in many cases acting directly and in others through AGE receptor-mediated mechanisms, as substantively illustrated in several recent reviews on the biochemistry and the biological effects of AGEs (Bucala et al, 1992; Vlassara et al, 1994b).

Early in AGE research it was speculated that a receptor-based system occurred whereby AGE products could be removed from tissues and sera, in vivo, thereby limiting their potentially toxic and harmful effects, and that imbalances caused to such a system could underlie cellular and tissue dysfunction in pathological situations such as diabetes. Work in this laboratory demonstrated that both in vivo formed or in vitro synthesized AGE proteins are recognized by a macrophage AGE-receptor system which is distinct from previously described scavenger receptors (Vlassara et al, 1986a; Vlassara et al, 1986b). Two AGE-binding proteins, approximately 60 kDa (p60) and 90 kDa (p90), isolated from rat liver membranes were initially identified (Yang et al, 1991; Radoff et al, 1990). The first, now referred to as AGE-R1 was shown to be homologous to an approximately 50 kDa protein component of the oligosaccharyltransferase complex (OST-48), (Patel & Kligman, 1987) while the 80–90 kDa, termed AGE-R2, is homologous to the protein kinase substrate 80K-H (Patel & Kligman, 1987; Sakai et al, 1989; Li et al, 1996). Both these proteins are expressed on the surface of many human cells, including endothelial cells, monocytes/macrophages, T lymphocytes, neural tissue, renal cells and smooth muscle cells (Li et al, 1996) (Table 12.1). While AGE-R1 likely serves as both cell surface and intracellular AGE-binding and transporting protein, AGE-R2 in its capacity as a substrate for protein kinase C, may have a role in intracellular signalling leading to activation, cytokine and growth factor secretion associated with AGE-receptor binding (Vlassara et al, 1988; Kirstein et al 1992). Another well-known 32 kDa protein originally described as Galectin-3, Mac-2 or carbohydrate binding protein-35 (CBP-35), also exhibits high-affinity binding for AGE-ligands (Kd $3.5 \times 10^7 M^{-1}$) (Vlassara et al, 1995a) and is expressed on the surface of macrophages, lymphocytes, endothelial, renal and neuronal cells. AGE binding to Galectin-3 (henceforth designated AGE-R3) occurs within the 18 kDa C-terminal peptide, and appears capable of promoting high molecular weight complex formation with AGE ligands and with other membrane-associated receptor molecules on the cell surface. This complex formation is likely to involve the attack on a thiol ester of Galectin-3 by nucleophilic groups present on AGE proteins. The significance of the participation of high energy thiol ester bonds, although still under investigation, may reflect the need for efficient attachment and subsequent trafficking to intracellular degradative pathways of an abundant, heterogeneous class of AGE-modified structures. Furthermore, the AGE-R2 and AGE-R3 components are easily upregulated by AGE proteins, a response which likely accounts for increased ligand binding and endocytosis (Kirstein et al, 1992) as well as for specific gene overexpression (Vlassara et al, 1988; Kirstein et al, 1992).

Two additional cell surface binding proteins for AGE determinants have been identified and cloned from various tissues and cells, a 35 kDa member of the immunoglobulin superfamily of receptors, named RAGE (Schmidt et al, 1992; Neeper et al, 1992) also shown to serve as a receptor for amphoterin (Schmidt et al, 1992) and an 80 kDa protein, homologous to lactoferrin (Hori et al, 1995; Yan et al, 1994). RAGE has been functionally linked to AGE-mediated increased intracellular oxidant stress and NFκB activation (Yan et al, 1994).

Based on protein sequence, ligand specificity and functional differences between the AGE-binding polypeptides described above, it is speculated that there may exist a number of AGE-binding proteins, with or without 'receptor' characteristics, which may contribute to AGE removal, transport and/or processing as well as diverse cellular functions. Variability in the expression of any of these molecules may underlie genetic differences in the susceptibility to specific tissue sequelae among diabetic patients and thereby account for the observation that some diabetics develop a few complications, despite a long history of poor glucose control, while others suffer severe debilitating complications despite relatively good control.

The polyol pathway

Over the past 15 years, the polyol pathway has received extensive attention as an alternative route for glucose metabolism. In this pathway glucose is first reduced to sorbitol by aldose reductase and then oxidized to fructose by sorbitol dehydrogenase. In the presence of hyperglycaemia, sorbitol accumulation – and coordinate myo-inositol depletion (Schmidt et al, 1991a,b; Tesfamariam et al, 1993); are thought to play a major role in cellular dysfunction and organ damage (Orosz et al, 1981). Aldose reductase inhibition has been shown to prevent diabetes-induced increases in vascular permeability, and regional blood flow in tissues from diabetic rats (Williamson et al 1986, 1987; Tilton et al, 1989; Pugliese et al, 1990a,b). There have also been studies that did not reveal any beneficial effects of aldose reductase inhibitors (Engerman & Kern, 1993). These disappointing effects, mostly referring to diabetic humans and chronic studies in animals, may be partly explained by the fact that they were intervention trials: treatment was initiated years after tissue injury was induced (Pederson et al, 1991). Aldose reductase activity is much higher in rodents than in humans and the relevance of this mechanism in humans is still under debate.

Pseudohypoxia

Increased flux through the polyol pathway is also thought to have an effect on vascular function, particularly when it triggers an increased reduced to oxidized nicotinamide-adenine dinucleotide ($NADH/NAD^+$) ratio. At the onset of diabetes, increased blood flow and vasodilation occur as the vascular system's natural defence reaction to hyperglycaemia and tissue hypoxia. These vascular changes have been linked to impaired oxidation of NADH to NAD^+ and increased ratio of $NADH/NAD^+$, particularly in hyperglycaemic tissues, where an increased rate of reduction of NAD^+ to NADH can occur (Cheng & Gonzalez, 1986). Importantly, glucose to sorbitol rates of conversion increase with higher glucose levels in tissues not requiring insulin for glucose uptake. As glucose levels are elevated, sorbitol levels increase and trigger a higher rate of oxidation of sorbitol to fructose while causing a reduction in NAD^+ to NADH ratio. Glucose metabolism via the sorbitol pathway can account for one-third of glucose consumption by the lens and for as much as 10% by human erythrocytes (Williamson et al, 1967; Langunas et al, 1970; Travis et al, 1971; Cheng & Gonzalez, 1986).

Arrhythmia, increased blood flow and vascular permeation are all predicted outcomes when redox imbalance occurs. This change is mirrored in diabetic tissue as well and can include dysfunction, particularly in the retinal and nerve areas, muscle impairment, and further debilitating contractile functions of the heart and skeletal muscle. Although initial increases in blood flow occur when tissues experience mild or brief hypoxia or ischemia, the blood flow drops significantly after prolonged exposure. Again, the reaction is mirrored in the diabetic tissues: initial increased blood flow, followed by a steady decrease over time.

Renin–angiotensin system (RAS)

Renin–angiotensin inhibitors are considered effective in the prevention or delay of diabetic nephropathy. Renin activates conversion of angiotensinogen to angiotensin I. The presence of the angiotensin converting enzyme (ACE) causes its conversion to the vasoactive peptide angiotensin II (Dzau, 1988; Campbell, 1987). It has been amply demonstrated that angiotensin II effects mitogenic and hypertrophic smooth muscle cells in vivo and in vitro, the vascular extracellular matrix, as well as promoting vascular proliferation (Schelling et al, 1991). Drugs with the ability to inhibit ACE have been found effective in aiding the prevention or delay of diabetic nephropathy. Benefits of the presence of an inhibitor of this type can include reduction in urinary albumin excretion (Taguma et al, 1985) and decreased blood pressure (Passa et al, 1987). Treatment of IDDM normotensive patients with ACE inhibitors indicate that nephropathy can be delayed (Marre et al, 1988; Mathiesen et al, 1991).

Microangiopathy
Nephropathy

Diabetic nephropathy (DN), a conglomerate of lesions which occur concurrently in the kidney in up to 35–45% of diabetic patients with IDDM and NIDDM (Krolewski et al, 1988) represents the leading cause of End-Stage Renal Disease (ESRD) in the United States (URDS, 1992). This disease is characterized by increased glomerular basement membrane (BM) thickening (Osterby et al, 1983) and mesangial extracellular matrix (ECM) deposition, followed by mesangial hypertrophy, diffuse and nodular glomerulosclerosis (Osterby et al, 1983) and subsequent impairment of filtration capacity, culminating in complete renal failure (Mogensen, 1976).

Structural changes to the glomerulus during chronic diabetes are accompanied by multiple biochemical abnormalities, many of which have also been demonstrated in isolated glomerular endothelial and mesangial cells cultured in high glucose concentrations in vitro. Some of the reversible changes have been attributed to the polyol pathway and the associated alterations in the redox state of pyridine nucleotides (Tilton et al, 1989; Pugliese et al, 1990b) the de novo synthesis of diacylglycerol, which can lead to the activation of several isoforms of protein kinase C (Lee et al, 1989; Craven & DeRubertis, 1989), decreased cellular uptake of myoinositol leading to reduced Na^+/K^+-ATPase activity (Simmons & Winegrad, 1989) and intracellular protein glycation (Sensi et al, 1993; Garner et al, 1990). These mechanisms may cause transient alterations in blood flow, vascular permeability and intracellular imbalances of critical metabolites and cofactors but such effects are generally reversible upon normalization of glucose levels. Other changes, such as those due to advanced glycation, are more permanent and not readily reversed upon return to normoglycaemia (Bucala et al, 1992; Monnier & Cerami, 1981; Kohn et al, 1984; Vlassara et al, 1994; Reiser, 1991).

In vitro, glomerular mesangial cells bind AGEs through a specific AGE receptor complex (Skolnik et al, 1991) and respond to short-term exposure to AGEs by a receptor-mediated upregulation of mRNA and protein secretion of matrix proteins, such as $\alpha 1$ type IV collagen, laminin A, B1 and B2 (Doi et al, 1992). Significantly, the collagen $\alpha 1$ IV mRNA increase initiated by the AGE-receptor appeared to be mediated at least in vitro by PDGF (Doi et al, 1992).

Based on these and additional in vitro data, a unified basis was formulated regarding the role of different types of cells in tissue dysfunction, as might occur in diabetes and ageing. It was thus assumed that under conditions of cumulative AGE deposition, as occurs in diabetes, disturbances of cellular AGE receptor properties could potentially lead to widespread tissue dysfunction.

A subsequent study was undertaken to determine the direct contribution of cellular AGE-dependent responses to the intact glomerular structure in vivo, by examining selected molecular events involved in mesangial cell responsiveness, such as the induction of ECM or growth factor genes (Yang et al, 1994). The study focused on microdissected glomeruli following the injection of AGE-mouse serum albumin (MSA) for 3–4 weeks. A predominant increase in $\alpha 1IV$ collagen and laminin B1 mRNA was observed only in those mice receiving AGE-modified MSA (Yang et al, 1994). Of note, the mRNA of another growth-promoting molecule, TGF-$\beta 1$ was found significantly increased in the AGE-treated mice. Prolonged treatment of non-diabetic rats with AGEs resulted in glomerular hypertrophy, basement membrane thickening and mesangial ECM expansion, consistent with frank glomerulosclerosis, which was associated with significant proteinuria and albuminuria (Vlassara et al, 1994b). We have observed AGE immunoreactivity in kidney tissues from normal and, especially from diabetic rats, suggesting that glomerular BM and mesangium accumulate AGEs in diabetes. Of note, glomerular podocytes, Bowman's capsule parietal cells and renal tubules contained AGE deposits in their lysosomal compartment. These studies were consistent with reports showing gold-conjugated AGE-BSA binding to glomerular tissues of rats (Gugliucci & Bendayan, 1995a) and that AGE peptides are reabsorbed and catabolized by the renal proximal tubular cells (Gugliucci & Bendayan, 1995b).

Based on the available data, it has been speculated that peripheral tissues utilize this AGE receptor system as a principal degradation mechanism for AGE-modified tissues and cells, releasing small soluble AGE peptides, which, combined with extracellular proteolysis of matrix components, give rise to a class of circulating low molecular weight AGE-modified substances. Levels of these substances would likely depend on the underlying tissue levels and the activity of receptor and receptor-independent removal systems. These degradation products of AGE-modified proteins are presumably released into the circulation to be cleared by the kidneys, as in serum, the levels of AGE peptides correlate with renal function (Makita, 1991; Makita et al, 1994). Although diabetic individuals with normal renal clearance can also clear AGE peptides at the same rate, progressive loss of kidney function leads to a rise in circulating AGE levels, up to eight fold in diabetic patients with ESRD (Makita, 1991; Makita et al, 1994). This pronounced increase in AGE degradation products observed in the circulation of diabetic uraemic patients has raised the possibility that such uncleared AGEs may include reactive intermediates that can attach onto target tissues, e.g. kidney and vessel walls, as well as plasma components and accelerate ongoing vascular pathology (Fig. 12.1).

In vivo evidence of this 'reactivity' of serum AGE peptides was sought by measuring AGE levels on plasma proteins, such as Apo B LDL, a highly atherogenic macromolecule from patients with renal failure with or without diabetes. Marked elevations in AGE-Apo B were found in plasma samples from diabetic, as well as non-diabetic patients with renal failure, compared with normals, and diabetics with normal renal function (Bucala et al, 1994).

These studies point to an important side-effect of the normal turnover of AGE-

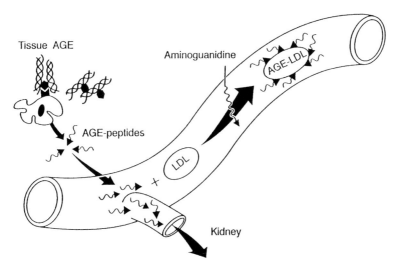

Fig. 12.1. Schematic representation of AGE turnover, generation of reactive degradation products (AGE-peptides, glycotoxins), and their reactive potential.

modified proteins and lipids, whether due to AGE receptor, or receptor independent mechanisms, the catabolic products of AGE macromolecules include highly reactive substances which, if not eliminated by the kidney, can irreversibly alter key structures in vascular tissues, perpetuating vascular dysfunction.

Retinopathy

Of the known vascular complications of diabetes, diabetic retinopathy (DR) is one of the most common and widespread. In diabetics with IDDM of 10 years duration, the prevalence of DR is about 80% and this increases to virtually 100% by 20 years duration (Klein et al, 1984a,b). DR is less frequent in NIDDM but this is accounted for by the later onset of this form of the disease. Nonetheless, DR remains among the leading causes of blindness in the USA (Kahn & Moorhead, 1973). DR is principally a disease of the intraretinal blood vessels and can be classified as two distinct types: non-proliferative and proliferative. Non-proliferative DR is by far the most common form and is manifested by a progressive increase in capillary permeability (Sander et al, 1994), BM thickening (Stitt et al, 1994), pericyte cell death (De Venicia et al, 1967), saccular microaneurysms, (Stitt et al, 1995b) endothelial cell death (Kohner & Henking, 1970) and thereby widespread non-perfusion (Garner, 1993). It is interesting that many of these pathological lesions occur secondary to subtle physiological and functional changes in the retinal vessels, such as increased blood flow (Kohner, 1993) or increased endocytic activity in the capillary endothelial cell (Gardiner et al, 1995; Stitt et al, 1995a). The retinal lesions characteristic of DR are often quite unique to the retinal vessels. The greatest risk for visual loss emerges with the proliferative phase of DR, with the development of widespread macular edema and retinal neovascularization, the former being a direct consequence of blood–retinal barrier breakdown, while the latter is due to widespread retinal ischaemia (Frank, 1995).

The pathogenesis of DR is complex and likely to be multifactorial in nature, but the DCCT trial points to the pivotal importance of prolonged hyperglycaemia (Diabetes Control and Complications Trial Research group, 1993). Significantly, Kern & Engerman have demonstrated that optimal glycemic control following an initial 2.5 year period of suboptimal control is not protective against DR progression (Engerman & Kern, 1987) and this strongly suggests that prolonged hyperglycaemia produces a chronic, largely irreversible functional abnormality in the retina of diabetics which is not easily reversed.

As a direct consequence of the hyperglycaemia experienced in diabetes, altered activity of the polyol pathway has been introduced as one explanation of this complication (Frank et al, 1983; Robison et al, 1983; Engerman & Kern, 1984). It is notable that because of its very high Km for glucose, sorbitol only accumulates under prolonged periods of hyperglycaemia and it can account for up to 30% of glucose metabolism under such conditions (Cheng & Gonzalez, 1986). Aldose reductase and sorbitol have been found at relatively high levels in the retinal vasculature (Kennedy et al, 1983) and both enzyme and its product have received considerable attention as contributory factors to diabetic retinopathy (Robison et al, 1995). This has remained controversial, however, while various aldose reductase intervention treatments have failed to prevent retinopathy, despite a modest benefit to diabetic peripheral nerve dysfunction (Engerman & Kern, 1993; Engerman et al, 1994). Another notable hypothesis on the pathogenesis of DR has focused on the increased microvascular pressure and blood flow in the retinal capillary bed early in diabetes, which results in endothelial injury, cell dysfunction and subsequent formation of microvascular lesions (Tooke, 1995).

Despite the strong links between AGEs and diabetic complications, e.g. with nephropathy, surprisingly few studies have investigated the role of AGEs in DR, especially in view of the fact that advanced glycation is a universal phenomenon, with AGE products widespread on vessel walls (Brownlee et al, 1988) or carried in the bloodstream at elevated levels in diabetics (Makita, 1991; Makita et al, 1994). The intrinsic fluorescent properties of AGEs have enabled the demonstration of AGE-crosslinking in the retinal vessels of diabetic rats, while the AGE inhibitor aminoguanidine was shown to prevent retinopathy in diabetic rats (Hammes et al, 1991). Interestingly, aminoguanidine does not prevent lesion formation in the initial phase of experimental diabetic retinopathy in rats (Hammes et al, 1995a); however, a secondary intervention study with this agent indicated that it could potentially retard disease progression (Hammes et al, 1995b). Recently, we have demonstrated a markedly increased AGE immunoreactivity in the retinal vessels of diabetic rats, a phenomenon which increased as a function of diabetes-duration (Stitt et al, 1996a). In the diabetic rats, AGEs appeared to accumulate intracellularly in the retinal pericytes after 8 months of experimental diabetes, a disease duration associated with pericyte toxicity and loss (Stitt et al, 1996b). In the same study, accumulation of AGEs within the pericytes was observed in normal rats infused with extrinsic AGEs in a distribution pattern which closely matched that of the AGE-receptors (R1 and R2) (Stitt et al, 1996b). An unequivocal link between AGEs and DR pathogenesis remains to be determined, however, the accumulation of these products within the pericytes during long-term diabetes and after AGE infusion provides an additional link between these products and the dysfunction that is characteristic of this complication.

Neuropathy

Diabetic neuropathy is a very diverse, multi focal disease which may affect the peripheral or the central nervous system of up to 40% of diabetics (Zeigler et al, 1993) and is characterized at its end-stage by axonal atrophy with segmental demyelination. Often occurring in diabetics as a subtle peripheral neuropathy, these patients experience a diminished sensation which may result in the development of ulcers that are slow to heal. Diabetic neuropathy can occur at the somatic, autonomic and central levels. Although chronic hyperglycaemia is almost certainly involved, the underlying cause of this complication remains controversial (Tesfaye et al, 1994). Although the accumulation of sorbitol (Tomlinson et al, 1994; Simmons et al, 1993), the depletion of myo-inositol (Simmons et al, 1993; Kamijo et al, 1994) and even the development of a humoral neurotoxic response have been proposed as likely causal factors, abnormalities in the peripheral nerve microvasculature have now been recognized as a major, underlying pathogenic mechanism (Dyck et al, 1985). In the microvascular supply of the peripheral neurons, the extent of capillary dysfunction and closure is widespread, leading to a so-called hypoxic or ischaemic neuropathy in which axonal transport is compromised (Vinik et al, 1992). Recently, the role of perivascular and vascular inflammation in diabetic neuropathy has been reported in diabetic patients, who responded favourably to anti-inflammatory and/or anti-immune therapy (Krendel et al, 1995). Significant correlations have been observed between the severity of neuropathy and chronic hyperglycaemia in diabetic patients and it suggests that the pathogenesis of this complication (Ryan et al, 1992) is related to that of diabetic nephropathy and retinopathy, via the common denominator of hyperglycemia.

Macroangiopathy

Atherosclerosis

Large vessel disease is significantly increased in diabetes and is accompanied by a greatly increased risk of cardiovascular mortality (Pyorala, 1990). Furthermore, diabetics are more likely to develop serious cerebrovascular disease, suffering more than twice the risk of stroke (Lithner et al, 1988). Atherosclerosis is marked not only by the complex nature of its pathogenesis but also by its involvement in many atherosclerosis-related pathologies, most notably myocardial and cerebral infarction. Atherosclerotic plaque formation is the pathophysiological hallmark of this disease process; the complex interactions between blood-borne proteins, growth factors and many distinct cell types culminate in the formation of the fatty streak and the dense plaque (Ross, 1993). Atheromatous lesions in diabetics are indistinguishable from those in non-diabetics (Ruderman & Haudenshild, 1984).

Accumulation of low density lipoprotein (LDL) species in the vessel wall leading to the formation of so-called 'fatty streaks' is of paramount importance in the initiation of atherosclerotic lesions. It has been widely speculated that oxidative modification of LDL (oxLDL) in vivo results in its reduced recognition by the LDL receptor, elevated serum LDL levels and increased uptake of the modified protein by scavenger receptors of macrophages and vascular smooth muscle cells. Glucose-derived AGEs are now recognized as important participants in the formation and acceleration of atherosclerotic lesions (Nakamura et al, 1993; Kume et al, 1995; Palinski et al, 1995; Stitt et al, 1996b). Studies in our own laboratory suggest that advanced glycation of both the lipid and ApoB components of the LDL molecule (lipid-AGE/ApoB-AGE) may represent a physiologically significant modification of lipoproteins (Bucala et al, 1993, 1994, 1995) which occurs concomitantly with oxLDL in vitro. In addition, chemical modification of ApoB has been shown to interfere with its recognition by the LDL receptor (Mahley et al, 1987, 1979) and lead to abnormally high levels of circulating LDL (Goldstein et al, 1979; Fogelman et al, 1980). ApoB is a relatively large protein with many potential lysine and arginine AGE modification sites, but the predominant site of AGE modification of

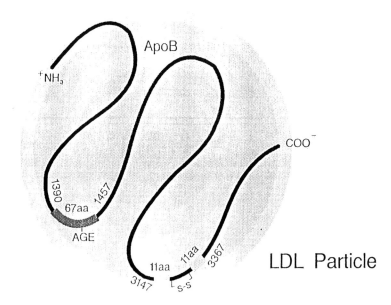

Fig. 12.2. AGE-modified domain of ApoB lies 1690 amino acids N-terminal to the LDL-receptor binding domain(s).

ApoB has now been confirmed to be at the amino acid sequence distal to the NH_2 group (Bucala et al, 1995) (Fig. 12.2). Using an in vivo model, it was demonstrated that presence of AGE-ApoB on circulating LDL, when injected into transgenic mice express-ing the human LDL receptor delays AGE-LDL clearance compared with native LDL (Bucala et al, 1994).

A significant correlation has recently been demonstrated between serum AGE-ApoB and tissue AGE levels in biopsies of carotid arteries from non-diabetic patients undergo-ing endarterectomy (Stitt et al, 1996). The macrovascular endothelium expresses recep-tors for AGEs (Li et al, 1996) and it is likely that high circulating levels of AGE-LDL can be transported via the endothelium directly onto the vessel wall. This has been sup-ported by a correlation between serum AGE-ApoB and vessel wall AGE levels in atheromatous lesions (Stitt et al, 1996a).

Significantly, AGE-R1 and AGE-R2 are coexpressed in several cellular components of human atherosclerotic plaque, where they colocalize with intracellular AGEs. Con-sistent with this, endocytic uptake of AGEs has been described in the endothelium, smooth muscle cells and macrophage/monocytes in vitro, and their expression in vivo supports an inherent capacity of these cells for binding and endocytosing AGEs. The latter suggests that the process may be active in normal life, being enhanced during atheromatous plaque formation and expected to accelerate even further under diabetic or hyperlipidemic conditions.

Blood rheology/hypertension

Alterations in the blood rheology and haemodynamics have substantially influence on the micro- and macrovascular complications of diabetes. Significantly altered blood rheology and blood haemodynamics have been described during diabetes (Megnien et al, 1992; Liu & Fung, 1992). For example, in diabetic patients, platelets demonstrate enhanced adhesiveness and aggregative capacity while the endothelium expresses increased levels of procoagulant substances such as von Willebrand factor (vWF) (Colwell et al, 1989; Porta et al, 1981). Hypertension is also widespread in diabetics, who are at least twice as likely to develop this complication (Barnett, 1994) that adds greatly to their risk for renal disease (Hoelscherr et al, 1995). A very strong correlation between hypertension and the onset of NIDDM has been shown, with more uncertain links between these and insulin resistance (Berger & Sawicki, 1994). As with other vascular complications of diabetes the pathogenesis of procoagulant changes and hypertension remains somewhat unclear; however, the use of non-steroidal anti-inflammatory drugs and calcium antagonists (Tse & Kendal, 1994) and ACE inhibitors (Hsueh & Anderson, 1992) has added not only to therapeutic intervention, but to an increased understanding of the complex underlying mechanisms of these complications.

A putative link between advanced glycation processes and blood rheological abnormalities and hypertension has been hypothesized. AGE adducts occur in diabetic and atherosclerotic vessels (Kakamura et al, 1993; Kume et al, 1995; Stitt et al, 1996b) and they can cause tissue ridgidity and a decrease in the susceptibility of proteins to enzymatic digestion. Moreover, AGEs can act as a trapping site for immunogobulins and LDL species (Brownlee et al, 1983) within the walls of arteries and arterioles. Such covalent protein crosslinking in the vessel wall has far-reaching implications, as it has been shown that AGE formation on the glomerular matrix components collagen and laminin leads to alteration of matrix heparin sulphate proteoglycan content and charge (Tsilibary et al, 1988; Charonis & Tsilibary, 1992). A disruption of the normally negative charge at the BM is thought to explain the increased permeability in the microvasculature.

With significance to atherosclerosis and diabetic hypertension, AGE adducts residing in the vessel wall are known to interfere with the vasodilatory action of endothelium-derived nitric oxide (NO), reacting directly to inactivate its bioactivity (Bucala et al, 1991). These important AGE-modulatory effects on NO have been further confirmed by the markedly abnormal vaso-relaxation responses following exogenous administration of AGE-modified proteins to healthy animals, a phenomenon which was inhibited by aminoguanidine (Vlassara et al, 1992). In addition, it has been shown that the normally antiproliferative effects of NO on smooth muscle cells are inhibited in vitro (Hogan et al, 1992).

Endothelial dysfunction leading to changes in blood rheology, procoagulant activity and inflammation may be modulated by exposure of endothelial cells to high glucose in vitro (Stern et al, 1991). Indeed the involvement of chronic hyperglycaemia may be largely reflected in the interaction of AGEs with the endothelium. A markedly enhanced pro-atherogenic potential was noted recently in AGE-infused rabbits, characterized by a significant increase in the expression of vascular cell adhesion molecule-1 (VCAM-1) and intercellular adhesion molecule-1 (ICAM-1) on the aortic endothelial surface (Vlassara et al, 1995b). These AGE-induced changes were significantly accelerated in animals placed briefly on a cholesterol-rich diet, manifested by multifocal atheroma formation within less than 2 weeks (Vlassara et al, 1995b). Also in cultured endothelial cells, AGEs can cause down regulation of the surface anticoagulant thrombomodulin, increased permeability (Esposito et al, 1989) and promote transendothelial migration of human monocytes (Kirstein et al, 1990). Taken together, it is apparent that AGEs can induce significant changes to the macrovascular endothelium in ways that predispose the vessel wall for the development of atherosclerotic lesions, hypertension and prothrombotic events.

Potential intervention therapies

One of the best characterized early steps of glycation is the Amadori product, forming from glucose reacting with free amino groups of proteins. As reviewed earlier, through a cascade of further reactions and rearrangement, this product is converted to the more reactive glycation intermediate and advanced and products (AGE). Thus, Amadori formation is, in a way, the basis of advanced glycosylation chemistry because progression to protein crosslinks requires slow rearrangement reactions to create 'reactive' intermediates that can react with amino groups before irreversible formation of AGEs. An important pharmacological strategy for inhibition of this process utilizes the nucleophilic compound aminoguanidine, which was shown to be a potent and specific inhibitor of glucose-mediated crosslinking and tissue damage in vivo (Brownlee et al, 1986) (Fig. 12.3). The terminal amino group of aminoguanidine, by virtue of its low pKa, reacts specifically with glucose-derived reactive intermediates and prevents protein-protein or protein-lipid crosslinks from forming. This mechanism of action of aminoguanidine has now been confirmed in numerous studies, in which it is shown to prevent diabetes-related vascular complications in experimental animals (Nichols & Mandel, 1989; Ellis & Good, 1991; Cho et al, 1991; Soulis-Liparota et al, 1991; Edelstein & Brownlee, 1992). From these and numerous other studies, it is apparent that aminoguanidine can be used to prevent advanced glycation and the AGE-mediated tissue in animal models of diabetes and ageing.

In humans, a phase I study of aminoguanidine measured advanced glycation-modified haemoglobin (AGE-Hb) in treated and untreated diabetic subjects and found that

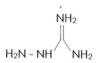

Fig. 12.3. The chemical structure of the first effective advanced glycation inhibitor identified, aminoguanidine.

AGE-Hb was significantly reduced in the treated group (Makita et al, 1992b). HbA_{1c} values were not affected by aminoguanidine treatment, pointing to the specificity of aminoguanidine for inhibition of post-Amadori, advanced glycosylation reactions. Of direct relevance to atherosclerosis, aminoguanidine therapy caused a 28% decrease in LDL-cholesterol, a 19% decrease in total cholesterol and a 19% decrease in triglycerides (Makita et al, 1992a). Aminoguanidine and related advanced glycosylation inhibitors may eventually find widespread use in diabetics or in individuals at risk of age-related vascular sequelae. Development of aminoguanidine is now at phase II/III efficacy trials.

It has been suggested that individuals with high levels of AGE-LDL in serum may actually be indicative of enhanced AGE deposition in vessel walls and may therefore be at increased risk of atheroma formation (Stitt et al, 1996). High levels of circulating AGEs in certain non-diabetic patients may even point to a dysfunction in their AGE receptor-mediated clearance mechanisms as receptor expression between individuals is likely to be highly variable. Therefore it may prove eventually prudent to test for serum AGEs at an early age, using the highly sensitive, AGE-specific immunochemical techniques (Makita et al, 1992b; Mitsuhashi, 1996) in unison with standard blood lipoprotein tests. Such an approach may provide useful warning for patients, especially those at risk to vascular complications and enable early therapeutic interventions.

Conclusions

Diabetic vascular complications consist of distinctive and progressive functional/structural alterations. It may be somewhat unrealistic to seek for a single determinant as the sole underlying cause of this large and diverse group of vasculopathies, as each tissue is distinct in its cell population and their unique requirements for homeostasis; however, the sequence of events leading to diabetic micro-and macroangiopathy may be linked by pathogenic factors such as hyperglycaemia and AGE accumulation, acting as common denominators. Furthermore, the gene expression and regulation of AGE receptors on various types of vascular cells, such as endothelium, mesangium, smooth muscle and pericytes, could also play a pivotal role in the development and progression of diabetic vascular complications.

References

Barnett, A. H. (1994). Diabetes and hypertension. *British Medical Bulletin*, **50**, 397–407.

Bensoussan, D., Levy-Toledano, S., Passa, P., Caen, J. & Canivet, J. (1975). Platelet hyperaggregation and increased plasma level of von Willebrand factor in diabetics with retinopathy. *Diabetologia*, **11**, 307–12.

Berger, M. & Sawicki, P. T. (1994). The clinical significance of insulin resistance in the treatment of hypertension. *European Journal of Histolology*, **15**(Suppl. C), 74–7.

Brownlee, M., Pongor, S. & Cerami, A. (1983). Covalent attachment of soluble proteins by non-enzymatic glycosylated collagen; role in the in situ formation of immune complexes. *Journal of Experimental Medicine*, **158**, 1739–44.

Brownlee, M., Vlassara, H. & Cerami, A. (1988). Advanced glycosylation end products in tissue and the biochemical basis of diabetic complications. *New England Journal of Medicine*, **318**, 1315–21.

Brownlee, M., Vlassara, H., Kooney, A., Ulrich, P. & Cerami, A. (1986). Aminoguanidine prevents diabetes-induced arterial wall protein crosslinking. *Science*, **232**, 1629–32.

Bucala, R., Makita, Z., Koschinsky, T., Cerami, A. & Vlassara, H. (1993). Lipid advanced glycosylation: pathway for lipid oxidation in vivo. *Proceedings of the National Academy of Sciences of the USA*, **90**, 6434–8.

Bucala, R., Makita, Z., Vega, G., Grundy, S., Koschinsky, T., Cerami, A. & Vlassara, H. (1994). Modification of LDL by advanced glycosylation endproducts contributes to the dyslipidemia of diabetes and renal insufficiency. *Proceedings of the National Academy of Sciences of the USA*, **91**, 9441–5.

Bucala, R., Mitchell, R., Arnold, K., Innerarity, T., Vlassara, H. & Cerami, A. (1995). Identification of the major site of apolipoprotein B modification by advanced glycation endproducts blocking uptake by the low density lipoprotein receptor *Journal of Biological Chemistry* **270**, 10828–32.

Bucala, R., Tracey, K. J. & Cerami, A. (1991). Advanced glycosylation products quench nitric oxide and mediate defective endotheium-dependent vasodilatation in experimental diabetes. *Journal of Clinical Investigation*, **87**, 432–8.

Bucala, R., Vlassara, H. & Cerami, A. (1992). Advanced glycosylation endproducts. In *Post Translational Modifications of Proteins*, vol. 2, ed. J. J. Harding & M. J. C. Crabbe, pp. 53–59. Boca Raton, Florida: CRS Press.

Campbell, D. J. (1987). Circulating and tissue angiotensin systems. *Journal of Clinical Investigation*, **79**, 1–6.

Charonis, A. S. & Tsilibary, E. C. (1992). Structural and functional changes of laminin and type IV collagen after nonenzymatic glycation. *Diabetes*, **41**(Suppl. 2), 49–51.

Cheng, H.-M. & Gonzalez, R. G. (1986). The effect of high glucose and oxidative stress on lens metabolism, aldose reductase and senile cataractogenesis. *Metabolism*, **35**(Suppl. 1), 10–14.

Cho, H. K., Kozu, H., Peyman, G. A., Parry, G. J. & Khoobehi, B. (1991). The effect of aminoguanidine on the blood-retinal barrier in streptozotocin-induced diabetic rats. *Ophthalmic Surgery*, **22**, 44–7.

Colwell, J. A., Wincour, P. D. & Lopes-Virella, M. F. (1989). Platelet function and platelet-plasma interactions in atherosclerosis and diabetes mellitus. In *Diabetes Mellitus: Theory and Practice*, ed. H. Rifkin & D. Porte, pp. 249–56. New York: Elsevier.

Craven, P. A. & DeRubertis, F. R. (1989). Protein kinase C is activated in glomeruli from streptozotocin diabetic rats. Possible mediation by glucose. *Journal of Clinical Investigation*, **83**, 1667–75.

De Venicia, G., Davis, M. D. & Engerman, R. L. (1967). Clinicopathologic correlations in diabetic retinopathy. I. Histology and fluorescein angiography of microaneurysms. *Archives of Ophthalmology*, **94**, 1766–73.

Diabetes Control and Complications Trial Research Group. (1993). The effect of intensive treatment of diabetes on the development and progression of long-term complications in insulin-dependent diabetes mellitus. *New England Journal of Medicine*, **329**, 977–86.

Doi, T., Vlassara, H., Kirstein, M., Yamada, Y., Striker, G. E. & Striker, L. J. (1992). Receptor-specific increase in extracellular matrix production in mouse mesangial cells by advanced glycosylation end products is mediated via platelet-derived growth factor. *Proceedings of the National Academy of Sciences of the USA*, **89**, 2873–7.

Donahue, R. P. & Orchard, T. J. (1992). Diabetes mellitus and microvascular complications. An epidemiological perspective. *Diabetes Care*, **15**, 1141–55.

Dyck, P. J., Hansen, S., Karnes, J., O'Brien, P., Yasuda, H., Windebank, A. & Zimmerman, B. (1985). Capillary number and percentage closed in human diabetic sural nerve. *Proceedings of the National Academy of Sciences of the USA*, **82**, 2513–17.

Dzau, V. J. (1988). Circulating versus local renin-angiotensin system in cardiovascular homeostasis. *Circulation* (Suppl. 1), **77**, 4–13.

Edelstein, D. & Brownlee, M. (1992). Mechanistic studies of advanced glycosylation endproduct inhibition by aminoguanidine. *Diabetes*, **41**, 26–8.

Ellis, E. N. & Good, B. H. (1991). Prevention of glomerular basement membrane thickening by aminoguanidine in experimental diabetes mellitus. *Metabolism*, **40**, 1016–19.

Engerman, R. L. & Kern, T. S. (1984). Experimental galactosemia produces diabetic-like retinopathy. *Diabetes*, **33**, 97–100.

Engerman, R. L. & Kern, T. S. (1987). Progression of incipient diabetic retinopathy during good glycemic control. *Diabetes*, **36**, 808–12.

Engerman, R. L. & Kern, T. S. (1993). Aldose reductase inhibition fails to prevent retinopathy in diabetic and galactosemic dogs. *Diabetes*, **42**, 820–5.

Engerman, R. L., Kern, T. S. & Larson, M. E. (1994). Nerve conduction and aldose reductase inhibition during 5 years of diabetes or galactosaemia in dogs. *Diabetologia*, **37**, 141–4.

Esposito, C., Gerlach, H., Brett, J., Stern, D. & Vlassara, H. (1989). Endothelial receptor-mediated binding of glucose-modified albumin is associated with increased monolayer permeability and modulation of cell surface coagulant properties. *Journal of Experimental Medicine*, **170**, 1387–407.

Fogelman, A. M., Haberland, M. E., Seager, J., Hokom, M. & Edwards, P. A. (1980). Factors regulating the activities of the low density lipoprotein receptor and the scavenger receptor on human monocytes-macrophages. *Journal of Lipid Research* **22**, 1131–41.

Frank, R. N. (1995). Diabetic retinopathy. In *Progress in Retinal and Eye Research*, **14**, pp. 361–92. Amsterdam: Elsevier Science.

Frank, R. N., Keirn, R. J., Kennedy, A. & Frank, K. W. (1983). Galactose-induced retinal capillary basement membrane thickening: prevention by sorbinil. *Investigations in Ophthalmology and Vision Science*, **24**, 1519–24.

Gardiner, T. A., Stitt, A. W. & Archer, D. B. (1995). Retinal vascular endothelial cell endocytosis increases in early diabetes. *Laboratory Investigation*, **72**, 439–44.

Garner, A. (1993). Histopathology of diabetic retinopathy in man. *Eye*, **7**, 250–3.

Garner, M. H., Bahador, A. & Sachs, G. (1990). Nonenzymatic glycation of Na, K-ATPase. Effects of ATP hydrolysis and K^+ occlusion. *Journal of Biological Chemistry*, **265**, 15058–66.

Goldstein, J. L., Ho, Y. K., Basu, S. K. & Brown, M. S. (1979). Binding site on macrophages that mediates uptake and degradation of acetylated low density lipoproteins producing massive cholesterol deposition. *Proceedings of the National Academy of Sciences of the USA*, **76**, 333–7.

Gugliucci, A. & Bendayan, M. (1995a). Reaction of advanced glycation endproducts with renal tissue from normal and streptozotocin-induced diabetic rats. An ultrastructural study using colloidal gold cytochemistry. *Journal of Histochemistry and Cytochemistry* **43**, 591–600.

Gugliucci, A. & Bendayan, M (1995b). Renal fate of circulating advanced glycation end products (AGE): evidence for reabsorption and catabolism of AGE-peptides by renal proximal tubular cells. *Diabetologia*, **39**, 149–60.

Hammes, H. P., Martin, S., Federlin, K., Geisen, K. & Brownlee, M. (1991). Aminoguanidine treatment inhibits the development of experimental diabetic retinopathy. *Proceedings of the National Academy of Sciences of the USA*, **88**, 11555–8.

Hammes, H. P., Ali, S. S., Uhlmann, M., Weiss, A., Federlin, K., Geisen, K. & Brownlee, M. (1995a). Aminoguanidine does not inhibit the initial phase of experimental diabetic retinopathy in rats. *Diabetologia*, **38**, 269–73.

Hammes, H. P., Strodter, D., Weiss, A., Bretzel, R. G., Federlin, K. & Brownlee, M. (1995b). Secondary intervention with aminoguanidine retards the progression of diabetic retinopathy in the rat model. *Diabetologia*, **38**, 656–60.

Hoelscherr, D. D., Weir, M. R. & Bakris, G. L. (1995). Hypertension in diabetic patients: an update of interventional studies to preserve renal function. *Journal of Clinical Pharmacology*, **35**, 73–80.

Hogan, M., Cerami, A. & Bucala, R. (1992). Advanced glycosylation endproducts block the antiproliferative effect of nitric oxide. *Journal of Clinical Investigation*, **90**, 1110–15.

Hori, O., Brett, J., Slattery, T., Cao, R., Zhang, J., Chen, J. X., Nagashima, M., Lundh, E. R., Vijay, S., Nitecki, D. & Stern, D. (1995). The receptor for advanced glycation endproducts (RAGE) is a cellular binding site for amphoterin. Mediation of neurite outgrowth and co-expression of RAGE and amphoterin in the developing nervous system. *Journal of Biological Chemistry* **270**, 25752–61.

Hsueh, W. A. & Anderson, P. W. (1992). Hypertension, the endothelial cell, and the vascular complications of diabetes mellitus. *Hypertension*, **20**, 253–63.

Kahn, H. A. & Moorhead, H. B. (1973). *Statistics on blindness in the model reporting area, 1969–1970*, U.S. Department of Health, Education, and Welfare Publication No. (NIH) 73–427, U.S. Government Printing Office, Washington.

Kamijo, M., Basso, M., Cherian, P. V., Hohman, T. C. & Sima, A. A. (1994). Galactosemia produces ARI-preventable nodal changes similar to those of diabetic neuropathy. *Diabetes Research in Clinical Practice*, **25**, 117–29.

Kennedy, A., Frank, R. N. & Varma, S. D. (1983). Aldose reductase in retinal and cerbral microvessels and cultured vascular cells. *Investigations in Ophthalmology and Vision Science*, **24**, 1250–4.

Kirstein, M., Aston, C., Hintz, R. & Vlassara, H. (1992). Receptor -specific induction of insulin-like growth factor I in human monocytes by advanced glycosylation endproduct-modified proteins. *Journal of Clinical Investigation*, **90**, 439–46.

Kirstein, M., Brett, J., Radoff, S., Ogawa, S., Stern, D. & Vlassara, H. (1990). Advanced glycosylation endproducts induces transendothelial human monocyte chemotaxis and secretion of platelet-derived growth factor: role in vascular disease of diabetes and aging. *Proceedings of the National Academy of Sciences of the USA*, **87**, 9010–14.

Klein, R., Klein, B. E. K., Moss, S. E., Davis, M. D. & DeMets, D. L. (1984a). The Wisconsin Epidemiological study of Diabetic Retinopathy. II. Prevalence and risk of diabetic retinopathy when age at diagnosis is less than 30 years. *Archives of Ophthalmology*, **102**, 520–6.

Klein, R., Klein, B. E. K., Moss, S. E., Davis, M. D. & DeMets, D. L. (1984b). The Wisconsin Epidemiological study of Diabetic Retinopathy. III. Prevalence and risk of diabetic retinopathy when age at diagnosis is 30 or more years. *Archives of Ophthalmology*, **102**, 527–32.

Koenig, R. J. & Cerami, A. (1975). Synthesis of hemoglobin A1C in normal and diabetic mice: potential model of basement membrane thickening. *Proceedings of the National Academy of Sciences of the USA*, **72**, 3867–91.

Kohn, R. R., Cerami, A. & Monnier, A. (1984). Collagen aging in vitro by nonenzymatic glycosylation and browning. *Diabetes*, **33**, 57–9.

Kohner, E. M. (1993). The retinal blood flow in diabetes. *Diabetes Metabolism*, **19**, 401–4.

Kohner, E. M. & Henkind, P. (1970). Correlation of fluorescein angiogram and retinal digest in diabetic retinopathy. *American Journal of Ophthalmology*, **69**, 403–14.

Krendel, D. A., Costigan, D. A. & Hopkins, L. A. (1995). Successful treatment of neuropathies in patients with diabetes mellitus. *Archives of Neurology*, **52**, 1053–61.

Krolewski, A. S., Canessa, M., Warram, J. H., Laffel, L. M., Christlieb, A. R., Knowler, W. C.

& Rand, L. I. (1988). Predisposition to hypertension and susceptibility to renal disease in insulin-dependent diabetes mellitus. *New England Journal of Medicine*, **318**, 140–5.

Kume, S., Takeya, M., Mori, T., Araki, N., Suzuki, H., Horiuchi, S., Kodama, T., Miyauchi, Y. & Takahashi, K. (1995). Immunohistochemical and ultrastructural detection of advanced glycation endproducts in atherosclerotic lesions of human aorta with a novel specific monoclonal antibody. *American Journal of Pathology*, **147**, 654–67.

Langunas, R., McLean, P. & Greenbaum, A. L. (1970). The effect of raising the NAD + content on the pathways of carbohydrate metabolism and lipogenesis in rat liver. *European Journal of Biochemistry*, **15**, 179–90.

Lee, T. S., MacGregor, L. C., Fluharty, S. J. & King, G. L. (1989). Differential regulation of protein kinase C and (Na,K)-adenosine triphosphatase activities by elevated glucose levels in retinal capillary endothelial cells. *Journal of Clinical Investigation*, **83**, 90–4.

Li, Y. M., Wojciehowicz, D., Mitsuhashi, T., Gilmore, R., Shimizu, N., Li, J., Stitt, A. W., He, C. & Vlassara, H. (1996). Molecular identity and tissue distribution of advanced glycation endproduct receptors. Relationship of p60 to OST-48 and 80KH membrane proteins. *Proceedings of the National Academy of Sciences of the USA* (in press).

Lithner, F., Asplund, K., Eriksson, S., Hagg, E., Strand, T. & Wester, P. O. (1988). Clinical characteristics in diabetic stroke patients. *Diabetes Metabolism*, **14**, 15–19.

Liu, S. Q. & Fung, Y. C. (1992). Changes in the rheological properties of blood vessel tissue remodelling in the course of development of diabetes. *Biorheology*, **29**, 443–57.

Mahley, R. W., Innerarity, T. L., Pitas, R. E., Weisgraber, K. H., Brown, J. H. & Gross, E. (1987). Inhibition of lipoprotein binding to surface receptors of fibroblasts following selective modification of arginyl residues in apoprotein B. *Journal of Biology and Chemistry*, **252**, 7279–87.

Mahley, R. W., Innerarity, T. L., Weisgraber, K. N. & Oh, S. Y. (1979). Altered metabolism (in vivo and in vitro) of plasma lipoproteins after selective chemical modification of lysine residues of the apoprotein B. *Journal of Clinical Investigation*, **64**, 743–50.

Makita, Z. (1991). Clinical assessment and significance of advanced glycosylation in patients with diabetic nephropathy. *New England Journal of Medicine*, **325**, 836–42.

Makita, Z., Makita, Z., Bucala, R., Rayfield, E. J., Friedman, E. A., Kaufman, A. M., Kobet, S. M., Barth, R. H., Winston, J. A., Fuh, H., Monogue, K. R., Cerami, A. & Vlassara, H. (1994). Reactive glycosylation endproducts in diabetic uraemia and treatment of renal failure. *Lancet*, **343** (8912), 19–22.

Makita, Z., Vlassara, H., Cerami, A. & Bucala, R. (1992a). Immunological detection of advanced glycosylation end products in vivo. *Journal of Biological Chemistry*, **267**, 5133–8.

Makita, Z., Vlassara, H., Rayfield, E., Cartwright, K., Friedman, E., Rodby, R., Cerami, A. & Bucala, R. (1992b). Hemoglobin-AGE: a circulating marker of advanced glycosylation. *Science*, **258**, 651–3.

Marre, M., Chatellier, G. & Leblanc, H. (1988). Prevention of diabetic nephropathy with enalapril in normotensive diabetics with microalbuminuria. *British Medical Journal* **297**, 1092–5.

Mathiesen, E., Hommel, E., Giese, J. & Parving, H. (1991). Efficacy of captopril in postponing nephropathy in normotensive insulin dependent diabetic patients with microalbuminuria. *British Medical Journal*, **303**, 81–7.

Megnien, J. L., Simon, A., Valensi, P., Flaud, P., Merli, I. & Levenson, J. (1992). Comparative effects of diabetes mellitus and hypertension on physical properties of human large vessels. *Journal of American College of Cardiology*, **20**, 1562–8.

Mitsuhashi, T., Vlassara, H., Founds, H. & Li, Y. M. (1997). Standardizing the immunological measurement of advanced glycation endproducts using normal human serum *Journal of Immunological Methods*, **207**, 79–88.

Mogensen, C. E. (1976). Renal function changes in diabetes. *Diabetes*, **25** (Suppl. 2), 872–9.

Monnier, V. M. & Cerami, A. (1981). Non-enzymatic browning in vivo: possible process for aging of long-lived proteins. *Science* **211**, 491–4.

Nakamura, Y., Horii, Y., Nishino, T., Shiiki, H., Sakaguchi, Y., Kagoshima, T., Dohi, K., Makita, Z., Vlassara, H. & Bucala, R. (1993). Immunohistochemical localization of advanced glycosylation endproducts (AGEs) in coronary atheroma and cardiac tissue in diabetes. *American Journal of Pathology*, **143**, 1649–56.

Neeper, M., Schmidt, A. M., Brett, J., Yan, S. D., Wang, F., Pan, Y. C., Elliston, K., Stern, D. & Shaw, A. (1992). Cloning and expression of a cell surface receptor for advanced glycosylation endproducts of proteins. *Journal of Biological Chemistry*, **267**, 14998–5004.

Nichols, K. & Mandel, T. E. (1989). Advanced glycosylation endproducts in experimental murine diabetic nephropathy: Effect of iselt isografting and of aminoguanidine. *Journal of Laboratory Investigation*, **60**, 486–91.

Orosz, S. E., Townsend, S. F., Tornheim, P. A., Brownscheidle, C. M. (1981). Localization of aldose reductase and sorbitol dehydrogenase in the nervous system of normal and diabetic rats. *Acta Diabetol Lat*, **18**, 373–81.

Osterby, R. (1975). Early phases in the development of diabetic glomerulopathy. *Acta Medica Scandinavica* (Supp. 1)**574**, 13–77.

Osterby, R., Anderson, M. J. F., Gundersen, H. J. G., Jorgensen, H. E., Mogensen, C. E. & Parving, H. H. (1983). Quantitative study on glomerular ultrastructure in type I diabetes with incipient nephropathy. *Diabetic Nephropathy*, **3**, 95–100.

Palinski, W., Koschinsky, T., Butler, S. W., Miller, E., Vlassara, H., Cerami, A. & Witztum, J. L. (1995). Immunological evidence for the presence of advanced glycosylation endproducts products in atherosclerotic lesions of euglycemic rabbits. *Arteriosclerosis Thrombosis & Vascular Biology*, **15**, 571–82.

Passa, P., Leblanc, H. & Marre, M. (1987). Effects of enalapril in insulin-deptendent diabetic subjects with mild to moderate hypertension. *Diabetes Care*, **10**, 200–4.

Patel, J. & Kligman, D. (1987). Purification and characterization of an Mr87,000 protein kinase C substrate from rat brain. *Journal of Biological Chemistry*, **262**, 16686–91.

Pedersen, M. M., Christiansen, J. S. & Mogensen, C. E. (1991). Reduction of glomerular hyperfiltration in normoalbuminuric IDDM patients by 6 months of aldose reductase inhibition. *Diabetes*, **40**, 527–31.

Porta, M., Townsend, C., Clover, G. M., Nanson, M., Alderson, A. R., McCraw, A. & Kohner, E. M. (1981). Evidence for functional endothelial cell damage in early diabetic retinopathy. *Diabetologia*, **20**, 597–601.

Pugliese, G., Tilton, R. G., Speedy, A., Santarelli, E., Eades, D., Province, M. A., Kilo, K., Sherman, W. R. & Williamson, J. R. (1990a). Modulation of hemodynamic and vascular filtration changes in diabetic rats by dietary myo-inositol. *Diabetes*, **39**, 312–22.

Pugliese, G., Tilton, R. G., Speedy, A., Chang, K., Province, M. A., Kilo, C. & Williamson, J. R. (1990b). Vascular filtration function in galactose-fed versus diabetic rats: the role of polyol pathway activity. *Metabolism*, **39**, 690–7.

Pyorala, K. (1990). Diabetes and coronary artery disease: what a coincidence? *Journal of Cardiovascular Pharmacology*, **16**, S8–S14.

Radoff, S., Cerami, A. & Vlassara, H. (1990). Isolation of surface binding protein specific for advanced glycosylation endproducts from mouse murine macrophage-derived cell line RAW 264.7. *Diabetes*, **39**, 1510–18.

Reiser, K. M. (1991). Nonenzymatic glycation of collagen in aging and diabetes. *Proceedings of the Society of Experimental Biological Medicine*, **196**, 17–29.

Robison, W. G. Jr, Kador, P. F. & Kinoshita, J. H. (1983). Retinal capillaries: basement membrane thickening by galactosemia prevented with aldose reductase inhibitor. *Science*, **221**, 1177–9.

Ross, R. (1993). The pathogenesis of atherosclerosis: a perspective for the 1990s. *Nature*, **362**, 801–9.

Robison, W. G. Jr, Laver, N. M. & Lou, M. F. (1995). The role of aldose reductase in diabetic retinopathy: prevention and intervention studies. In *Progress in Retinal and Eye Research*, 14, 593–640. Amsterdam: Elsevier Science.

Ruderman, N. B. & Haudenshild, C. (1984). Diabetes as an atherogenic factor. *Progress in Cardiovascular Disease*, **26**, 373–412.

Ryan, C. M., Williams, T. M., Orchard, T. J. & Finegold, D. N. (1992). Psychomotor slowing is associated with distal symmetrical polyneuropathy in adults with diabetes mellitus. *Diabetes*, **41**, 107–13.

Sakai, K., Hirai, M., Minoshima, S., Kudoh, J., Fukuyama, R. & Shimizu, N. (1989). Isolation of cDNAs encoding a substrate for protein kniase C: nucleotide sequence and chromosomal mapping of the gene for a human 80K protein. *Genomics*, **5**, 309–15.

Sander, B., Larsen, M., Engler, C., Lund-Anderson, H. & Parving, H. H. (1994). Early changes in diabetic retinopathy: capillary loss and blood-retina barrier permeability in relation to metabolic control. *Acta Ophthalmology*, **72**, 553–9.

Schelling, P., Fischer, H. & Ganten, D. (1991). Angiotensin and cell growth: a link to carediovascular hypertrophy. *Journal of Hypertension*, **9**, 3–15.

Schmidt, R. E., Plurad, S. B., Sherman, W. R., Williamson, J. R. & Tilton, R. G. (1991a). Effects of aldose reductase inhibitor sorbinil on neuroaxonal dystrophy and levels of myo-inositol and sorbitol in sympathetic autonomic ganglia of streptozocin-induced diabetic rats. *Diabetes*, **38**, 569–79.

Schmidt, R. E., Plurad, S. B., Coleman, B. D., Williamson, J. R. & Tilton, R. G. (1991b). Effects of sorbinil, dietary myo-inositol supplementation, and insulin on resolution of neuroaxonal dystrophy in mesenteric nerves of streptozocin-induced diabetic rats. *Diabetes*, **40**, 574–82.

Schmidt, A. M., Vianna, M., Gerlach, M., Brett, J., Ryan, J. & Kao, J. (1992). Isolation and characterization of two binding proteins for advanced glycosylation end products from bovine lung which are present on the endothelial cell surface. *Journal of Biological Chemistry*, **256**, 14987–97.

Sensi, M., De Rossi, M. G., Celi, F. S. et al. (1993). D-lysine reduces the non-enzymatic glycation of proteins in experimental diabetes mellitus in rats. *Diabetologia*, **36**, 797–801.

Simmons, D. A. & Winegrad, A. I. (1989). Mechanism of glucose-induced (Na^+, K^+) -ATPase inhibition in aortic wall of rabbits. *Diabetologia*, **32**, 402–8.

Simmons, D., Ng, L. L. & Bomford, J. (1993). Relationship between myoinositol influx and lipids in diabetic neuropathy. *Acta Diabetologie*, **30**, 233–7.

Skolnik, E. Y., Yang, Z., Makita, Z., Radoff, S., Kirstein, M. & Vlassara, H. (1991). Human and rat mesangial cell receptors for glucose-modified proteins: potential role in knidney tissue remodelling and diabetic nephropathy. *Journal of Experimental Medicine*, **174**, 931–9.

Soulis-Liparota, T., Cooper, M., Papazoglou, D., Clarke, B. & Jerums, G. (1991). Retardation by aminoguanidine of development of albuminuria, mesangial expansion, and tissue fluorescence in streptozotocin-induced rat. *Diabetes*, **40**, 1328–34.

Stern, D., Esposito, C., Gerlach, H., Gerlach, M., Ryan, J., Handley, D. & Nawroth, P. (1991). Endothelium and regulation of coagulation. *Diabetes Care*, **14**, 160–6.

Stitt, A. W., Anderson, H. R., Gardiner, T. A. & Archer, D. B. (1994). Diabetic retinopathy: quantitative variation in capillary basement membrane thickening in arterial and venous environments. *British Journal of Ophthalmology*, **78**, 133–7.

Stitt, A. W., Friedman, S., Scher, L., Rossi, P., Ong, H., Founds, H., Bucala, R. & Vlassara, H. (1996a). Carotid artery advanced glycation endproducts and their receptors correlate with severity of lesion and with plasma AGE-ApoB levels in non-diabetic patients. *FASEB Journal*, **10**, A616.

Stitt, A. W., Chakravarthy, U., Archer, D.B. & Gardiner, T. A. (1995a). Increased endocytosis in retinal vascular endothelial cells grown in high glucose medium is modulated by inhibitors of nonenzymatic glycosylation. *Diabetologia*, **38**, 1271–5.

Stitt, A. W., Gardiner, T. A. & Archer, D. B. (1995). A histological and ultrastructural investigation of retinal microaneurysm development in diabetic patients. *British Journal of Ophthalmology*, **79**, 362–5.

Stitt, A. W., Li, Y. M., Gardiner, T. A., Bucala, R., Archer, D. B. & Vlassara, H. (1997). Advanced glycation endproducts (AGEs) co-localize with AGE-receptors in the retinal vasculature of diabetic and of AGE-infused rats. *American Journal of Pathology*, **150**, 523–31.

Taguma, Y., Kilamot, I. & Futaki, G. (1985). Effects of captopril on heavy proteinuria in azotemic diabetes. *New England Journal of Medicine*, **313**, 1617–20.

Tesfamariam, B., Palacino, J. J., Weisbrod, R. M. & Cohen, R. A. (1993). Aldose reductase inhibition restores endothelial cell function in diabetic rabbit aorta. *Journal of Cardiovascular Pharmacology*, **21**, 205–11.

Tesfaye, S., Malik, R. & Wardm, J. D. (1994). Vascular factors in diabetic neuropathy. *Diabetologia*, **37**, 847–54.

Tilton, G. R., Chang, K., Pugliese, G., Eades, D. M., Province, M. A., Sherman, W. R., Kilo, C. & Williamson, J. R. (1989). Prevention of hemodynamic and vascular albumin filtration changes in diabetic rats by aldose reductase inhibitors. *Diabetes*, **38**, 1258–70.

Tilton, R. G., Chang, K., Nyengaard, J. R., Van den Enden, I. Y. & Williamson, J. R. (1995). Inhibition of sorbitol dehydrogenase. Effects on vascular and neural dysfunction in streptozotocin diabetic rats. *Diabetes*, **44**, 234–42.

Tomlinson, D. R., Stevens, E. J. & Diemel, L. T. (1994). Aldose reductase inhibitors and their potential for the treatment of diabetic complications. *Trends in Pharmacological Science*, **15**, 293–7.

Tooke, J. E. (1995). Microvascular function in human diabetes. A physiological perspective. *Diabetes*, **44**, 721–6.

Travis, S. F., Morrison, A. D., Clements, R. S., Winegrad, A. L. & Oski, F. A. (1971). Metabolic alterations in the human erythrocyte produced by increases in glucose concentration: the role of the polyol pathway. *Journal of Clinical Investigation*, **50**, 2104–12.

Tse, W. J. & Kendal, M. (1994). Is there a role beta-blockers in hypertensive diabetic patients. *Diabetic Medicine*, **11**, 137–44.

Tsilibary, E. C., Koliakos, G. G., Charonis, A. S., Vogel, A. M., Reger, L. A. & Furcht, L. T. (1988). Heparin type IV collagen interactions: equilibrium binding and inhibition of type IV collagen self-assembly. *Journal of Biological Chemistry*, **263**, 19112–18.

URDS (1992). Improvements in data quality in the USRDS database: determining treatment modalities. *American Journal of Kidney Disease*, **20** (Suppl. 2), 89–94.

Vinik, A. I., Holland, M. T., Le Beau, J. M., Liuzi, F. J., Stansberry, K. B. & Colen, L. B. (1992). Diabetic neuropathies. *Diabetes Care*, **15**, 1926–75.

Vlassara, H., Brownlee, M. & Cerami, A. (1986a). Novel macrophage receptor for glucose modified proteins is distinct from previously described scavenger receptors. *Journal of Experimental Medicine*, **164**, 1301–9.

Vlassara, H., Valinsky, J., Brownlee, M., Cerami, C., Nishimoto, S. & Cerami, A. (1986b). Advanced glycosylation endpoducts on erythrocyte cell surface induce receptor mediated phagocytosis by macrophages. A model for turnover of aging cells. *Journal of Experimental Medicine*, **166**, 539–49.

Vlassara, H., Brownlee, M., Manogue, K. R., Dinarello, C. & Pasagian, A. (1988). Cachectin/TNF and IL-1 induced by glucose modified proteins: role in normal tissue remodelling. *Science*, **240**, 1546–8.

Vlassara, H., Bucala, R. & Striker, L. (1994a). Pathogenic effects of advanced glycosylation endproducts: biochemical, biologic, and clinical implications for diabetes and aging. *Laboratory Investigation*, **70**, 138–51.

Vlassara, H., Fuh, H., Makita, Z., Krungkrai, S., Cerami, A. & Bucala, R. (1992). Exogenous advanced glycosylation endproducts induce complex vascular dysfunction in normal animals: a model for diabetic and aging complications. *Proceedings of the National Academy of Sciences of the USA*, **89**, 12043–7.

Vlassara, H., Li, Y. M., Imani, F., Wojciechowicz, D., Yang, Z., Liu, F. & Cerami, A. (1995a). Identification of Galectin-3 as a high affinity binding protein for advanced glycation endproducts (AGE): a new member of the AGE-receptor complex. *Molecular Medicine*, **1**, 634–46.

Vlassara, H., Fuh, H., Donnelly, T. & Cybulsky, M. (1995b). Identification of the major site of apolipoprotein-B modification by advanced glycation endproducts (AGEs) promote adhesion molecule (VCAM-1, ICAM-1) expression and atheroma formation in normal rabbits. *Molecular Medicine*, **1**, 447–56.

Vlassara, H., Striker, L. J., Teichberg, S., Fuh, H., Li, Y. M. & Steffes, M. (1994b). Advanced glycosylation endproducts induce glomerular sclerosis and albuminuria in normal rats. *Proceedings of the National Academy of Sciences of the USA*, **91**, 11704–8.

Williamson, D. H., Lund, P. & Krebs, H. A. (1967). The redox state of free nicotinamide-adenine dinucleotide in the cytoplasm and mitochondria of rat liver. *Biochemistry Journal*, **103**, 514–27.

Williamson, J. R., Chang, K., Rowold, E., Kilo, C. & Lace, P. E. (1986). Islet transplants in diabetic Lewis rats prevent and reverse diabetes-induced increases in vascular permeability and prevent but do not reverse collagen solubility changes. *Diabetologia*, **29**, 392–6.

Williamson, J. R., Chang, K., Tilton, R. G., Prater, C., Jeffrey, J. R., Weigel, C., Sherman, W. R., Eades, D. M. & Kilo, C. (1987). Increased vascular permeability in spontaneously diabetic BB/W rats and in rats with mild versus severe streptozocin-induced diabetes. Prevention by aldose reductase inhibitors and castration, *Diabetes*, **36**, 813–21.

Yan, S. D., Schmidt, A. M., Anderson, G., Zhang, J., Brett, J., Zou, Y. S., Pinsky, D. & Stern, D. (1994). Enhanced cellular oxidant stress by the interaction of advanced glycation endproducts with their receptors/binding proteins. *Journal of Biological Chemistry*, **269**, 9889–97.

Yang, C. W., Vlassara, H., Peten, E. P., He, C. J., Striker, G. E., Striker, L. J. (1994). Advanced glycosylation endproducts up-regulate gene expression found in diabetic glomerular disease. *Proceedings of the National Academy of Sciences of the USA*, **91**, 9436–40.

Yang, Z., Makita, Z., Horii, Y., Brunelle, S., Cerami, A., Sehajpal, P., Suthanthiran, M. & Vlassara, H. (1991). Two novel rat liver membrane proteins that bind advanced glycosylation endproducts: relationship to macrophage scavenger receptor for glucose-modified proteins. *Journal of Experimental Medicine*, **174**, 515–24.

Zeigler, D., Gries, F. A., Spuler, M. & Lessmann, F. (1993). The epidemiology of diabetic neuropathy. *Diabetic Medicine*, **10**(Suppl. 2), 82S–86S.

Part 3

Other clinical pathological problems of the vascular system

13

Wound healing: laboratory investigation and modulating agents

N. L. OCCLESTON and P. T. KHAW

Introduction

The past several years has seen a considerable increase in our understanding of the cellular and molecular mechanisms underlying the wound healing process. This process consists of a series of events involving interactions between different cell types, the extracellular matrix and a number of chemical mediators and has been the subject of many excellent reviews. As the field of wound healing research has become too large to cover in depth in a single chapter, we try to highlight crucial components of the wound healing process, methods of investigating these components and finally ways in which the healing process can be modulated.

Wound healing: an overview

The repair of lost or damaged adult tissue is achieved by the production of scar tissue. The healing response generally consists of a series of ordered events, some of which occur concurrently, involving several cell types, regulators of cell function and ultimately the production and remodelling of new tissue (Fig. 13.1). Variations in the processes involved in this response can result in inadequate or excessive healing, both of which may result in the impairment or loss of tissue or organ function. Inappropriate response to injury in particular is a major cause of clinical morbidity, for example in atherosclerosis, restenosis following angioplasty and vein graft disease; following thermal, chemical or radiation burns; following injury or surgery, e.g. internal adhesions, intestinal blockage and keloids; and scarring due to disease, e.g. cirrhosis and scleroderma. In addition to this, the scarring response plays an extremely important role in the pathogenesis or failure of treatment of many visually disabling or blinding conditions in the world today including cataracts, trachoma, glaucoma, burns, proliferative vitreoretinopathy (following retinal detachment or diabetes) and age-related macular degeneration.

For simplicity and discussion in the following chapter, the multistage healing process has been arbitrarily divided into early, central and late events.

197

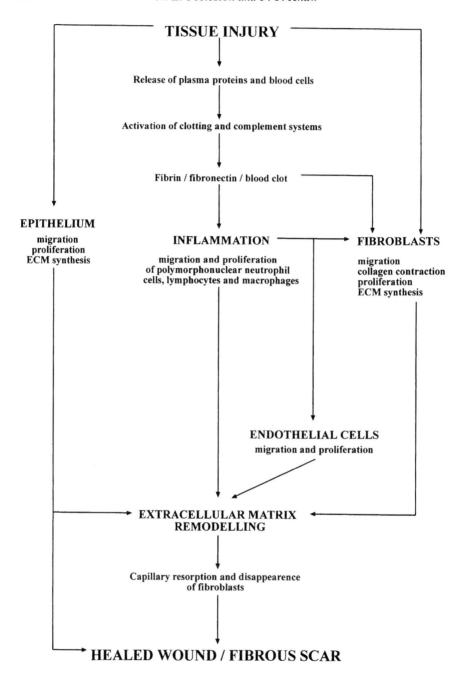

Fig. 13.1. Wound healing response

Wound healing: early events

Role of the blood and clotting systems

One of the earliest factors thought to be involved in the healing process are platelets and the coagulation system. The clotting cascade is activated following vascular damage, resulting in the formation of a clot containing fibrin, fibronectin and blood cells. Fibrin derived from plasma fibrinogen cross-links and clots to fill the wound site, following contact with a variety of coagulation factors (Clark et al, 1983). Fibronectin then covalently cross-links to fibrin forming a fibrin–fibronectin matrix (Kurkinen et al, 1980; Grinnell, 1984), probably serving as a framework on which collagen is later laid down (McDonald et al, 1982; Grinnell, 1984). In addition to this, platelets and extravascular coagulation promoting factors (Maynard et al, 1975; Dvorak et al, 1985) promote the rapid clotting of trapped plasma and blood proteins. Platelets aggregate and attach via interactions with collagen fibrils and von Willebrand factor (factor VIII), to damaged blood vessels which is then followed by platelet degranulation (Samuelsson et al, 1978). A variety of factors are released from platelets including platelet derived growth factor (PDGF), epidermal growth factor (EGF), and transforming growth factor beta (TGF-β) (Ross et al, 1986), which have been reported to stimulate the chemotaxis of monocytes (Deuel et al, 1982), fibroblasts (Seppa et al, 1982) and vascular smooth muscle cells (Heldin & Westermark, 1984; Ross, 1989).

Role of inflammatory cells

The first inflammatory cells entering the wound site are granulocytes, appearing within 24 hours after-injury (Burger et al, 1983). Following this, neutrophils enter the site via the chemotactic effects of various factors released from platelets and the complement cascade. Monocytes are the next cells to appear in the wound site (Issekutz et al, 1981), which then differentiate into macrophages. Once at the wound site, macrophages (which do not differentiate into fibroblasts) not only produce a whole range of regulatory factors which influence the control of the following healing process (Knighton et al, 1984; Riches, 1988; Knighton & Fiegel, 1989), but also phagocytose and breakdown cellular debris and bacteria.

Wound healing: central events

Roles of the fibroblast

The fibroblast is the key player in the wound healing process, carrying out a number of crucial functions including: migration, wound contraction, proliferation, synthesis of new extracellular matrix (ECM) and remodelling of this new matrix. As such, work in our and many other laboratories has concentrated on understanding the mechanisms underlying the regulation of fibroblast function. In a few specialized parts of the body other cells carry out this pivotal part of the healing function, e.g. retinal pigmented epithelial cells in the retina, glia in the central nervous system and vascular smooth muscle cells in the vasculature.

Migration

The movement of fibroblasts to the wound site is mediated by various polypeptides including inflammatory cell products (Postlethwaite et al, 1976; Sobel & Gallin, 1979; Postlethwaite & Kang, 1980), complement (Postlethwaite et al, 1979), platelet-derived growth factor (PDGF) (Seppa et al, 1982), TGF-β (Postlethwaite et al, 1987), and extracellular matrix (ECM) components including collagen (Postlethwaite et al, 1978), elastin (Senior et al, 1984), fibronectin (Joseph et al, 1987) and fibrinogen derivatives (Senior et al, 1986). These polypeptides (termed chemoattractants) are regarded as stimulating migration through the process of chemotaxis. Chemotaxis has been defined as the directed migration of cells in response to a concentration gradient of a soluble chemoattractant (McCarthy et al, 1988) and is regarded as the major mechanism by which cellular migration is controlled. In addition to chemotaxis, the movement of cells independently of the chemoattractant gradient (termed chemokinesis; Zigmond & Hirsch, 1973), haptotaxis (the movement of cells via a substratum bound gradient of a particular matrix constituent (Harris, 1973) and contact guidance (the tendency of cells to align and move along discontinuities in the ECM (Weiss, 1945, 1958) may also contribute to the migration of cells into the wound site.

A number of in vitro assay systems have been used to study cellular migration including Boyden migration chambers (Boyden, 1962), two compartment Boyden chambers (Zigmond & Hirsch, 1973), orientation chambers (Zigmond, 1977), under agarose (Nelson et al, 1978) and modified 48 microwell two tiered blindwell Boyden migration chambers. We use 48 microwell modified Boyden chambers to study the effects of varying concentrations of growth factors including TGF-β_1, EGF, basic fibroblast growth factor (bFGF) and insulin-like growth factor-1 (IGF-1) on ocular fibroblast migration. In addition to Boyden chambers, we have also found 24 well Transwell tissue culture inserts (see Fig. 13.2) a useful way of studying cellular migration, as have other studies investigating vascular smooth muscle cell migration (Okada et al,

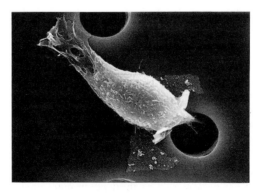

Fig. 13.2. Cell migration assay. Photograph shows an ocular fibroblast migrating through a Transwell pore, by scanning electron microscopy.

1995; Noda-Heiny & Sobel, 1995). Although the use of Transwells reduces the technical difficulty of the migration assay, the volume of chemoattractant required is approximately 20 times greater than used in the modified Boyden chamber. When using any of the above assay systems to study migration, it should be borne in mind that although they allow quantitation of cellular migration and the study of individual chemoattractants, the conditions are obviously very different to those *in vivo*. In the in vivo situation, not only are cells moving through their surrounding ECM during migration, but also that this process is probably under the control of not one but several regulatory signals acting in concert.

Extracellular matrix contraction

The contraction of collagen containing tissues is fundamental not only to the wound healing process (Grinnell, 1994) but also morphogenesis (Stopak & Harris, 1982; Lewis, 1984) and development (Brenner et al, 1989). ECM contraction was originally thought to be due to the actions of specialised cells exhibiting smooth muscle cell characteristics – myofibroblasts (Gabbiani et al, 1972); however, this process is now regarded as resulting from the tractional forces exerted by migrating fibroblasts upon their substratum (Harris et al, 1981; Ehrlich & Rajaratnam, 1990, also see Fig. 13.3).

We and many other groups have been using an in vitro model of collagen contraction consisting of fibroblasts entrapped within a three-dimensional collagen matrix, which was originally described by Bell et al (1979). The cells within this matrix reorganize and subsequently contract the matrix over a period of several days (Fig. 13.3), the morphological characteristics of these cells resembling those seen in vivo (Tomasek & Hay, 1984). Studies using this model consisting of fibroblasts seeded within or upon three-dimensional collagen matrices (Bell et al, 1979; Schor, 1980; Guidry & Grinnell, 1985), have demonstrated that contraction is dependent upon a variety of factors including collagen concentration and cell number (Bell et al, 1979; Allen & Schor, 1983; Buttle & Ehrlich, 1983; Occleston et al, 1994), an intact actin cytoskeleton (Bell et al, 1979; Guidry & Grinnell, 1985), attachment of cells to their surrounding matrix (Schiro et al, 1991; Klein et al, 1991), and protein synthesis (Guidry & Grinnell, 1985). In addition to this, the contraction of collagen has been shown to be stimulated by a variety of growth factors including EGF, TGFβ, IGF-I, PDGF and bFGF, and to involve intracellular signalling cascades (Guidry, 1993).

Although much research upon the process of collagen contraction has been carried out, the exact mechanisms underlying this process are currently unclear. Such mechanisms include the elucidation of how fibroblasts within a three-dimensional matrix migrate, are signalled to start and stop contraction, and how these cells respond to changes in biophysical forces within granulation tissue. Studies in our laboratory have suggested that the matrix metalloproteinases (MMPs) play an essential role in the contraction of collagen lattices in vitro. We have demonstrated that fibroblasts markedly increase their production of MMPs both at the mRNA level, using a quantitative competitive RT-PCR (QCRT-PCR) technique developed by our colleagues at the Institute for Wound Research, University of Florida (Tarnuzzer et al, 1996), and at the

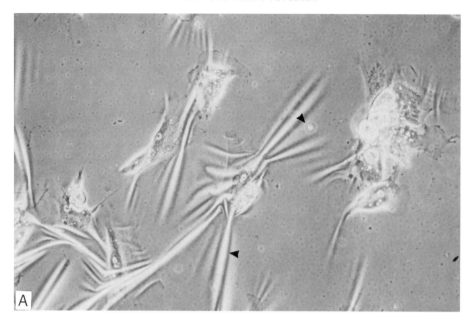

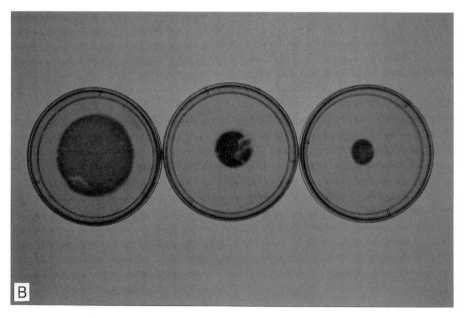

Fig. 13.3. Models of in vitro contraction. (A) Silicon sheets. Fibroblasts migrating on ultrathin silicon sheets produce tractional forces (arrows). (B) Collagen lattices. Fibroblasts seeded within three-dimensional collagen matrices reorganize and subsequently contract their surrounding matrix over several days.

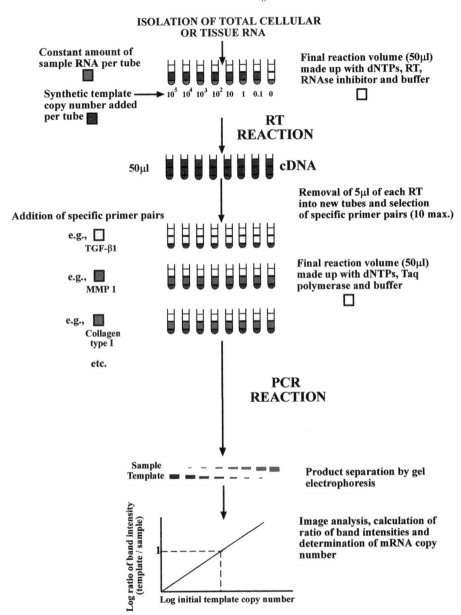

Fig. 13.4. Quantitative competitive reverse transcriptase polymerase chain reaction (QCRT-PCR) technique. This technique allows the quantitation of mRNA levels from cells or tissues for a variety of growth factors, growth factor receptors, ECM components, ECM degrading enzymes and their inhibitors.

protein level. This QCRT-PCR technique is extremely powerful as we are able to quantitate the levels of mRNA in cells or tissue for a variety of MMPs, ECM components, growth factors and growth factor receptors (Tarnuzzer et al, 1996; also see Fig. 13.4), from the same sample and using only small amounts of RNA. From further experiments in our laboratory, it appears that the MMPs allow fibroblasts to penetrate / invade their surrounding collagen matrix and then move through this matrix. It is this penetration of the matrix and subsequent movement through the matrix which ultimately results in its contraction. In addition to the above techniques, our colleagues at the Phoenix Tissue Repair Unit, University College London have developed a novel system for studying fibroblast behaviour in ECM – the Culture Force Monitor (CFM; Fig. 13.5). The original prototype of the CFM allowed accurate, sensitive and reproducible measurement of the contractile forces generated by cells within a collagen matrix (Eastwood et al, 1994). Other instruments have now been developed at the Phoenix Tissue Repair Unit to investigate the effects of biophysical forces on cellular behaviour in ECM (tension CFM) and the formation of adhesions between tissue interfaces in vitro (adhesion CFM; Cacou et al, 1996).

Proliferation

Following the migration of fibroblasts to the wound site and the resultant contraction of the ECM, they then proliferate reaching maximal numbers within 1–2 weeks post injury (Ross & Odland, 1968). The proliferation of fibroblasts at the wound site is important in order for the cell number to be sufficient to allow adequate healing. As for fibroblast migration and ECM contraction, the proliferation of these cells is stimulated by a number of growth factors including EGF, TGFβ, IGF-I, PDGF and bFGF; however, these growth factors also have inhibitory as well as stimulatory effects on cellular functions related to wound healing, depending upon the cell type studied (see Table 13.1). The quantitation of proliferation in response to a variety of stimuli has been achieved using several methods including ^{3}H-thymidine assays (Freshney, 1987), counted cell number e.g. haemocytometer, Coulter counter and colourimetric assays e.g. MTT and WST assays based upon cellular matabolic activity (Mosmann, 1983; Kawase et al, 1995), and the methylene blue assays based upon dye binding to the cell monolayer (Finlay et al, 1984).

Role of endothelial cells

Neovascularization of the wound occurs simultaneously with the migration into and the proliferation of fibroblasts at the wound site. The process of formation of capillary beds via the influx of microvessel buds from the surrounding tissue vasculature (angiogenesis) is a central component of the wound healing process. Angiogenesis is a complex process and is thought to involve several stages including migration, growth and capillary tube formation. As for the other stages of wound healing, angiogenesis is regulated by several factors including chemical mediators (see Role of growth factors in wound healing) and the reader is referred to Chapter 1 for a more extensive review of this process.

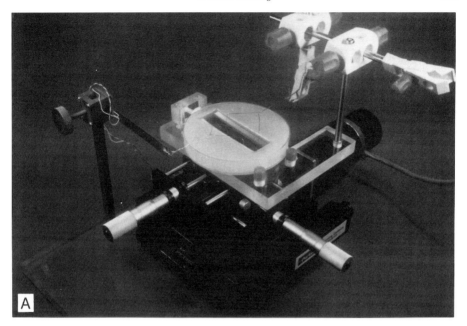

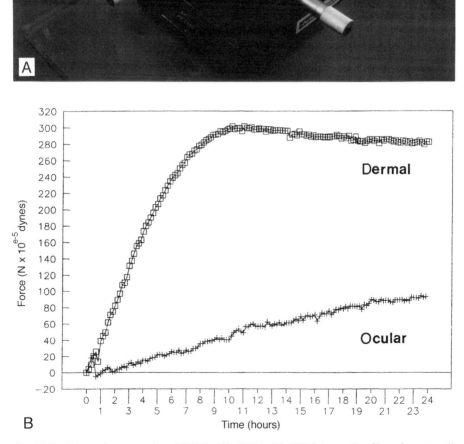

Fig. 13.5. Culture force monitor (CFM). (A) CFM. (B) CFM trace. Profiles of contractile forces generated over 24 h by dermal and ocular (Tenon's capsule) fibroblasts within a collagen lattice.

Table 13.1. *Role of growth factors in wound healing*

Growth factor	Molecular weight (kDa)	Found in	Reported effects on cellular functions related to wound healing Fibroblasts	Endothelial cells	Epithelial cells	Vascular smooth muscle cells
EGF	6	Almost all body fluids, Platelets	Stimulates migration ECM contraction proliferation, ECM synthesis	Stimulates proliferation angiogenesis	Stimulates migration proliferation	Stimulates proliferation
TGF-α	5–20	Macrophages Eosinocytes Keratinocytes	see effects of EGF above			
TGF-β	25	Platelets Macrophages Lymphocytes Fibroblasts Keratinocytes	Stimulates migration ECM contraction proliferation ECM synthesis	Inhibits proliferation migration Stimulates angiogenesis	Inhibits proliferation migration Stimulates ECM synthesis	Inhibits proliferation (normal cells) Stimulates proliferation ECM synthesis (cells from vascular lesions)
IGF-1	7.5	Most tissues Macrophages Fibroblasts	Stimulates migration ECM contraction proliferation ECM synthesis	Stimulates migration proliferation	Stimulates migration proliferation	Stimulates migration proliferation
PDGF	28–35	Platelets Macrophages Fibroblasts Endothelial Cells	Stimulates migration proliferation	Stimulates proliferation	Stimulates proliferation	Stimulates migration proliferation
VEGF	45	Pituitary Cells Vascular Smooth Muscle Cells		Stimulates proliferation angiogenesis		
FGF (acidic and basic)	16–18	Fibroblasts Endothelial Cells	Stimulates migration ECM contraction proliferation ECM synthesis	Stimulates migration proliferation ECM synthesis angiogenesis	Stimulates migration ECM synthesis	Stimulates migration proliferation
KGF	28	Fibroblasts			Stimulates proliferation migration	

Note: EGF: epidermal growth factor; FGF: fibroblast growth factor; IGF-1: insulin-like growth factor-1; KGF: keratinocyte growth factor; PGDF: platelet-derived growth factor; TGF: transforming growth factor; VEGF: vascular endothelial growth factor.

Interestingly recent work has suggested a role for the MMPs in angiogenesis (Galardy et al, 1994), and the modulation of this process and other inhibitors of angiogenesis are highlighted in this section on Modulation of wound healing.

Role of epithelial cells

Re-epithelialiation is an important factor in the closure of wounds. Two different mechanisms have been reported to be involved in the re-epithelialiation of wounds. Studies by Martin & Lewis (1992) and Bement et al (1993), have suggested a purse string closure mechanism involving the formation of an actin cable in foetal epithelial healing and gastrointestinal epithelial healing. In addition, it is also thought that basal epithelial cells migrate directionally across the wound defect pulling the upper layers of the epidermis passively along, followed by proliferation and finally deposition of a new basement membrane and restratification of the epidermis (Mackenzie & Fusenig, 1983). Recently, this migration of epithelial cells across a wound defect has been shown to involve the action of MMPs (Woodley et al, 1986; Saarialho et al, 1993; Iwasaki et al, 1994; Saarialho-Kere et al, 1995). Once re-epithelialization has occurred, the remodelling and maturation phases of the healing process begin (ECM production and remodelling).

Wound healing: late events
ECM production and remodelling

The reformation of the ECM begins simultaneously with the formation of granulation tissue by inflammatory cells, fibroblasts and endothelial cells. Initially high levels of fibronectin and hyaluronic acid are deposited at the wound site, disappearing as the matrix matures over several weeks with increasing wound collagen and proteoglycan content. In addition to repairing the ECM damage, the production of collagen types I and III as well as fibronectin and fibrin provides support for epithelial cell migration (Clark et al, 1982; Woodley et al, 1985) and thus re-epithelialisation of the wound. The production of new ECM at the wound site involves several cell types involved in the healing process. For example, fibronectin is derived from macrophages, endothelial cells, fibroblasts and some epithelial cells (Oh et al, 1981; Clark et al, 1982), while proteoglycans have been shown to be produced by fibroblasts, smooth muscle and endothelial cells (Lane et al, 1986; Paulsson et al, 1986).

It is the fibroblast which is the major producer of new ECM, these cells secreting a number of ECM molecules including fibronectin, glycosaminoglycans, hyaluronic acid and collagen types I and III (Barnes et al, 1976; Williams et al, 1984). Collagen is the major component of the wound matrix and as such two members of this large family of proteins, collagen types I and III, are highlighted here as the roles of these in wound healing is best defined. The first collagen to be laid down at the wound site is collagen type III (Gabbiani et al, 1976; Guber & Ross, 1978) in close association with pre-existing fibrin networks, and are subsequently stabilized by mucopolysaccharides (Ross &

Odland, 1968). Following the regression of both fibroblasts and endothelial cells, collagen type III is replaced by collagen type I (Dvorak, 1986). The procollagen molecule, consisting of three helical polypeptides (Gabbiani & Montandon, 1977), is secreted into the extracellular space forming the collagen precursor tropocollagen, via the loss of NH_2 and COOH domains (Gabbiani & Montandon, 1977). This tropocollagen molecule is then cross-linked by lysyl oxidase, the degree of cross-linking reflecting the strength of the healed tissue (Chvapil & Koopmann, 1984). A number of growth factors have been shown to stimulate ECM synthesis including PDGF (Grotendorst et al, 1985), TGF-β (Sporn et al, 1983; Ignotz & Massague, 1986), EGF, IGF-I and bFGF (Table 13.1).

Several degradative enzymes play crucial roles in the remodelling of the exisiting and newly synthesized ECM throughout the healing process. For discussion, these enzymes have been divided into two groups: plasminogen activators (PAs) and MMPs. The PAs include urokinase (u-PA) and tissue-type (t-PA) and are capable of activating plasminogen to plasmin, which has been shown to be involved in the degradation of fibrin clots (Robbins et al, 1981). u-PA has been shown to be produced by inflammatory cells (Gordon et al, 1974; Vassalli et al, 1984) and it is thought that in conjunction with t-PA derived from vessel disruption, leads to the degradation of the fibrin clot. Plasmin has also been shown to degrade fibronectin (Werb et al, 1980) and to activate the latent forms of MMPs (Werb et al, 1977). PAs have also been implicated in the migration of fibroblasts and endothelial cells, although the exact mechanisms of this process are unclear, as well as the proliferative process during arterial repair (Wysocki et al, 1996).

The other major group of ECM degrading enzymes are the MMPs, which are involved in the degradation of collagens (types I – V and VII – XI), gelatin (denatured collagen), fibronectin, laminin, elastin and proteoglycan core protein (for reviews see Woessner, 1991; Matrisian, 1992; Birkedal-Hansen et al, 1993; Birkedal-Hansen, 1995). There are several members of the MMP family which share a number of structural and functional features including a Zn^{2+} binding site and may be regarded as derivatives (formed by deletion or addition of domains) of the modular structure of collagenases and stromelysins (see chapter on extracellular matrix for further details). Members of this family include MMP-1 (collagenase), MMP-2 (72 kD gelatinase), MMP-3 (stromelysin), MMP-7 (PUMP-1, putative metalloproteinase-1), MMP-8 (neutrophil collagenase), MMP-9 (92 kD gelatinase), MMP-10 (stromelysin-2), MMP-11 (stromelysin-3) and elastase. Individual MMPs tend to cleave specific ECM substrates, although there is some overlap in the substrate specificity of these enzymes. These enzymes are initially secreted in an inactive or proform, and are subsequently activated extracellularly. MMPs have been reported to be produced by a variety of cells involved in the wound healing process including neutrophils, macrophages, fibroblasts, endothelial cells, keratinocytes and vascular smooth muscle cells (Birkedal-Hansen et al, 1993; Pauly et al, 1994), their production being regulated by a number of external stimuli including growth factors. Another characteristic of these enzymes is that their activity is regulated by the tissue inhibitors of matrix metalloproteinases (TIMPs), of which three forms have currently been reported (TIMP-1, 2 and 3). The degree of degradation of the

ECM is dependent upon the balance between the ratio of MMPs : TIMPs, a relative increase in MMPs or a decrease in TIMPs resulting in an overall increase in degradation and vice versa. An example of the importance of the balance of these two systems in ECM turnover has been highlighted in restenosis, where Tyagi et al (1995) reported an increase in ECM production and a decrease in MMP activity compared to normal artery. Studies performed by Newby et al (1994) have also suggested that the MMPs may be involved in the proliferation and outgrowth of vascular smooth muscle cells in atherosclerosis.

In addition to these secreted MMPs two members of a novel subclass of the MMP family, membrane type-matrix metalloproteinases (MT-MMPs) 1 and 2, have recently been reported (Sato et al, 1994; Takino et al, 1995). Although the exact roles of MT-MMPs in wound healing are currently unclear, it is thought that they may play a role in MMP activation at the cell surface (Takino et al, 1995; Lewalle et al, 1995; Strongin et al, 1995).

We have successfully used a variety of techniques for studying ECM production and MMP/TIMP expression. These include QCRT-PCR (quantitative reverse transcriptase-polymerase chain reaction), zymography, reverse zymography, Western blotting, enzyme linked immunosorbent assays (ELISAs) and immunocytochemistry.

Role of growth factors in wound healing

Several growth factors have been implicated in the wound healing process including members of the EGF, TGF-β, IGF, PDGF and FGF families. These growth factors are thought to play many key roles not only in the initiation but also in sustaining the wound healing process, the properties and molecular biology of these factors being the subject of several reviews (Bennett & Schultz, 1993a,b; Clark & Henson, 1988). The roles of growth factors include the stimulation or inhibition of several cellular functions including proliferation, migration, ECM contraction and ECM synthesis. The effects of these growth factors on cell function regulation relating to wound healing are summarised in Table 13.1, and the reader is referred to the above references for a more comprehensive treatise. Although the effects and roles of individual growth factors have been extensively studied in vitro, their interactions and roles in vivo during the wound healing process are obviously extremely complex and as yet are incompletely elucidated.

A number of techniques have been used in our laboratory to quantitate growth factor and growth factor receptor expression. These include QCRT-PCR for quantitation at the mRNA level, and ELISAs, radioreceptor assays and immunocytochemistry at the protein levels for members of the EGF, TGF-β, IGF, PDGF and FGF families.

Modulation of wound healing

The wound healing process as illustrated above is a complex array of cellular, ECM and chemical mediator interactions. As a result, wound healing can be modulated at various stages as shown in Fig. 13.6. Many antiscarring therapies have been available for several

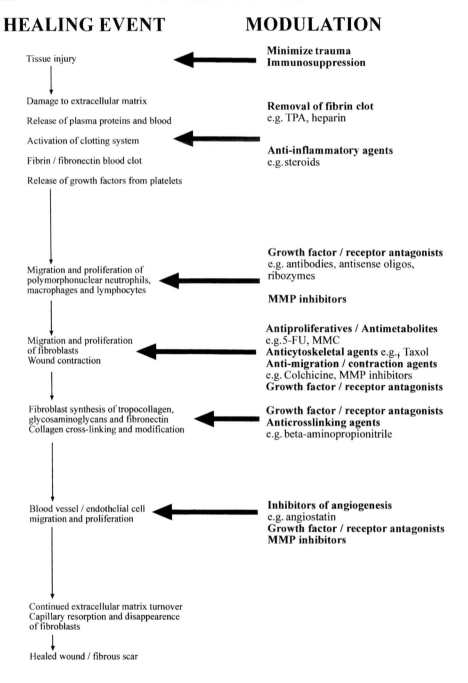

Fig. 13.6. Modulation of wound healing.

years, but it is only recently that our increase in knowledge of the mechanisms underlying the healing process in both adult and foetal tissue (which does not scar), that therapy refinement and the development of potential therapies have been achieved. In addition to this, the application of both basic science and therapeutic findings from different fields of wound healing research may prove not only essential but also successful. Some of the recent advances in our understanding of the healing process, agents available for modifying healing (and their modes of action) and new/potential methods for modulating healing are outlined below.

Attempts have been made to particularly target specific cell functions during the wound healing process, many of the agents used having effects on several cell functions and types. For simplicity of discussion, these agents have been divided into immunosuppressives/anti-inflammatories, antimigration/anticytoskeletal agents, antiproliferative/antimetabolic agents, inhibitors of angiogenesis, agents affecting ECM synthesis and degradation and agents affecting growth factors and growth factor receptors.

Immunosuppressives/anti-inflammatories

These agents affect the early phases of the wound healing process. As the influx of inflammatory cells into the wound site is thought to play a role in the stimulation of later healing events, the use of corticosteroids and other immunosuppressives have been shown to not only impair inflammatory cell chemotaxis but also subsequent angiogenesis, fibroblast proliferation and matrix synthesis (Wahl, 1989) resulting in reduced scarring in tissues such as the conjunctiva (Roth et al, 1988). Recently, the extravasation of inflammatory cells both in vitro and in vivo (Gijbels et al, 1994; Leppert et al, 1995) has been shown to involve the MMPs suggesting a potential role for potent, broad spectrum MMP inhibitors in the modulation of the inflammatory response and subsequent scarring (also see below).

Antimigration/anticytoskeletal agents

Examples of these agents include colchicine, cytochalasin b and particularly taxol, which has been shown to inhibit the ability of fibroblasts to migrate towards a chemical stimulus (Metcalfe & Weetman, 1994). Colchicine has been shown to inhibit vascular smooth muscle cell proliferation in vitro (Voisard et al, 1995), while taxol has also been shown to inhibit fibroblast proliferation and to reduce scarring in an aggressive *in vivo* model (Jampel et al, 1990), as well as restenosis following angioplasty (Sollott et al, 1995). As described earlier in wound healing: central events, the ability of cells to contract the ECM appears to be dependent upon the migration of these cells, as it is the subsequent generation of tractional forces upon their substratum via cell movement which ultimately results in contraction of the ECM. We have been using collagen type I matrices populated with fibroblasts as an in vitro model of wound contraction. Upon stimulation with serum or growth factors, the fibroblasts contract these matrices. We have demonstrated that the degree of collagen contraction can be significantly inhibited upon single, 5 minute exposures to the antiproliferative / antimetabolic agents 5-fluorouracil (5-FU) and mitomycin-C (MMC), without cell death (Occleston et al, 1994). Observations made during this study suggested that the MMPs may play a major role in the process of collagen contraction. Subsequent work in our laboratory has shown that the MMPs are essential to the process of collagen contraction and that this process can be significantly inhibited using specific MMP inhibitors. In addition, we have found that the requirement of MMPs for contraction may be a ubiquitous mechanism, not only throughout different tissue sites (cornea, conjunctiva, dermis, synovial sheath and endotendon) but also species (human, rabbit and rat). These findings may have important therapeutic implications as we have also demonstrated that the effects of MMP inhibitors on collagen contraction are specfic, non-toxic and can be applied to or removed from tissue constructs to control the degree of contraction. MMPs have also been implicated in the migration of a variety of other cell types through basement membrane in vitro including inflammatory cells, endothelial cells and vascular smooth muscle cells (Pauly et al, 1994; Leppert et al, 1995; Taraboletti et al, 1995), the inhibition of these enzymes also reducing angiogenesis in vivo (Galardy et al, 1994; Taraboletti et al, 1995), suggesting a potential role for MMP inhibitors in the modulation of these healing related processes.

Antiproliferative/antimetabolic agents

Much of the antiscarring research in ophthalmology has concentrated on the use of these agents, primarily to reduce cell division. Blumenkranz and colleagues established that 5-FU inhibited the proliferation of fibroblasts in vitro and ocular scarring in vivo (1982, 1984). Following these findings, an antiscarring regimen involving subconjunctival 5-FU injections after glaucoma filtration surgery was developed in Miami, Florida, USA, resulting in a multicentre trial (The Fluorouracil Filtering Surgery Study Group. 1989). Largely unnoticed, Chen et al (1983, 1990) had been using single applications of the agent MMC for more than a decade. Further research in our laboratory demonstrated that 5-FU and MMC had long-term antiproliferative effects on fibroblasts, with single exposures as short as 5 minutes (Khaw et al, 1991, 1992b). We subsequently showed that effective suppression of proliferation in excess of 36 days, without cell death, could be achieved (Khaw et al, 1992b,c). These single, 5 minute treatments were also found to be effective in vivo, being titratable in terms of length of action (Doyle et al, 1993; Khaw et al, 1993b) and focal (Khaw et al, 1992a, 1993a). These single intraoperative, 5 minute exposures to 5-FU and MMC are now the standard treatment for patients undergoing glaucoma filtration surgery at Moorfields Eye Hospital (Fig. 13.7), and are currently the subject of a 5 year MRC clinical trial. The main advantage of these agents is that they can be applied relatively focally and then washed out. MMC has also been shown to inhibit vascular smooth muscle cell migration and proliferation in vitro (Tanaka et al, 1994), perhaps suggesting a role for these agents in the modulation of restenosis. Additionally, we have demonstrated that applications of β-radiation have similar antiproliferative effects as the agents above in vitro (Khaw et al,

1991) and focal applications result in reduced scarring in vivo (Miller & Rice, 1991). These findings are similar to the reported effects of β-radiation on restenosis in animal models (Waksman et al, 1995; Verin et al, 1995; Laird et al, 1996).

Inhibitors of angiogenesis

As highlighted earlier, angiogenesis plays a crucial role in the formation of granulation tissue during wound healing. Although several studies have revealed important targets for the inhibition of angiogenesis and subsequent inhibitors, e.g. inhibitors of VEGF/ FGF, angiostatin, urokinase receptor antagonists and scatter factor inhibitors, their use in modulating the wound healing response is still unclear. In addition to this, MMPs have been implicated in endothelial cell migration in vitro and subsequently the inhibition of MMP activity has been shown to reduce angiogenesis *in vivo* (Galardy et al, 1994).

Agents affecting ECM synthesis and degradation

Examples of agents which affect ECM synthesis include the lathyrogenic agent β-aminopropionitrile, which is thought to have its clinical effect (McGuigan et al, 1986, 1987; Moorhead et al, 1990) by inhibiting the enzyme lysyl oxidase and thus preventing collagen cross-linking (Siegel, 1977). As discussed in ECM production and remodelling, the ECM present in wounds is the product of both synthesis and degradative processes. Major players in the degradation of the ECM are the MMPs and their inhibitors (TIMPs). As such, interfering with either of these families of molecules may have profound effects on the healing process. Potential modulating agents include chemical inhibitors of the MMPs, MMP/TIMP neutralising antibodies, antisense oligonucleotides or ribozymes to MMPs or TIMPs (also see Agents affecting growth factor/growth factor receptors below), which may have future uses in healing modulation. These molecules (MMPs/TIMPs) are of particular importance in the modulation of wound healing as they appear to play crucial roles throughout the healing response as shown in earlier sections, and as such are receiving considerable attention.

Agents affecting growth factors and growth factor receptors

As highlighted earlier, growth factors and their receptors play a central regulatory role in the wound healing process. Consequently, both the growth factors, the receptors through which they elicit their effects, and the intracellular signalling cascades involved are extremely good candidates for therapeutic intervention. In the following paragraph the modulation of one of the pivotal growth factor families in wound healing at many tissue sites, TGF-β, will be used as an example.

Several approaches to the modulation of TGF-β in wound healing have been or are currently being investigated. These include the neutralisation of TGF-β activity using antibodies or TGF-β_3, which have been shown to reduce scarring *in vivo* (Shah et al,

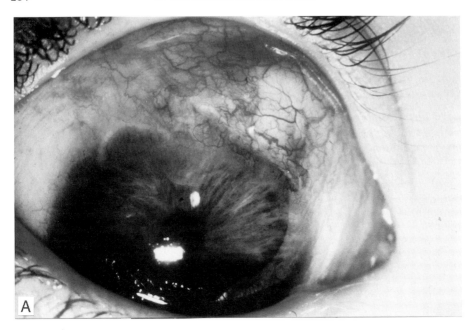

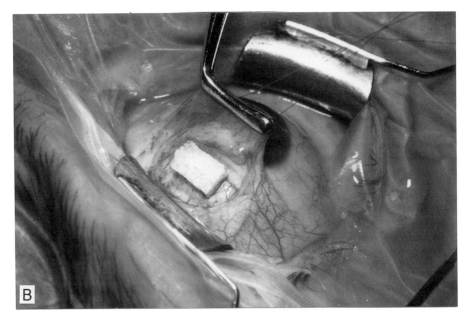

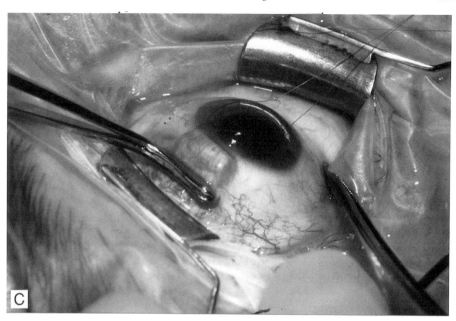

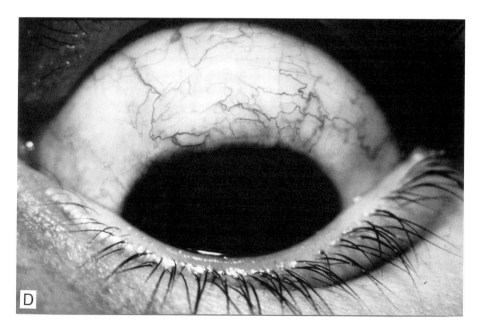

Fig. 13.7. Reduction of postoperative scarring using short, single applications of anti-proliferatives. (A) Scarring and tissue contraction following unsuccessful glaucomafiltration surgery. (B and C) Intraoperative application of a sponge soaked in antiproliferative/antimetabolite. (D) Reduction in scarring following a short, single application of anti-proliferative/antimetabolite, resulting in successful filtration surgery.

1992, 1994, 1995). In addition to this, there is a potential antiscarring role for TGF-β receptor antagonists. Studies have shown that the sugar mannose-6-phosphate (which competitively binds to the mannose-6-phosphate/IGF receptor) reduces cutaneous scarring by inhibiting the activation of latent TGF-β (M. W. Ferguson, personal communication). In addition to this, Indolfi et al (1995) have recently demonstrated that the inhibition of ras (which are key players in the transduction of growth factor signals from the cell surface to the nucleus) prevents smooth muscle cell proliferation in vivo following vascular injury. Another possible approach to interfering with TGF-β protein production at the wound site would be the local application of specific antisense oligonucleotides to TGF-β mRNA, although their use is still in the early stages (M. W. Ferguson, personal communication). A related, potential way of modulating TGF-β production would be the use of ribozymes. These are RNA molecules that have been shown to cleave other RNA molecules (Bartel & Szostak, 1993; Moore, 1995; Wilson & Szostak, 1995). Like antisense oligonucleotides, ribozymes can be designed to attach to a specific mRNA of choice. There are however, significant advantages of ribozyme technology over antisense. Once the ribozyme has attached to the 'target' mRNA, it cleaves the mRNA and is then free to attach to and cleave another 'target' mRNA. So theoretically, the actions of ribozymes unlike antisense oligonucleotides should not be concentration or time dependent. The use of ribozymes as RNA directed gene therapies has been shown (Altman, 1993; Dorai et al, 1994) although their use as antiscarring agents is still to be fully investigated. Current work in our laboratory, in conjunction with our collaborative colleagues at the University of Florida, is investigating the use of ribozymes directed against TGF-β_1 and the TGF-β type II receptor in the modulation of ocular scarring.

In summary, we now have a variety of techniques available to investigate the basic science of the cellular and molecular mechanisms underlying the wound healing process. Our recent advances in understanding have directly led to methods to modulate healing, several of which are now entering clinical trial or are used routinely in the clinic (e.g. single, short exposures to 5-FU or MMC). It is only by gaining an even deeper understanding of the basic cellular and molecular biology of the healing response throughout the body, that we will be able to achieve our ultimate goal: safe, effective control of healing with retention of both function and aesthetics.

References

Allen, T. D. & Schor, S. L. (1983). The contraction of collagen matrices by dermal fibroblasts. *Journal of Ultrastructural Research*, **83**, 205–19.

Altman, S. (1993). RNA enzyme-directed gene therapy. *Proceedings of the National Academy of Sciences of the USA*, **90**, 10898–900.

Barnes, M. J., Morton, L. F., Bennett, R. C., Bailey, A. J. & Sims, T. J. (1976). Presence of type III collagen in guinea-pig dermal scar. *Biochemistry Journal*, **157**, 263–6.

Bartel, D. P. & Szostak, J. W. (1993). Isolation of new ribozymes from a large pool of random sequences. *Science*, **261**, 1411–18.

Bell, E., Ivarsson, B. & Merrill, C. (1979). Production of a tissue-like structure by contraction of collagen lattices by human fibroblasts of different proliferative potential in vitro. *Proceedings of the National Academy of Sciences of the USA*, **76**, 1274–8.

Bement, W. M., Forscher, P. & Mooseker, M. S. (1993). A novel cytoskeletal structure involved in purse string wound closure and cell polarity maintenance. *Journal of Cell Biology*, **121**, 565–78.

Bennett, N. T. & Schultz, G. S. (1993a). Growth factors and wound healing: Biochemical properties of growth factors and their receptors. *American Journal of Surgery*, **165**, 728–37.

Bennett, N. T. & Schultz, G. S. (1993b). Growth factors and wound healing: Part II. Role in normal and chronic wound healing. *American Journal of Surgery*, **166**, 74–81.

Birkedal-Hansen, H. (1995). Proteolytic remodeling of extracellular matrix. *Current Biology*, **7**, 728–35.

Birkedal-Hansen, H., Moore, W. G. I., Bodden, M. K., Windsor, L. J., Birkedal-Hansen, B., DeCarlo, A. & Engler, J. A. (1993). Matrix metalloproteinases: a review. *Critical Reviews of Oral Biology and Medicine*, **4**, 197–250.

Blumenkranz, M. S., Claffin, A. & Hajek, A. S. (1984). Selection of agents for intraocular proliferative disease. *Archives of Ophthalmology*, **102**, 598–604.

Blumenkranz, M. S., Ophir, A., Claffin, A. & Hajek, A. S. (1982). Fluorouracil for the treatement of massive periretinal proliferation. *American Journal of Ophthalmology*, **94**, 458–67.

Boyden, S. (1962). The chemotactic effect of mixtures of antibody and antigen on polymorphonuclear leucocytes. *Journal of Experimental Medicine*, **115**, 453–66.

Brenner, C. A., Adler, R. R., Rappolee, D. A., Pdersen, R. A. & Werb, Z. (1989). Genes for extracellular matrix-degrading metalloproteinases and their inhibitor TIMP, are expressed during early mammalian development. *Genes Develoment*, **3**, 848–59.

Burger, P. C., Chandler, D. B. & Klintworth, G. K. (1983). Corneal neovascularisation as studies by scanning electron microscopy of vascular casts. *Journal of Clinical Investigation*, **48**, 169–80.

Buttle, D. J. & Ehrlich, H. P. (1983). Comparative studies of collagen lattice contraction utilizing a normal and a transformed cell line. *Journal of Cell Physiology*, **116**, 159–66.

Cacou, C., Eastwood, M., McGrouther, D. A. & Brown, R. A. (1996). Culture force monitor for investigating the formation of adhesions between tissue interfaces in vitro. *Cellular Engineering*, **1**, 109–14.

Chen, C. W. (1983). Enhanced intraocular pressure controlling effectiveness of trabeculectomy by local application of mitomycin C. *Trans Asia Pacific Academy of Ophthalmology* **9**, 172–7.

Chen, C., Huang, H., Bair, J. S. & Lee, C. (1990). Trabeculectomy with simultaneous topical application of mitomycin C in refractory glaucoma. *Journal of Ocular Pharmacology*, **6**, 175–82.

Chvapil, M. & Koopmann, C. F. (1984). Scar formation: physiology and pathology states. *Otolaryngeal Clinics of North America*, **17/2**, 265–72.

Clark, R. A. F. & Henson, P. M. (1988). *The Molecular and Cellular Biology of Wound Repair*. New York: Plenum Press.

Clark, R. A., DellaPelle, P., Manseau, E., Lanigan, J. M., Dvorak, H. F. & Colvin, R. B. (1982a). Blood vessel fibronectin increases in conjunction with endothelial cell proliferation and capillary ingrowth during wound healing. *Journal of Investigative Dermatology* **79**, 269–76.

Clark, J. G., Kahn, C., McDonald, J. A. & Mecham, R. P. (1983). Lung connective tissue. *International Review of Connective Tissue Research*, **10**, 249–331.

Clark, R. A. F., Lanigan, J. M., DellaPelle, P., Manseau, E., Dvorak, H. F. & Colvin, R. B. (1982b). Fibronectin and fibrin provide a provisional matrix for epidermal cell migration during wound reepithelialization. *Journal of Investigative Dermatology,* **79**, 264–9.

Deuel, T. F., Senior, R. M., Huang, J. S. & Griffin, G. L. (1982). Chemotaxis of monocytes and neutrophils to platelet derived growth factor. *Journal of Clinical Investigation,* **69**, 1046–9.

Dorai, T., Kobayashi, H., Holland, J. F. & Ohnuma, T. (1994). Modulation of platelet-derived growth factor-beta mRNA expression and cell growth in a human mesothelioma cell line by a hammerhead ribozyme. *Molecular Pharmacology,* **46**, 437–44.

Doyle, J. W., Sherwood, M. B., Khaw, P. T., McGorray, S. & Smith, M. F. (1993). Intraoperative 5-fluorouracil for filtration surgery in the rabbit. *Investigative Ophthalmology and Vision Science,* **34**, 3313–19.

Dvorak, H. F., Senger, D. R., Dvorak, A. M., Harvey, V. S. & McDonagh, J. (1985). Regulation of extravascular coagulation by microvascular permeability. *Science.* **227**, 1059–61.

Eastwood, M., McGrouther, D. A. & Brown, R. A. (1994). A culture force monitor for measurement of contraction forces generated in human dermal fibroblast cultures: evidence for cell-matrix mechanical signalling. *Biochimica et Biophysica Acta,* **1201**, 186–192.

Ehrlich, H. P. & Rajaratnam, J. B. M. (1990). Cell locomotion forces versus cell contraction forces for collagen lattice contraction: an in vitro model of wound healing. *Tissue Cell,* **22**, 407–17.

Finlay, G. J., Baguley, B. C. & Wilson, W. R. (1984). A semiautomated microculture method for investigating growth inhibitory effects of cytotoxic compounds on exponentially growing carcinoma cells. *Analytical. Biochemistry,* **139**, 272–7.

Fluorouracil Filtering Surgery Study Group. (1989). Fluorouracil filtering surgery study one-year follow-up. *American Journal of Ophthalmology,* **108**, 625–35.

Freshney, R. I. (1987). *Culture of Animal Cells. A Manual of Basic Technique. 2nd edn.* New York: Alan R. Liss.

Gabbiani, G., Hirschel, B. J., Ryan, G. B. et al. (1972). Granulation tissue as a contractile organ. A study of structure and function. *Journal of Experimental Medicine,* **135**, 719–34.

Gabbiani, G., Lelous, M., Bailey, A. J. & DeLauney, A. (1976). Collagen and myofibrils of granulation tissue. A chemical, ultrastructural and immunologic study. *Virchows Archives (Cellular Pholology),* **21**, 133–45.

Gabbiani, G. & Montandon, D. (1977). Reparative processes in mammalian wound healing: the role of contractile phenomena. *International Reviews of Cytology,* **48**, 187–219.

Galardy, R. E., Grobelny, D., Foellmer, H. G. & Fernandez, L. A. (1994). Inhibition of angiogenesis by the matrix metalloprotease inhibitor N-[2R-2-(hydroxamidocarbonymethyl)-4-methylpentanoyl)]-L-tryptophan methylamide. *Cancer Research,* **54**, 4715–18.

Gijbels, K., Galardy, R. E. & Steineman, L. (1994). Reversal of experimental autoimmune encephalomyelitis with a hydroamate inhibitor of matrix metalloproteases. *Journal of Clinical Investigation,* **94**, 2177–82.

Gordon, S., Unkeless, J. C. & Cohn, Z. A. (1974). Induction of macrophage plasminogen activator by endotoxin stimulation and phagocytosis. *Journal of Experimental Medicine,* **140**, 995–1010.

Grinnell, F. (1984). Fibronectin and wound healing. *Journal of Cellular Biochemistry,* **26**, 107–16.

Grinnell, F. (1994). Mini-review on the cellular mechanisms of disease: Fibroblasts, myofibroblasts and wound contraction. *Journal of Cell Biolology,* **124**, 401–4.

Grotendorst, G. R., Martin, G. R., Pencev, D., Sodek, J. & Harvey, A. K. (1985). Stimulation of granulation tissue by platelet derived growth factor in normal and diabetic rats. *Journal of Clinical Investigation*, **762**, 2323–9.

Guber, S. & Ross, R. (1978). The myofibroblast. *Surgery, Gynecology and Obstetrics*, **146**, 641–9.

Guidry, C. (1993). Fibroblast contraction of collagen gels requires activation of protein kinase C. *Journal of Cellular Physiology*, **155**, 358–67.

Guidry, C. & Grinnell, F. (1985). Studies on the mechanism of hydrated collagen gel reorganization by human skin fibroblasts. *Journal of Cellular Science*, **79**, 67–81.

Harris, A. K. (1973). The behaviour of cultured cells on substrata of variable adhesiveness. *Experimental Cell Research*, **77**, 285–97.

Harris, A. K., Stopak, D. & Wild, P. (1981). Fibroblast traction as a mechanism of for collagen morphogenesis. *Nature*. **290**, 249–51.

Heldin, C. H. & Westermark, B. (1984). Growth factors: mechanism of action and relation to oncogenes. *Cell*. **37**, 9–20.

Ignotz, R. & Massague, J. (1986). Transforming growth factor beta stimulates the expression of fibronectin and their incorporation into the extracellular matrix. *Journal of Biological Chemistry*, **261**, 4337–45.

Indolfi, C., Avvedimente, E. V., Rapacciuolo, A., Di-Lorenzo, E., Esposito, G., Stabile, E., Feliciello, A., Mele, E., Giuliano, P. & Condorelli, G. (1995). Inhibition of cellular ras prevents smooth muscle cell proliferation after vascular injury in vivo. *Nature Medicine*, **1**, 541–5.

Issekutz, T. B., Issekutz, A. C. & Movat, H. Z. (1981). The in vivo quantitation kinetics of monocyte migration into acute inflammatory tissue. *Journal of Pathology*, **103**, 47–55.

Iwasaki, T., Chen, J. D., Kim, J. P., Wynn, K. C. & Woodley, D. T. (1994). Dibutyryl cyclic AMP modulates keratinocyte migration without alteration of integrin expression. *Journal of Investigative Dermatology*, **102**, 891–7.

Jampel, H. D., Leong, K. W., Koya, P. & Quigley, H. A. (1990). The use of hydrophobic drugs incorporated into polyanhydrides in experimental glaucoma surgery. *Investigative Ophthalmology and Vision Science* (*Suppl.*), **31**, 2.

Joseph, J. P., Grierson, I. & Hitchings, R. A. (1987). Normal rabbit aqueous humour, fibronectin and fibroblast conditioned medium are chemoattractant to Tenon's capsule fibroblasts. *Eye*, **1**, 585–92.

Kawase, T., Ogata, S., Orikasa, M. & Burns, D. M. (1995). 1,25-dihydrocyvitamin D3 promoted prostaglandin E1-induced differentiation of HL-60 cells. *Calcified Tissue International*, **57**, 359–66.

Khaw, P. T., Doyle, J. W., Sherwood, M. B., Grierson, I., Schultz, G. S. & McGorray, S. (1993a). Prolonged localized tissue effects from 5-minute exposures to fluorouracil and mitomycin C. *Archives of Ophthalmology*, **111**, 263–7.

Khaw, P. T., Doyle, J. W., Sherwood, M. B., Smith, F. M. & McGorray, S. (1993b). Effects of intraoperative 5-fluorouracil or mitomycin C on glaucoma filtration surgery in the rabbit. *Ophthalmology*, **100**, 367–72.

Khaw, P. T., Sherwood, M. B., Doyle, J. W., Smith, M. F., Grieson, I., McGorray, S. & Schultz, G. S. (1992a). Intraoperative and post operative treatment with 5-Fluorouracil and mitomycin-C: long-term effects in vivo on subconjunctival and scleral fibroblasts. *International Ophthalmology*, **16**, 381–5.

Khaw, P. T., Sherwood, M. B., MacKay, S. L. D., Rossi, M. J. & Schultz, G. S. (1992b). Five-minute treatments with fluorouracil, floxuridine, and mitomycin have long-term effects on human Tenon's capsule fibroblasts. *Archives of Ophthalmology*, **110**, 1150–4.

Khaw, P. T., Ward, S., Grierson, I. & Rice, N. S. C. (1991). The effects of beta-radiation on proliferating human Tenon's capsule fibroblasts. *British Journal of Ophthalmology*, **75**, 580–3.

Khaw, P. T., Ward, S., Porter, A., Grierson, I., Hitchings, R. A. & Rice, N. S. C. (1992c). The long-term effects of 5-fluorouracil and sodium butyrate on human Tenon's fibroblasts. *Investigative Ophthalmology and Vision Science*, **33**, 2043–52.

Klein, C. E., Dressel, D., Steinmayer, T., Mauch, C., Eckes, B., Krieg, T., Bankert, R. B. & Weber, L. (1991). Integrin a2β1 is upregulated in fibroblasts and highly aggressive melanoma cells in three-dimensional collagen lattices and mediates the reorganization of collagen I fibrils. *Journal of Cell Biology*, **115**, 1427–36.

Knighton, D. R., Siver, I. A. & Hunt, T. K. (1984). Studies on inflammation and wound healing: Angiogenesis and collagen synthesis stimulated in vivo by resident and activated wound macrophages. *Surgery*, **96**, 48–54.

Knighton, D. R. & Fiegel, V. D. (1989). The macrophage: effector cell wound repair. In ed. J. C. Passmore, S. M. Reichard, D. G. Reynolds & J. Traber, *Perspectives in Shock Research: Metabolism, Immunology, Mediators and Models*, pp. 211–26. New York: Alan R. Liss.

Kurkinen, M., Vaheri, M., Roberts, P. J. & Stenman, S. (1980). Sequential appearance of fibronectin and collagen in experimental granulation tissue. *Laboratory Investigation*, **43**, 47–51.

Laird, J. R., Carter, A. J., Kufs, W. M., Hoopes, T. G., Farb, A., Nott, S. H., Fischell, R. E., Fischell, D. R., Virmani, R. & Fischell, T. A. (1996). Inhibition of neointimal proliferation with low-dose irradiation from a beta particle-emitting stent. *Circulation*, **93**, 529–36.

Lane, D. A., Pejler, G., Flynn, A. M., Thompson, E. A. & Lindahl, U. (1986). Neutralization of heparin-related saccharides by histidine-rich glycoprotein and platelet factor 4. *Journal of Biological Chemistry*, **261**, 3980–6.

Leppert, D., Waubant, E., Galardy, R. E., Bunnett, N. W. & Hauser, S. L. (1995). T cell gelatinases mediate basement membrane transmigration in vitro. *Journal of Immunology*, **154**, 4379–89.

Lewalle, J. M., Munaut, C., Pichot, B., Cataldo, D., Baramova, E. & Foidart, J. M. (1995). Plasma membrane-dependent activation of gelatinase A in human vascular endothelial cells. *Journal of Cell Physiology*, **165**, 475–83.

Lewis, J. (1984). Morphogenesis by fibroblast traction. *Nature*, **307**, 413–14.

Mackenzie, I. C. & Fusenig, N. E. (1983). Regeneration of organized epithelial structure. *Journal of Investigative Dermatology*, **81**, 1895–1945.

McCarthy, J. B., Sas, D. F. & Furcht, L. T. (1988). Mechanisms of parenchymal cell migration into wounds. In *The Molecular and Cellular Biology of Wound Repair*, ed. R. A. F. Clark and P. M. Henson, pp. 281–319. New York: Plenium Press.

McDonald, J. A., Kelley, D. G. & Broekelmann, T. J. (1982). Role of fibronectin in collagen deposition. Fab1 antibodies to the gelatin-binding domain of fibronectin inhibits both fibronectin and collagen organization in fibroblast extracellular matrix. *Journal of Cell Biology*, **92**, 485–92.

McGuigan, L. J. B., Cook, D. J. & Yablonski, M. E. (1986). Dexamethasone, D-penicillamine, and glaucoma filtering surgery in rabbits. *Investigative Ophthalmology and Vision Science*, **27**, 1755.

McGuigan, L. J. B., Mason, R. P., Sanchez, R. & Quigley, H. A. (1987). D-penicillamine and beta-aminopropionitrile effects on experimental filtering surgery. *Investigative Ophthalmoogy and Vision Science*, **28**, 1625–9.

Martin, P. & Lewis, J. (1992). Actin cables and epidermal movement in embryonic wound healing. *Nature*, **360**, 179–82.

Matrisian, L. M. (1992). The matrix-degrading metalloproteinases. *Bioessays*, **14**, 455–63.

Maynard, J. R., Heckman, C. A., Pitlick, F. A. & Namerson, Y. A. (1975). Association of tissue factor activity with the surface of cultured cells. *Journal of Clinical Investigation*, **55**, 814–24.

Metcalfe, R. A. & Weetman, A. P. (1994). Stimulation of extraocular muscle fibroblasts by cytokines and hypoxia: possible role in thyroid-associated ophthalmology. *Clinical Endocrinology*, **40**, 67–72.

Miller, M. & Rice, N. (1991). Trabeculectomy combined with B radiation for congenital glaucoma. *British Journal of Ophthalmology*, **75**, 584–90.

Moore, M. J. (1995). Exploration by lamp light. *Nature*, **374**, 766–7.

Moorhead, L. C., Stewart, R. H., Kimbrough, P. L., Gross, R. L., Cyrlin, M. N., LeBlanc, R. P., Shields, M. B. & Kapetansky, F. N. (1990). Use of beta-aminopropiononitrile following glaucoma filtering surgery. *Investigative Ophthalmology and Vision Science*, **31** (Supp.), 3.

Nelson, R. D., McCormack, R. T. & Fiegel, V. D. (1978). Chemotaxis of human leukocytes under agarose. In *Leukocyte Chemotaxis*, ed. J. I. Gallin and P. C. Quie, pp. 25–42. New York: Raven Press.

Newby, A. C., Southgate, K. M. & Davies, M. (1994). Extracellular matrix degrading metalloproteinases in the pathogenesis of arteriosclerosis. *Basic Research in Cardiology*, **89**, 59–70.

Noda-Heiny, H. & Sobel, B. E. (1995). Vascular smooth muscle cell migration mediated by thrombin and urokinase receptor. *American Journal of Physiology*, **268**, C1195–C1201.

Occleston, N. L., Alexander, R. A., Mazure, A., Larkin, G. & Khaw, P. T. (1994). Effects of single exposures to antiproliferative agents on ocular fibroblast mediated collagen contraction. *Investigative Ophthalmology and Vision Science*, **35**, 3681–90.

Oh, E., Pierschbacher, M. & Ruoslahti, E. (1981). Deposition of plasma fibronectin in tissues. *Proceedings of the National Academy of Sciences of the USA*. **78**, 3218–21.

Okada, S. S., Kuo, A., Muttreja, M. R., Hozakowska, E., Weisz, P. B. & Barnathan, E. S. (1995). Inhibition of human vascular smooth muscle cell migration and proliferation by beta-cyclodextrin tetradecasulfate. *Journal of Pharmacological Experimental Therapy*, **273**, 948–54.

Paulsson, M., Fujiwara, S., Dziadek, M., Timpl, R., Pejler, G., Backstrom, G., Lindahl, U. & Engel, J. (1986). Structure and function of basement membrane proteoglycans. In *Functions of the Proteoglycans*, ed. D. Evered and J. Whelan, pp. 189–203. New York: John Wiley.

Pauly, R. R., Passaniti, A., Bilato, C., Monticone, R., Cheng, L., Papadopoulos, N., Gluzband, Y. A., Smith, L., Weinstein, C., Lakatta, E. G. & Crow, M. T. (1994). Migration of cultures vascular smooth muscle cells through a basement membrane barrier requires type IV collagenase activity and is inhibited by cellular differentiation. *Circulation Research*, **75**, 41–54.

Postlethwaite, A. E. & Kang, A. H. (1980). Characterization of guinea pig lymphocyte-derived chemotactic factor for fibroblasts. *Journal of Immunology*, **124**, 1426–66.

Postlethwaite, A. E., Keski-Oja, J., Moses, H. L. & Kang, A. H. (1987). Stimulation of the chemotactic migration of human fibroblasts by transforming growth factor beta. *Journal of Experimental Medicine*, **165**, 251–6.

Postlethwaite, A. E., Seyer, J. M. & Kang, A. H. (1978). Chemotactic attraction of human fibroblasts to type I, II and III collagens and collagen-derived peptides. *Proceedings of the National Academy of Sciences of the USA*, **75**, 871–5.

Postlethwaite, A. E., Snyderman, R. & Kang, A. H. (1976). The chemotactic attraction of human fibroblasts to a lymphocyte derived factor. *Journal of Experimental Medicine*, **144**, 1188–203.

Postlethwaite, A. E., Snyderman, R. K. & Kang, A. H. (1979). Generation of a fibroblast chemotactic factor in serum by activation of complement. *Journal of Clinical Investigation*, **64**, 1379–85.

Riches, D. W. (1988). The multiple roles of macrophages in wound healing. In *The Molecular and Cellular Biology of Wound Repair*, ed. R. A. F. Clark and P. M. Henson, pp. 213. New York: Plenum Press.

Robbins, K. C., Summaria, L. & Wohl, R. (1981). *Human plasmin. Methods in Enzymology*, **80**, 379–87.

Ross, R. (1989). Platelet-derived growth factor. *Lancet*, **8648**, 1179–81.

Ross, R. & Odland, G. (1968). Human wound repair. II. Inflammatory cells, epithelial mesenchymal interrelations and fibrogenesis. *Journal of Cell Biology*, **39**, 152–68.

Ross, R., Raines, E. W. & Bowen-Pope, D. F. (1986). The biology of platelet derived growth factor. *Cell*, **46**, 155–69.

Roth, S. M., Starita, R. J., Spaeth, G. L., Steinmann, W. C. & Paryzees, E. M. (1988). The effects of postoperative corticosteroids on trabeculectomy: long-term follow-up. *Investigative Ophthalmology and Vision Science*, Suppl. 367.

Saarialho, U. K., Kovacs, S. O., Pentland, A. P., Olerud, J. E., Welgus, H. G. & Parks, W. C. (1993). Cell–matrix interactions modulate interstitial collagenase expression by human keratinocytes actively involved in wound healing. *Journal of Clinical Investigation*, **92**, 2858–66.

Saarialho-Kere, U. K., Vaalamo, M., Airola, K., Niemi, K., Oikarinen, A. I. & Parks, W. C. (1995). Interstitial collagenase is expressed by keratinocytes that are actively involved in reepithelialization in blistering skin diseases. *Journal of Investigative Dermatology*, **104**, 982–8.

Samuelsson, B., Golyne, M., Granstrom, E., Hamberg, M., Hammarstrom, S. & Malmsten, C. (1978). Prostaglandins and thromboxanes. *Annual Reviews in Biochemistry*, **47**, 997–1029.

Sato, H., Takino, T., Okado, Y., Cao, J., Shinagawa, A., Yamamoto, E. & Seiki, M. (1994). A matrix metalloproteinase expressed on the surface of invasive tumour cells. *Nature*, **370**, 61–5.

Schiro, J. A., Chan, B. M. C., Roswit, W. T., Kassner, P. D., Pentland, A. P., Hemler, M. E., Eisen, A. Z. & Kupper, T. S. (1991). Integrin a2β1 (VLA-2) mediates reorganization and contraction of collagen matrices by human cells. *Cell*, **67**, 403–10.

Schor, S. L. (1980). Cell proliferation and migration on collagen substrata in vitro. *Journal of Cell Science*, **41**, 159–75.

Senior, R. M., Griffin, G. L. & Mechan, R. P. (1984). Val-Gly-Val-Ala-Pro-Gly: a repeating peptide in elastin, is chemotactic for fibroblasts and monocytes. *Journal of Cell Biology*, **99**, 870–4.

Senior, R. M., Skogen, W. F., Griffin, G. L. & Wilner, G. D. (1986). Effects of fibrinogen derivatives upon the inflammatory response. *Journal of Clinical Investigation*, **77**, 1014–19.

Seppa, H. E. J., Grotendorst, G. R., Seppa, S. I., Schiffmann, E. & Martin, G. R. (1982). Platelet-derived growth factor is chemotactic for fibroblasts. *Journal of Cell Biology*, **92**, 584–8.

Shah, M., Foreman, D. M. & Ferguson, M. W. J. (1992). Control of scarring in adult wounds by neutralising antibody to transforming growth factor beta. *Lancet*, **339**, 213–14.

Shah, M., Foreman, D. M. & Ferguson, M. W. J. (1994). Neutralising antibody to TGF-beta1,2 reduces cutaneous scarring in adult rodents. *Journal of Cell Science*, **107**, 1137–57.

Shah, M., Foreman, D. M. & Ferguson, M. W. J. (1995). Neutralisation if TGF-beta1 and TGF-beta2 or exogenous additon of TGF-beta 3 to cutaneous rat wounds reduces scarring. *Journal of Cell Science*, **108**, 985–1002.

Siegel, R. C. (1977). Collagen cross-linking effect of D-penicillamine on cross-linking in vivo. *Journal of Biological Chemistry*, **252**, 254.

Sobel, J. D. & Gallin, J. I. (1979). Polymorphonuclear leukocyte and monocyte chemoattractants produced by human fibroblasts. *Journal of Clinical Investigation*, **63**, 609–18.

Sollott, S. J., Cheng, L., Pauly, R. R., Jenkins, G. M., Monticone, R. E., Kuzuya, M., Froelich, J. P., Crow, M. T., Lakatta, E. G., Rowinsky, E. K. & Kinsella, J. L. (1995). Taxol inhibits neointimal smooth muscle cell accumulation after angioplasty in the rat. *Journal of Clinical Investigation*, **95**, 1869–76.

Sporn, M. B., Roberts, A. B., Shull, J. H., Smith, J. M., Ward, J. M. & Sodek, J. (1983). Polypeptide transforming growth factor isolated from bovine sources and used for wound healing in vitro. *Science*, **219**, 1329–31.

Stopak, D. & Harris, A. K. (1982). Connective tissue morphogenesis by fibroblast traction. I. Tissue culture observations. *Develoments in Biology*, **90**, 383–98.

Strongin, A. Y., Collier, I., Bannikov, G., Marmer, B. L., Grant, G. A. & Goldberg, G. I. (1995). Mechanism of cell surface activation of 72-kDa type IV collagenase. *Journal of Biological Chemistry*, . **270**, 5331–8.

Takino, T., Sato, H., Shinagawa, A. & Seiki, M. (1995). Identification of the second membrane-type matrix metalloproteinase (MT-MMP-2) gene from a human placenta cDNA library. *Journal of Biological Chemistry*, **270**, 23013–20.

Tanaka, K., Honda, M., Kuramochi, T. & Morioka, S. (1994). Prominent inhibitory effects of tranilast on migration and proliferation of and collagen synthesis by vascular smooth muscle cells. *Atherosclerosis*, **107**, 179–85.

Tarnuzzer, R. W., Macauley, S. P., Farmerie, W. G., Caballero, S., Ghassemifar, M. R., Anderson, J. T., Robinson, C. P., Grant, M. B., Humphreys-Beher, M. G., Franzen, L., Peck, A. B. & Schultz, G. S. (1996). Competitive RNA templates for detection and quantitation of growth factors, cytokines, extracellular matrix compnents and matrix metalloproteinases by RT-PCR. *Biotechniques*, **20**, 670–4.

Tomasek, J. J. & Hay, E. D. (1984). Analysis of the role of microfilaments and microtubules in acquisition of bipolarity and elongation of fibroblasts in hydrated collagen gels. *Journal of Cell Biology*, **99**, 536–49.

Tyagi, S. C., Meyer, L., Schmaltz, R. A., Reddy, H. K. & Voelker, D. J. (1995). Proteinases and restenosis in the human coronary artery: extracellular matrix production exceeds the expression of proteolytic activity. *Atherosclerosis*, **116**, 43–57.

Verin, V., Popowski, Y., Urban, P., Belenger, J., Redard, M., Costa, M., Widmer, M. C., Rouzaud, M., Nouet, P. & Grob, E. (1995). Intra-arterial beta irradiation prevents neointimal hyperplasia in a hypercholesterolemic rabbit restenosis model. *Circulation*, **92**, 2284–90.

Voisard, R., Seitzer, U., Baur, R., Dartsch, P. C., Osterhues, H., Hoher, M. & Hombach, V. (1995). A prescreening system for potential antiproliferation agents: implications for local treatment strategies of postangioplasty restenosis. *International Journal of Cardiology*, **51**, 15–28.

Wahl, S. M. (1989). Glucocorticoids and wound healing. In *Antiinflammatory Steroid Action*: *Basic and Clinical Aspects*, ed. R. P. Scleimer and E. Claman, pp. 280–302. New York: Academic Press.

Waksman, R., Robinson, K. A., Crocker, I. R., Wang, C., Gravanis, M. B., Cipolla, G. D., Hillstead, P. A. & King, S. B. I. (1995). Intracoronary low-dose beta-irradiation inhibits neointima formation after coronary artery balloon injury in the swine restenosis model. *Circulation*, **92**, 3025–31.

Weiss, P. (1945). The problem of specificity in growth and development. *Yale Journal of Biology and Medicine*, **19**, 239–78.

Weiss, P. (1958). Cell contact. *International Reviews in Cytology*, **7**, 391–423.

Werb, Z., Banda, M. J. & Jones, P. A. (1980). Degradation of connective tissue matrics by macrophages. I. Proteolysis of elastin glycoproteins and collagen by proteinases isolated from macrophages. *Journal of Experimental Medicine*, **152**, 1340–57.

Werb, Z., Mainardi, C., Vater, C. A. & Harris, E. D. J. (1977). Endogenous activation of latent collagenase by rheumatoid synovial cells. Evidence for a role of plasminogen activator. *New England Journal of Medicine*, **296**, 1017–23.

Williams, I. F., McCullagh, K. G. & Silver, I. A. (1984). The distribution of types I and III collagen and fibronectin in the healing equine tendon. *Connective Tissue Research*, **12**, 211–27.

Wilson, C. & Szostak, J. W. (1995). In vitro evolution of a self-alkylating ribozyme. *Nature*. **374**, 777–82.

Woessner, J. F. J. (1991). Matrix metalloproteinases and their inhibitors in connective tissue remodeling. *FASEB J*, **5**, 2145–54.

Woodley, D. T., Kalebec, T., Banes, A. J., Link, W., Prunieras, M. & Liotta, L. (1986). Adult human keratinocytes migrating over nonviable dermal collagen produce collagenolytic enzymes that degrade type I and type IV collagen. *Journal of Investigative Dermatology*, **86**, 418–23.

Woodley, D. T., O'Keefe, E. J. & Prunieras, M. (1985). Cutaneous wound healing: A model for cell-matrix interactions. *Journal of the American Academy of Dermatology*, **12**, 420–33.

Wysocki, S. J., Zheng, M., Fan, Y., Lamawansa, M. D., House, A. K. & Norman, P. E. (1996). Expression of transforming growth factor-beta1 (TGF-beta1) and urokinase-type plasminogen activator (u-PA) genes during arterial repair in the pig. *Cardiovascular Research*, **31**, 28–36.

Zigmond, S. H. & Hirsch, J. G. A. (1973). Leukocyte locomotion and chemotaxis: new methods for evaluation and demonstration of a cell derived chemotactic factor. *Journal of Experimental Medcine*, **137**, 387–410.

Zigmond, S. H. (1977). Ability of polymorphonuclear leukocytes to orient in gradients of chemotactic factors. *Journal of Cell Biology*, **75**, 606–16.

14

Endothelial function in inflammation, sepsis, reperfusion and the vasculitides

B. J. HUNT and K. M. JURD

Introduction

The endothelium is much more than the inert lining to blood vessels that it was originally considered to be, but is a highly specialized, metabolically active, organ. Resting endothelial cells which form a monolayer maintaining a barrier between blood constituents and the extravascular space, also exert multifunctional homeostatic effects (Table 14.1). Although only one cell thick, the endothelium constitutes a dynamic interface between the blood and the rest of the body. It is also increasingly recognized that endothelial cells are heterogeneous, in that the function and phenotype of endothelial cells is specialized according to their particular site, for example cerebral endothelial cells lack thrombomodulin (see below), and not all endothelial cells constitutively express histocompatibility locus A(HLA) class II molecules.

The quiescent endothelium maintains a status quo, but under the stimulation of certain agents such as interleukin 1 (IL-1) and tissue necrosis factor (TNF) it undergoes a series of metabolic changes and participates in the inflammatory process; this is known as *endothelial cell activation* (ECA) and is a central pathophysiological event.

The term endothelial cell activation was coined in the late 1960s when Willms-Kretshmer (Willms-Kretchmer et al, 1967) noted that in delayed hypersensitivity reactions venules became leaky and their endothelial cell linings became plump and protruded into the lumen. These endothelial cells also displayed increased quantities of biosynthetic organelles (such as endoplasmic reticulum). He referred to these endothelial cells as being 'activated', implying that there was a functional consequence to the altered morphology. In the 1970s this view of the endothelium having a dynamic function was ignored and the endothelium was considered to be inert and passive.

In the 1980s, however, there was growing realization that when endothelial cells were exposed in vitro to cytokines which mediate the inflammatory response, they exhibited new surface molecules and biological functions. To emphasize that this process did not represent sublethal injury with consequent dysfunction, Pober reintroduced the term ECA with the following definition: 'a quantitative change in the level of expression of certain gene products (i.e. proteins) that, in turn, endow endothelial cells with the new

Table 14.1. *Functions of the vascular endothelium*

Maintenance of selective permeability
Integration and transduction of blood–borne signals
Regulation of inflammatory and immune reactions
Regulation of vascular tone
Maintenance of thromboresistance
Modulation of leukocyte interactions with tissues
Regulation of vascular growth

capacities that cumulatively allow endothelial cells to perform new functions' (Pober, 1988).

Today the extraordinary multifunctional ability of endothelial cells to control and mediate inflammation is recognized at both basic science and clinical scientific meetings. Few scientists study all aspects of ECA but concentrate on the area relevant to them. Meetings on endothelial cells are characterized by the diversity of approaches used to study these multifunctional cells. Due to the complexity of the subject many are working on one aspect without being aware of the other areas. To an immunologist ECA means upregulation of MHC class II antigens, the expression of cell adhesion molecules and the production of certain cytokines. To those involved in thrombosis, ECA produces a change in phenotype from antithrombotic to prothrombotic. To the vascular biologist there is alteration in tone, due to changes in prostacyclin and nitric oxide (NO), which also promote platelet aggregation. In fact all these changes are present in ECA; biological functions cannot be pigeon holed and are often mutually dependent and interactive. For example, the haemostatic and immunological responses of the endothelium are intergrated; immunoregulatory cytokines such as IL-1 stimulate tissue factor (TF) expression, while thrombin, a molecule central in haemostasis has a number of bioregulatory roles, including chemotaxis, platelet activation and fibrinogen cleavage. Hence proinflammatory and prothrombotic responses are interlinked as part of host defence and the physical and biological behaviour of cells involved in these mechanisms can be dramatically affected by interactions between them.

ECA plays a central pathophysiological role in a number of diseases (Table 14.2). In this chapter the various aspects of the current understanding of endothelial cell activation are reviewed and the changes in specific states discussed.

Agents causing ECA include the cytokines IL-1 and TNF, bacterial endotoxin, i.e. lipopolysaccharide, complement, viral infections and immune complexes. Knowledge concerning ECA is largely based on in vitro stimulation by IL-1, TNF or lipopolysaccharide (LPS). Pober & Cotran (1991) have distinguished two types of endothelial cell response. The first 'endothelial cell stimulation', or type I ECA, does not require de novo protein synthesis or gene upregulation (e.g. the release of von Willebrand factor), and the second 'endothelial cell activation', or Type II ECA, which does. Thus ECA requires a period of time for the stimulating agent to cause an effect (e.g. expression of tissue factor

Table 14.2. *Diseases where the endothelium is critically involved*

Adult respiratory distress syndrome
Atherosclerosis
Diabetic vasculopathy
Haemolytic uraemic syndrome
Kawasaki's syndrome
Thrombotic thrombocytopenic purpura
Transplant rejection, both allograft and xenograft
Systemic inflammatory response syndrome
Vasculitis

by endothelial cells in culture occurs after 4–6 h), whereas in endothelial cell stimulation the response occurs within seconds.

Type I activation involves retraction of endothelial cells from one another, exposing underlying subendothelium. This is accompanied by expression of P-selectin, release of von Willebrand factor and secretion of platelet activating factor (PAF). Type II activation includes progressive induction, at the level of transcription, of many genes including leukocyte adhesion molecules (E-selectin, ICAM-1 and VCAM-1), cytokines (IL-1, IL-6, IL-8) and monocyte chemoattractant protein (MCP), and tissue factor which is the main initiator of coagulation. Thrombomodulin and other functionally important molecules are lost from the surface of endothelial cells (Bach et al, 1995).

Changes in endothelial cell activation

There are five main changes associated with ECA: loss of vascular integrity; expression of leukocyte adhesion molecules; secretion of cytokines; prothrombotic changes and upregulation of HLA molecules. They are reviewed below and summarized in Fig. 14.1.

Loss of vascular integrity

In type I ECA, after stimulation with agents such as thrombin or histamine, endothelial cells retract from one another leaving gaps that allow cells and proteins to pass from the intravascular space to the underlying tissue space.

Expression of leukocyte adhesion molecules

The key molecules are the integrins, E-selectin, P-selectin. Leukocyte–endothelial interactions (for recent reviews see Adams & Shaw, 1994; Carlos & Harlan, 1994), involve four sequential steps of tethering, triggering, strong adhesion and migration (Fig. 14.2). Tethering of circulating leukocytes to the endothelium results in their rolling along the vessel wall. Triggering agents, mainly cytokines, activate leukocyte adhesion molecules

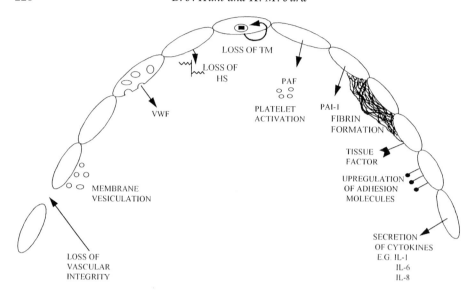

Fig. 14.1. Changes associated with endothelial cell activation. TM: thrombomoduline; HS: heparan sulphate; VWF: von Willebrand factor; PAF: Platelet activating factor; PAI-1: Plasminogen activator inhibitor type 1.

such as integrins. This step is vital as integrins on circulating leukocytes do not bind to endothelium until activated. Integrin-mediated binding to endothelial adhesion molecules following triggering results in strong adhesion and flattening of leukocytes which then become motile and migrate into the tissues. This sequence of events can be viewed as a cascade reaction similar to the complement and coagulation cascades.

Tethering is mediated by the selectins. E-selectin is synthesized and expressed by endothelial cells when activated by cytokines. P-selectin is expressed by activated endothelium and by platelets. It is present on the inner surface of intracellular storage bodies, known as Weibel Palade bodies, in the cytoplasm of endothelial cells and alpha granules of platelets. These bodies store von Willebrand factor. On stimulation of endothelial cells the Weibel Palade bodies fuse with the endothelial cell surface membrane, discharging their contents and exposing P-selectin. Surface expression of P-selectin is rapid and transient, peaking at 10 min and returning to normal by 20–30 min; however, more recent studies have demonstrated surface expression of P-selectin which lasts for hours rather than minutes when stimulated by thrombin or oxygen radicals. L-selectin is constitutively expressed on most leukocytes. Each selectin recognizes specific carbohydrate motifs on either endothelial cells or leukocytes. The endothelial cell selectins extend beyond the surrounding glycocalyx so allowing capture of circulating leukocytes that express the appropriate receptor. This loose association of leukocyte and endothelium allows exposure to triggering factors which activate leukocyte integrins.

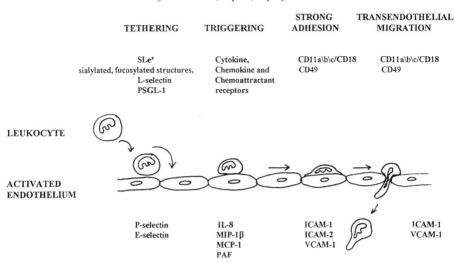

TETHERING	TRIGGERING	STRONG ADHESION	TRANSENDOTHELIAL MIGRATION
SLe^x sialylated, fucosylated structures, L-selectin PSGL-1	Cytokine, Chemokine and Chemoattractant receptors	CD11a\b\c/CD18 CD49	CD11a\b\c/CD18 CD49

LEUKOCYTE

ACTIVATED ENDOTHELIUM

| P-selectin E-selectin | IL-8 MIP-1β MCP-1 PAF | ICAM-1 ICAM-2 VCAM-1 | ICAM-1 VCAM-1 |

Fig. 14.2. Leukocyte adhesion. Simplified representation of leukocyte–endothelial adhesion reactions. Tethering of leukocytes to activated endothelium is mediated by low-affinity interactions between selectins. Strong adhesion and transendothelial migration are dependent on higher affinity reactions involving integrins and the IgG supergene family of adhesion molecules. PSGL-1: P-selectin glycosylation ligand 1; IL-8: interleukin 8; MIP 1β: monocyte inducible protein 1β; MCP-1: monocyte chemotactic protein 1; PAF, platelet activating factor; ICAM-1, intercellular adhesion molecule 1; VCAM-1: vascular cell adhesion molecule 1. The interactions shown are simplified and are not exclusive.

Integrins consist of α and β subunits and can be grouped according to their β subunit. At least four leukocyte integrins mediate strong adhesion. These are the β2 integrins CD11a/b/c, CD11a on lymphocytes and Mac-1 (CD11b) on neutrophils and monocytes, and β1 integrin CD49d on lymphocytes and monocytes. Activation of leukocytes triggers an increase in avidity caused by a conformational change in the integrin heterodimer. Once activated the leukocyte integrins bind to counter receptors on the endothelium, endothelial cell adhesion molecules, which are members of the immunoglobulin gene superfamily. β2 integrins bind to intercellular adhesion molecule 1 (ICAM-1) and ICAM-2. ICAM-2 is constitutively expressed on the endothelium, but ICAM-1 is increased with endothelial cell activation and inflammation. The β1 integrin mediates binding of lymphocytes and monocytes to vascular cell adhesion molecule 1 (VCAM-1) which is induced by proinflammatory cytokines. Important triggering factors for expression of integrins are IL-8, produced by the endothelium itself or underlying inflammatory cells; PAF, a phospholipid that is rapidly produced by endothelium in response to thrombin, histamine or leukotrienes; MIP-1β, bound to endothelial proteoglycans, bacterial wall components, and complement activation products. Following strong adhesion to the endothelium, leukocytes migrate into the tissues. Many of the cytokines that trigger strong adhesion are also chemotactic. IL-8 induces adhesion and chemotaxis of neutrophils and MIP-1β induces adhesion and migration of T cells.

In addition to host defence, endothelial–leukocyte interactions contribute to pathological inflammatory conditions such as reperfusion injury after ischaemia, autoimmunity, graft rejection and allergic reactions. Diseases characterized by acute inflammation and neutrophil infiltration show increased expression of E and P-selectin, whereas in chronic lymphocytic inflammation there is increased VCAM-1 expression. E-selectin, ICAM-1 and VCAM-1 are transcriptionally regulated by cytokines, LPS and other inflammatory mediators. Different combinations of cytokines can differentially modulate their induction. There are also differences in the ability to express these molecules between endothelium in large vessels and the microvasculature.

Cytokine production

Cytokines are important mediators of inflammation. They promote innate immunity and host defence in infectious disease, but also augment the pathogenesis of noninfectious inflammatory states contributing to tissue injury. In addition to acting as a target for the action of cytokines, the endothelium is an important source of these molecules (Table 14.3). Endothelium stimulated with IL-1, TNF, IFN or LPS produces cytokines. Endothelial cells synthesise large amounts of IL-6 that affects the proliferation of T and B cells and regulates production of acute phase proteins in the liver. Stimulation of the endothelium with LPS, TNF or IL-1, itself, induces IL-1 production by endothelial cells which amplifies the inflammatory response. The endothelium also releases chemoattractants such as IL-8 and MCP-1 (Mantovani & Dejana, 1989).

Prothrombotic changes

The antithrombotic effects of the resting endothelium can be separated into antiplatelet, anticoagulant and fibrinolytic. The prothrombotic effects of the endothelium are due to loss of antithrombotic effects and expression of prothrombotic molecules. These changes are reviewed below.

Antiplatelet/vasodilator effects

The key molecules are nitric oxide, prostacyclin, platelet activating factor (PAF), endothelin, ecto-ADPase.

EC exhibit an antithrombotic effect by reducing platelet reactivity by synthesizing and releasing prostacyclin (PGI_2), nitric oxide (NO), and also ecto-ADPase (for recent reviews see Davies et al, 1995; Marcus et al, 1991; Marcus, 1994; Bach et al, 1994; Hamblin, 1990).

Prostacyclin is a potent inhibitor of platelet aggregation and a powerful vasodilator. It is transiently and rapidly secreted in response to a variety of agonists including thrombin, histamine and adenosine diphosphate (ADP) thereby acting locally to inhibit the spread of thrombus.

Nitric oxide is a potent inhibitor of platelet aggregation and works synergistically with prostacyclin. The vascular relaxant and platelet inhibitory action of NO are

Table 14.3. *Cytokines produced by the endothelium*

Cytokine	Function
IL-1	Lymphocyte activation: Local and systemic inflammation Acute phase response Haematopoiesis
IL-6	Lymphocyte activation Acute phase response Haematopoiesis
CSFs	Leukocyte recruitment and activation Haematopoiesis Endothelial cell proliferation
Chemotactic factors (MCP-1, IL-8)	Leukocyte recruitment and activation
PDGF	Smooth muscle cell proliferation

Note: CSFs: colony stimulating factors; IL: interleukin; MCP: monocyte chemoattractant protein; PDGF: platelet-derived growth factor.

mediated via stimulation of soluble guanylate cyclase, thus elevating cyclic GMP levels in smooth muscle cells and platelets. This contrasts with the biological actions of prostacyclin, many of which are mediated via elevation of cyclic adenosine monophosphate (AMP) levels. Unlike prostacyclin, NO also inhibits platelet adhesion to subendothelium.

NO is synthesized by NO synthase (NOS). There are different classes of NO synthetase, one is constitutively (cNOS) expressed by endothelial cells, neuronal cells and several other cell types and is regulated by Ca^{2+} and calmodulin (Chapter 3). NO is released from the endothelium under basal conditions, and also in response to a number of physiological stimuli such as shear stress, circulating hormones (noradrenaline, vasopressin, bradykinin) and various autacoids (acetylcholine, histamine, substance P). Shear stress, in particular, appears to be a major stimulus for NO release, for NO activity is highest in largest diameter arteries that are subject to greater variation in pulsatile flow and shear stress.

The other class of NO syntase is an inducible enzyme (iNOS) which is found in macrophages and neutrophils. It is induced after cytokine exposure and is capable of generating far greater quantities of NO than cNOS; for at high concentrations NO is cytotoxic and thus plays a key role in the immune response to bacteria and other pathogens.

Rapid production of PAF is induced by many of the agonists that induce prostacyclin synthesis and causes platelet secretion and aggregation. Activated platelets release ATP and ADP from their dense granules. Adenine nucleotides are relatively stable and a system to degrade them is provided by ectonucleotidases at the endothelial cell surface, thus endothelial cells inhibit platelet aggregation, in part, by ecto-ADPase activity.

Ecto-ADPase catalyses hydrolysis of ATP and ADP to AMP and orthophosphate. ECs converts AMP to adenosine which has an antiaggregating effect. When endothelial cells are activated in vitro, platelet aggregation occurs associated with loss of ecto-ADPase activity, which will permit accumulation of ADP, a potent stimulus to platelet thrombosis.

Endothelin is the most potent vasoconstrictor known, and produces contraction of isolated arteries and veins. It is released in response to hypoxia, thrombin, transforming growth factor β (TGF-β) and noradrenaline. After binding to specific receptors endothelin promotes influx of calcium ions and release of calcium from intracellular stores, resulting in phosphorylation of myosin light chains and initiation of smooth muscle contraction (Chapter 3). It also has mitogenic properties, stimulating DNA synthesis in vascular smooth muscle, and more recently has been shown to stimulate neutrophil adhesion to endothelial cells through an effect on CD11/CD18. A critical balance exists between NO and endothelin: this may be a major determinant in the regulation of local and systemic haemodynamic function and cellular proliferation.

Anticoagulant pathways

The key molecules are antithrombin III (now known as antithrombin), heparan sulphate; thrombomodulin, tissue factor pathway inhibitor.

Aortic, venous and microvascular endothelium exert a profound anticoagulant effect by expressing heparan sulphate proteoglycans, consisting of a protein core to which heparan sulphate glycosaminglyocan chains are attached. Heparan sulphate potentiates antithrombin (AT) activity, which is a major physiological anticoagulant. Antithrombin is an irreversible inhibitor of not only thrombin as the name suggests, but of the majority of intrinsic coagulation proteases. Heparan sulphate, expressed on EC surfaces *in vivo*, acts as an endogenous catalyst for the anticoagulant actions of AT.

Heparan sulphate proteoglycans are the predominating proteoglycans of the endothelium. Cytokines stimulate synthesis of the glycosaminoglycans whilst physical injury, hypoxia and viral infection decrease its synthesis (Ihrcke et al, 1996). During inflammation heparan sulphate is released from the endothelium. Mechanisms causing this release include cleavage of the glycosaminoglycan chains by heparanases, produced by many cell types including activated platelets, activated endothelial cells and activated T cells. Proteases from activated T cells and neutrophil elastase may also cause heparan sulphate release through proteolysis of the protein core. The binding of antibodies to endothelial cells and the activation of complement also causes rapid release of heparan sulphate.

Apart from its anticoagulant function heparan sulphate is also important in maintaining vascular integrity and its loss from the surface may result in oedema and exudation of plasma proteins. There is also evidence that heparan sulphate can influence cellular immune responses through interactions with antigen presenting cells. Heparan sulphate tethers extracellular superoxide dismutase (SOD) to the vessel wall. The loss of heparan sulphate during ECA thus results in loss of both anticoagulant and anti-free radical mechanisms.

Thrombomodulin is an endothelial cell surface expressed glycoprotein, which is a critical receptor in the protein C anticoagulant system (Esmon & Owen, 1989). This system is activated when coagulation is initiated and thrombin is generated. Thrombin bound to thrombomodulin on the surface of endothelial cells allows it to bind and activate protein C. (Thrombin once bound to thrombomodulin loses its coagulant activity and is no longer able to convert fibrinogen to fibrin, or activate platelets.) Activated protein C, together with its cofactor protein S, act as an anticoagulant by inactivating factors Va and VIIIa thus limiting further thrombin generation.

ECA results in the loss of thrombomodulin from the endothelial cell surface. This is due to internalization of thrombomodulin, decreased transcription of mRNA and subsequent downregulation of thrombomodulin synthesis (Moore et al, 1989). Interestingly thrombomodulin is absent from the human cerebral endothelium. Other anticoagulant pathways such as protease nexin II may be important here.

Tissue factor pathway inhibitor (TFPI) is produced by the endothelium and inhibits the first steps of the extrinsic coagulation pathway by inhibiting FXa and the tissue factor/VIIa complex (Rapaport, 1991). Much of circulating TFPI is bound to lipoprotein, and platelets carry about 10% of circulating TFPI which they release upon activation. TFPI is also released into the circulation in response to heparin (Sandset et al, 1988) and other glycosaminoglycans to a lesser degree. It has been suggested that TFPI is bound to endothelial cell glycosaminoglycans, but this not certain. The main physiological role of TFPI appears to be in the inhibition of small amounts of tissue factor and is thus probably essential for maintaining a normal haemostatic balance. The effect of ECA on TFPI levels is uncertain, but it is increased in plasma by endotoxin suggesting it may be upregulated at the same time as tissue factor.

Procoagulant effects

The key molecules are von Willebrand factor, tissue factor, vesicles with prothrombinase activity.

von Willebrand factor is stored in Weibel Palade bodies in endothelial cells and in alpha granules in platelets, and is also present free in plasma and anchored in the subendothelium (Wagner, 1990). When platelets are activated it acts as the ligand for platelet adhesion by binding to a specific platelet receptor, glycoprotein Ib. Following type 1 ECA, Weibel Palade bodies fuse with the endothelial cell membrane releasing von Willebrand factor. The inner surface of the Weibel Palade bodies is coated with P-selectin, which is thus expressed on the endothelial cell surface. In the plasma von Willebrand factor is also the carrier for factor VIII, thus levels of factor VIII and von Willebrand factor are reduced in von Willebrand's disease. Levels of von Willebrand factor have been used as a marker of disease activity in the vasculitides; but they are not ideal because von Willebrand factor also behaves as an acute phase protein.

Tissue factor (TF) is an integral membrane component that serves as the essential cofactor for coagulation factor VII/VIIa which subsequently activates factor X, but has also been shown to activate factor IX. Tissue factor is strongly expressed on all solid tissues especially vascular adventitial cells, forming a haemostatic envelope around blood vessels. Thus if a vessel is injured extra-endothelial TF initiates coagulation (Drake et al, 1989). It is not expressed on endothelium, but in vitro expression is induced on monocytes and endothelium 2–6 h after stimulation with IL-1, TNF or LPS and will thus cause activation of coagulation and clot formation (Bevilacqua et al, 1984).

Stimulation of platelets or endothelium by complement results in deposition of C5-9 and subsequent vesiculation of their membranes. These vesicles are endowed with prothrombinase activity. This phenomenon also occurs with ECA.

Fibrinolytic

The fibrinolytic system is responsible for clot breakdown and thus healing. Plasmin is produced from its inactive precursor plasminogen by the action of tissue plasminogen activator (t-PA) which with its inhibitor, plasminogen activator inhibitor type I (PAI-1), is produced by the endothelium. Stimulation of endothelial cells with cytokines such as TNF or LPS leads to unaltered or decreased secretion of t-PA, but enhanced PAI-1 release. Thus overall there is a a reduction of fibrinolytic activators resulting in reduced fibrinolytic potential (Nawroth & Stern, 1986; Emeiss & Kooistra, 1986; Schleef et al, 1988).

Upregulation of expression of class I and II HLA molecules, allowing endothelial cells to act as antigen presenting cells and a target for cytotoxic T lymphocytes

The term 'antigen presenting cell' means that the cell is able to present antigen to resting T cells in a form they recognize as foreign and thus cause activation of T-cells. T cells recognize antigens as foreign in two ways: 'direct' recognition is when they see and are activated by major histocompatibility complex (MHC) molecules of a different type from their own; while 'indirect' recognition occurs when a foreign antigen is processed and 'presented' to them by self MHC molecules. Thus in transplant rejection recipient T cells will see MHC molecules on donor cells as foreign and become activated. This is discussed in Chapter 15 as is the controversy over whether endothelial cells can act as antigen presenting cells.

Major histocompatibility loci (MHC) are the major target of immune response following allograft rejection. It has also been suggested that aberrant expression of autologous MHC is involved in the pathogenesis of some autoimmune diseases. MHC expression is not a constant feature of endothelial cells as they can be induced by cytokines. Moreover an increase in expression will alter the magnitude of the immune response. Thus the distribution and the MHC will determine both the target and the strength of the immune response. Under standard culture conditions human endothelial cells express class I MHC molecules (HLA-A, B and C) but not class II (HLA-DR, DP. DQ). Treatment of cultured endothelial cells with interferon-β, interferon-α, TNF, lymphotoxin or CD40 ligand increases the level of expression of class I molecules without inducing class II molecules. Interferon gamma also increases the level of class I MHC molecule expression and, on human endothelial cells, is uniquely able to induce expression of class II MHC molecules. In general the MHC patterns of expression in vivo are the same as exhibited by cultured endothelial cells. Human endothelial cells are uniformly positive for class I molecules. Class II MHC molecules are expressed constitutively on some endothelial cells, including most postcapillary venules, veins and some arteries. This expression is altered at sites of inflammation and rejection, e.g. on quiescent pulmonary endothelium HLA class II MHC are variably expressed; however in chronic rejection there is enhanced and consistent expression of class II on endothelial cells (for a review see Pober et al, 1996).

The intracellular mechanisms underlying endothelial cell activation

The diverse effects of ECA share a common intracellular control mechanism which 'switch on' the facets of ECA by altering gene transcription (Baldwin, 1996). After a stimulating agent attaches to its receptor on the endothelial cell surface, the message is transmitted intracellularly to a transcription factor nuclear factor κB (NF-κB). Most inducible transcriptional activators are activated by a limited number of physiological agents, but NF-κB, however, is activated by a large variety of agents representing a threat to the organism. The genes which are upregulated during endothelial cell activation (e.g. tissue factor, plasminogen activator inhibitor, E-selectin) contain binding sites for NF-κB in their promoter area. NF-κB is stored in an inactive form in the cytoplasm, and is activated by the removal of an inhibitory subunit, IκB. This is initiated by phosphorylation followed by proteolysis (Henkel et al, 1993). In the absence of IκB, exposed sequences on the NF-κB dimer composed of p50 and p65 (RelA) subunits are recognized by a receptor and transported into the nucleus where binding to DNA regulatory sequences initiates transcription of the genes involved in ECA. NFκB binding sites are found in the regulatory region of essentially all the genes studied that are induced as part of EC activation (Collins et al, 1993). Control of NFκB activation may therefore enable ECA to be suppressed.

Endothelial cell activation in disease

Systemic inflammatory response syndrome (SIRS)

SIRS is defined as the clinical response to a non-specific insult resulting in two or more of the following: (1) temperature greater than 38°C or less than 36°C, (2) heart rate greater than 90 beats per minute, (3) respiratory rate greater than 20 breaths per minute or a pCO$_2$ less than 32 mm Hg, or (4) white blood cell count greater than $12.0 \times 10^9/l$ or less than $4.0 \times 10^9/l$ or the presence of more than 10% immature neutrophils. Sepsis refers to the presence of SIRS in association with a confirmed infectious process. Septic shock is defined as sepsis with hypotension in spite of adequate fluid resuscitation, or hypoperfusion (manifest as lactic acidosis, oliguria or altered mental status). Epidemiological evidence suggests that these occur sequentially and that a clinical progression from SIRS to sepsis to septic shock occurs. A stepwise increase in mortality rates exists for the hierarchy of SIRS, sepsis and septic shock: 7%, 16% and 46%, respectively. The likelihood of end organ dysfunction (adult respiratory distress syndrome (ARDS), acute renal failure, disseminated intravascular coagulation (DIC) increases directly as two, three and four criteria for SIRS are met (Rangel-Frauso et al, 1995). Overwhelming infection with Gram-negative bacteria results in the release of endotoxin, a LPS component of bacterial cell walls that stimulates production of proinflammatory cytokines. Widespread endothelial activation in response to the sequential release of TNF, IL-1, IL-6 and IL-8 is thought to be the mechanism underlying SIRS and its sequelae (Van Zee et al, 1991).

Excess NO production may mediate the hypotension and myocardial depression associated with septic shock. LPS and subsequent cytokine generation is capable of initiating iNOS production in macrophages and vascular SMCs. Once synthesized iNOS produces abundant amounts of NO resulting in vasodilation and hypotension (Petro et al, 1991). As NO is centrally involved in the pathophysiology of septic shock several treatments have been used to counteract NO overproduction. L-arginine analogues have been used (Gross et al, 1990). Glucocorticoids prevent endotoxin-induced upregulation of iNOS. Methylene blue (a guanylate cyclase inhibitor) reverses hypotension secondary to sepsis in association as well as normalizing plasma NO levels (Keaney et al, 1994). Although it appears that NO inhibition may be an effective therapy for the treatment of hypotension secondary to sepsis, there is no evidence that NOS inhibitors reduce mortality, and there is concern that complete, non-selective inhibition of NO synthesis may have deleterious side effects, as in animal models of sepsis, higher doses of an NOS inhibitor led to a higher mortality and glomerular thrombosis (Nava et al, 1992; Shultz & Raij, 1992). Therefore NO release during sepsis may be necessary to ensure adequate local perfusion to vital organs and to prevent vascular thrombosis in small arterioles by both minimising vascular resistance and impairing platelet activation.

Inducing septicaemia in primates results in widespread expression of E-selectin, especially in the kidney, lung and liver, organs that are all involved at an early stage of the development of multiorgan failure. There is also a rapid influx of neutrophils into lungs and central organs which parallels the expression of E-selectin (see Dinarello et al, 1993 for a review of animal models of SIRS).

Infusion of endotoxin into healthy volunteers results in early rises in TNF levels (at 30 min) followed by rises in IL-1 and IL-6 (Van Deventer et al, 1990; Suffredini et al, 1989). There is an increase in coagulation activation as measured by thrombin–antithrombin in complexes and prothrombin fragment 1.2, and also an increase in t-PA activity (soon to be offset by the release of PAI-1). Rises in plasma von Willebrand factor are also observed. These changes are consistent with endothelial cell activation type I and type II.

DIC is common during SIRS. DIC is a strong predictor of death and multiple organ failure in the setting of SIRS. Non-survivors of septic shock have a stronger activation of coagulation and a more marked inhibition of fibrinolysis than survivors (Lorente et al, 1993; Gando et al, 1995). Upregulation of tissue factor on endothelium and monocytes may be the initiator of activation of coagulation. Treatment with antithrombin concentrates and Protein C concentrates have been used to negate the effects of activation of coagulation, but the studies have been small and poorly controlled (Fourier et al, 1993;

Taylor et al, 1987). Following a bacterial infusion into baboons the administration of tissue factor pathway inhibitor resulted in the prolongation of survival time and attenuation of coagulopathy (Creasey et al, 1993). In addition, the use of a monoclonal antibody specific for tissue factor resulted in inhibition of an endotoxin induced coagulopathy in chimpanzees (Levi et al, 1994). As yet there are no comprehensive studies of their use in humans.

Anti-cytokine strategies aimed at TNF and IL-1 have been employed in animal models of SIRS (for a review see Dinarello et al, 1993). Specific blockade of TNF by soluble forms of the TNF receptor or neutralizing antibodies reduces mortality and severity of disease. Similar results have been obtained with IL-1 receptor antagonists and soluble IL-1 receptors. Clinical studies have demonstrated that blockade of these cytokines may also be useful in treating human SIRS (Boermeester et al, 1995), but the outcome is not always beneficial and further studies are needed.

Ischaemia/reperfusion injury

Ischaemia/reperfusion injury contributes to the pathophysiology of a number of clinical disorders. These include stroke and myocardial infarction, organ preservation, the use of fibrinolytic agents and surgery where blood vessels are cross clamped. The length of time a tissue can survive oxygen deprivation varies but all ischaemic tissue becomes necrotic eventually. For recent reviews of ischaemia/reperfusion see Cohen, 1995; Grace, 1994.

Cell damage following ischaemia is biphasic, with injury being initiated during ischaemia and exacerbated during reperfusion. Ischaemic injury has been well characterized: the cell is deprived of the energy needed to maintain ionic gradients and homeostasis, and failure of enzyme systems leads to cell death. Reperfusion is obviously necessary for recovery from ischaemic injury and for removal of toxic metabolites; however the return of toxic metabolites to the circulation may have serious metabolic consequences and paradoxically, reperfusion of ischaemic tissue may induce further local tissue injury. Reperfusion injury is mediated by the interaction of free radicals, neutrophils and activated endothelial cells (see Fig. 14.3 for a simplified series of events).

A free radical is an unstable molecule containing one or more unpaired electrons. The hydroxyl radical is formed via the iron catalyzed Haber–Weiss reaction. Superoxide radicals (a byproduct of normal cellular metabolism and produced by xanthine oxidase in postischaemic tissue) release iron from ferritin which in turn reacts with hydrogen peroxide to produce hydroxyl radicals. Hydroxyl radicals and superoxide are probably responsible for most of the cellular damage that occurs from free radicals (Weiss, 1986). The most damaging effect of free radicals is lipid peroxidation which produces structural and functional cell damage.

Reperfusion leads to accumulation of neutrophils in the microvasculature; neutrophil–endothelial cell interactions are a prerequisite for the microvascular injury of ischaemia–reperfusion. Neutrophils adhere to and migrate across the endothelium via adhesion molecules and cause local damage by releasing free radicals, proteolytic enzymes and peroxidase.

Aerobic metabolism interrupted and metabolites accumulate

⇓

Oxygen becomes available with reperfusion

⇓

Aerobic metabolism resumes with generation of O_2- and H_2O_2

⇓

Antioxidant system overwhelmed

⇓

Oxidative cell damage including lipid peroxidation

⇓

Endothelial cell activation

⇓

Leukocytes attack reperfused tissue

⇓

"Post ischaemia syndrome"-

cytokines released into systemic circulation

Fig. 14.3. Likely sequence of events in ischaemia reperfusion injury.

In ischaemia–reperfusion NO release is impaired or released NO is immediately inactivated by haemoglobin or oxygen-derived free radicals before it can exert its vasodilator effects. It has also been suggested that NO may react with superoxide to yield secondary cytotoxic species via peroxynitrite ($ONOO^-$). Some animal work has actually suggested that it may be causally involved in myocardial reoxygenation injury. Endothelin may also play a role in the pathogenesis of ischaemic injury. Increased circulating plasma endothelin concentrations have been found in vivo in arterial injury and in the early hours after myocardial infarction, with sustained increase in patients with continuing ischaemia. Watanabe and colleagues demonstrated that administration of endothelin antibody reduced myocardial infarct size in rats (Watanabe et al, 1991). Endothelial damage and impaired NO release occur during ischaemia, resulting in inhibition of vasodilation. Ischaemia stimulates endothelin release, which in turn results in vasoconstriction, continuing ischaemia and further infarction.

There are different opportunities to reduce the damage. The first is to directly prevent the generation of free radicals and hydrogen peroxide. Allopurinol inhibits the production of xanthine oxidase, and has been shown to reduce infarct size in animal models and in some clinical trials. Desferrioxamine is a powerful iron-chelating agent; because iron is essential for the Haber–Weiss reaction and production of the free radical it has been used with beneficial effects during ischaemia–reperfusion injury (Ambrosia et al, 1987).

A second option is to enhance the tissues' capacity to trap free radicals. A number of antioxidants and free radical scavengers have been investigated. Recombinant superoxide dismutase (SOD) is an enzyme that detoxifies O_2^-. Results of its use in clinical trials have so far been variable.

The use of monoclonal antibodies against key cytokines, IL-1 and TNF, reduced leg muscle injury in a rat leg model of ischaemia–reperfusion; while antibodies to adhesion molecules in animals have also shown success (see reviews see Cohen, 1995; Grace, 1994).

Ischaemic preconditioning is a term used to cover the phenomenon whereby resistance of a tissue to lethal period of ischaemia is enhanced by a preceding period of sublethal ischaemia. Ischaemic preconditioning from animal experiments, appears to be a biphasic phenomenon: there is an early phase of protection that lasts for about 2 h after the preconditioning stimulus, and a second window of protection that occurs 24 h later (Marber et al, 1993). Adenosine and heat shock proteins are implicated in this phenomenon.

Heat shock proteins are produced by all living organisms in response to adverse changes in the environment. This defensive process, called the heat-shock response, occurs in response to a wide range of stimuli including ischaemia preconditioning (Lindquist, 1986). How they work is unclear; experimental work suggests they are associated with increased production of free radical scavengers, especially catalase and superoxide dismutase (Karmazyn et al, 1990).

Adenosine is a ubiquitous product of ischaemia. The early phase of ischaemic preconditioning appears to be effected by the intervention of A_1 receptors and protein kinase C in myocytes, for if adenosine receptors are blocked then preconditioning does not have an effect. Similar effects are seen with inhibitors and agonists of the protein kinase C pathway (Cophen & Downey, 1993).

Currently there is no clear cut solution to the management of ischaemia–reperfusion injury. The future may be in the use of combination therapy with better techniques for reperfusion, and the use of antioxidants with neutrophil inhibitors.

Endothelium in the systemic vasculitides

The vasculitides are a heterogeneous group of diseases characterised by inflammation of blood vessels. They are typically multisystemic disorders. Classification of the vasculitides is difficult as long as the aetiology and pathogenesis are unclear. The most clinically useful classification remains that based on the size of blood vessels involved (Jeanette et al, 1994). The pathogenesis of most types of vasculitis remains poorly defined. Different aspects of the immune response have been described as being the main causative mediators of different types of vasculitis: antiendothelial cell antibodies, immune complexes and cytotoxic lymphocytes. Viruses have been implicated as initiators of the immune response in some cases. Potential pathogenic mechanisms underlying the vasculitides will be briefly described and the current understanding of one type of vasculitis – Wegener's granulomatosis – will then be reviewed with particular reference to endothelial interactions in more detail.

Antiendothelial cell antibodies

Studies in many conditions suggest a pathogenic role for antiendothelial antibodies. They have been reported in patients with different connective tissue disorders and autoimmune states, Behçet's disease, retinal vasculitis, Kawasaki's disease, haemolytic uraemic syndrome, inflammatory bowel disease, multiple sclerosis, acute preeclampsia and some viral infections; however, no definite conclusions have been drawn about their clinical significance or pathogenic role. All studies should be reviewed carefully, especially the method section for it is difficult to identify true antiendothelial cell antibodies. The endothelium is bathed in plasma containing antibodies and many antiendothelial cell assays are based on measuring binding of antibodies to endothelial cells. Thus binding of low titre immunoglobulins may have little pathological significance. In addition assays are often performed in vitro on human umbilical vein endothelial cells following three or more passages in vitro. This can alter the endothelial cell surface phenotype or the response to standard stimuli. Finally, there is enormous endothelial cell heterogeneity, depending on their site, so antiendothelial cell antibodies could be specific for certain antigens present only on a few types of endothelium.

Antiendothelial cell antibodies have been described in active systemic lupus erythematosis (Meroni et al, 1995). In culture they bind to endothelium, deposit complement, cause platelets to adhere and disrupt the endothelial cell monolayer. The addition of peripheral blood mononuclear cells has been shown to induce endothelial cell cytotoxicity in combination with antiendothelial cell antibodies. One study has shown that antibodies in sera from patients with systemic lupus erythematosus (SLE) could induce tissue factor on cultured endothelial cells (Tannenbaum et al, 1986).

Immune complexes

Normally the mononuclear phagocytic system is an efficient scavenger of immune complexes. Under certain circumstances, however, immune complexes apparently escape the system and are deposited on tissues causing inflammation. The association of serum sickness with systemic necrotising vascultis is widely recognized. Animal models have formed the basis of our current understanding (for a review see Cochrane & Koffler, 1973).

If antigen is injected into the skin of sensitized animals then this is followed by a vasculitis mediated by the formation of immune complexes (the Arthus reaction). These immune complexes are removed within 24–48 h by neutrophils. Activated neutrophils release proteases that digest proteins and they also generate free radicals. These cause endothelial cell detachment and lysis with vessel wall damage and occlusion (Kniker & Cochrane, 1965).

SLE is considered a prototype disease mediated by immune complexes. Serum complement levels are reduced in active lupus and improve with treatment (Schur & Sandson, 1968). Complement deposition has been identified in inflamed tissues (Tann & Kunkel, 1966). Anti-double stranded DNA antibodies (anti-dsDNA) are considered to be a marker of lupus activity, and DNA and anti-DNA antibodies are found in renal tissue and skin (Fournie, 1988); although there are some patients with very high serum levels and apparently inactive disease and visa versa.

Immune complex -mediated vasculitis occurs with hepatitis B infection. Cases of polyarteritis nodosa associated with chronic carriage of hepatitis B were first described in 1970 (Gocke et al, 1970). The circulating immune complexes from patients with vasculitis in association with chronic hepatitis B contain viral antigen, and the vasculitis is accompanied by low complement levels, cryoglobulins and deposits of immunoglobulin and complement in affected vessel walls (Shusterman & London, 1984). In vitro studies would suggest this would cause local endothelial cell activation. Cryoglobulins can cause vasculitis due to the deposition of immune complexes (Ferri et al, 1995). Cryoglobulins precipitate reversibly at temperatures below 37°C. They can be found in infections, immunological and neoplastic disorders. They are classified according to their associated immunoglobulin clonality: type I is the presence of an isolated monoclonal immunoglobulin. Type II and type III contain polyclonal IgG and mono- or polyclonal IgM with rheumatoid factor activity, respectively. 'Essential' mixed cryoglobulinaemia is diagnosed when there is no other systemic disorder. Recent studies have shown that hepatitis C infection is present in the majority of these patients.

Many drugs have been implicated in the development of vasculitis including sulphonamides, penicillin and streptokinase. In some cases immune complexes and cryoglobulins containing the drug and antibodies have been demonstrated in sera from patients with vasculitis (Davies et al, 1990).

Non-specific markers such as C-reactive protein and erythrocyte sedimentation rate are used to monitor vasculitic activity. Von Willebrand factor levels are also elevated in the systemic vasculitides and there is some evidence to show that plasma levels reflect disease activity; many authors feel that levels reflect the extent of ECA but it must be remembered that levels are also increased as part of the acute phase response (Nusinow et al, 1984).

Cytotoxic lymphocytes

Occasionally vasculitis is marked by a perivascular lymphocytic infiltration and absence of neutrophils. This area remains poorly understood, (for a review see Altmann, 1995).

Wegener's granulomatosis

Wegener's granulomatosis is due to a necrotizing vasculitis of small arteries, venules and capillaries. Commonly the process involves inflammation of the upper and lower respiratory tract and kidneys. It is associated with the presence of antineutrophil cytoplasm antibodies (ANCA), although the use of this assay in making a diagnosis without histology is not reliable (Rao et al, 1995).

Ultrastructural renal biopsies have shown endothelial cell swelling and increase in cytoplasmic organelles (Weiss & Crissman, 1984). In addition endothelial cells may become necrotic and separated from the basement membrane. Thrombosis may develop prior to any inflammatory infiltrate, this may reflect intense early ECA by cytokines or other inflammatory mediators.

Immunofluoresence studies of neutrophils show that there are two patterns of binding of ANCA, granular cytoplasmic (c-ANCA) and perinuclear (P-ANCA) The predominant antigen for c-ANCA is proteinase 3 (PR3) (Goldschmeding et al, 1989). Cytokines induce the expression of PR3 on the surface of human neutrophils in vitro and also their presence was shown on ex vivo neutrophils from patients with Wegener's granulomatosis (Csernok et al, 1994). ANCA can activate neutrophils (Falk et al, 1990), promote their adhesion to the endothelium and induce neutrophil-mediated endothelial cell injury, for cytotoxicity assays on human umbilical endothelial cells have demonstrated that ANCA-mediated neutrophil activation can result in endothelial cell lysis (Savage et al, 1992), after priming of neutrophils by agents such as TNF. The incidence of antiendothelial cell antibodies in Wegener's granulomatosis has reportedly varied from 10 to 86%. Their role in the pathogenesis of the condition is not clear. It is not known whether binding of these antibodies to endothelial cells causes endothelial cell activation in Wegener's granulomatosis. ANCA has been shown to initiate some of the changes of endothelial cell activation for in vitro it induces E-selectin (Mayet & Meyer, 1993), increases neutrophil adhesion to the endothelium and via activation of neutrophils there is increased permeability of endothelial cell monolayers (Beynon et al, 1993).

Renal biopsies from patients with Wegener's granulomatosis show glomerular endothelial ICAM-1 expression with perhaps more intense staining that that seen in a normal kidney. In addition there is glomerular endothelial VCAM-1 staining which is not seen in the normal kidney. There are significantly increased levels of soluble ICAM-1 and soluble E-selectin in patients with active Wegener's, probably reflecting endothelial activation (Pall et al, 1994). Different studies have reported increased levels of TNF-α, IL-1, IL-6, interferon-γ and IL-8 in the circulation. IL-6 in the supernatant of peripheral blood mononuclear cells from the same patients was not increased compared with controls which suggests that circulating IL-6 probably originates from activated endothelium (for a review see Kekow et al, 1992).

Finally, there are a group of patients with Wegener's granulomatosis that remain persistently ANCA negative. It is possible that T cell-mediated injury may predominate in these patients. Histologically T cells are found in necrotizing small vessel vasculitis.

The aetiology of the primary systemic vasculitides remains obscure, although in Wegener's granulomatosis the evidence favours an autoimmune inflammatory response in which the endothelium is a target and a participator.

Conclusion

In conclusion, ECA appears to be an effector mechanism in the inflammatory response and thus a component of the pathophysiological response to injury. ECA may play an important role in the pathogenesis of many diseases; however it must be remembered that many of the mechanisms described here have only been observed in vitro or in animal models. There is considerable scope for future research.

In future there may be more fundamental approaches to switching off endothelial cell activation – at the level of NF-κB. Intriguingly glucocorticosteroids stimulate the production of I-κB, thus locking up NF-κB, while the glucocorticoid receptor complex binds to NF-κB, preventing it from binding to DNA and thus preventing increased gene activity (Marx, 1995). The design of a pharmaceutical agent behaving in the same way but without the side-effects of glucocorticoids would have obvious benefits. Aspirin, a widely used anti-inflammatory drug and platelet inhibitor, inhibits activation of NF-κB by preventing proteolytic degradation of I-κB (Kopp & Ghosh, 1994). Inhibition of NF-κB activation by antioxidants and specific protease inhibitors may also prove useful. Other approaches at switching off NF-κB are being actively explored. There is clearly great potential for interference with the mechanism of NF-κB activation and hence prevention of endothelial cell activation, which may aid in the treatment of many conditions.

References

Adams, D. H. & Shaw, S. (1994). Leucocyte-endothelial interactions and regulation of leucocyte migration. *Lancet*, **343**, 831–6.

Altmann, D. M. (1995). New concepts of mechanims in autoimmunity. In *Immunological Aspects of the Vascular Endothelium*, ed. C. O. Savage & J. D. Pearson. Cambridge: Cambridge University Press.

Ambrosia, G., Zweier, J., Jacobus, W. E. et al. (1987). Improvement of postischaemic myocardial function and metabolism induced by administration of desferoxamine at the time of reflow: the role of iron in the pathogenesis of reperfusion injury. *Circulation*, **76**, 906–15.

Bach, F. H., Robson, S. C., Ferran, C. Winkler, H., Mullan, M. T., Stuhlmeier, K. M.. (1994). Endothelial cell activation and thromboregulation during xenograft rejection. *Immunology Review*, **141**, 5–30.

Bach, F. H., Robson, S. C., Winkler, H., Ferran, C., Stuhlmeier, K. M., Wrighton, C. J. & Hancock, W. W. (1995). Barriers to xenotransplantation. *Nature Medicine*, **1**, 869–73.

Baldwin, A. S. (1996). The NF-κB and IκB proteins: New discoveries and insights. *Annual Review of Immunology*, **14**, 649–81.

Bevilacqua, M. P., Pober, J. S., Majeau, G. R., Cotran, R. S. & Gimbrone, M. A. Jr. (1984). IL-1 induces biosynthesis and cell surface expression of procoagulant activity in human vascular endothelial cells. *Journal of Experimental Medicine*, **160**, 618–23.

Beynon, H. L. C., Haskard, D. O., Davies, K. A., Haroutanian, R. & Walport, M. J. (1993). Combinations of low concentrations of cytokines and acute agonists synergise in increasing the permeability of endothelial monolayers. *Clinical and Experimental Immunology*, **91**, 314–19.

Boermeester, M. A., van Leewen, P. A. M., Coyle, S. M. et al. (1995). IL-1 blockade attenuates mediator relase and dysregulation of the haemostatic mechanism during human sepsis. *Archives of Surgery*, **130**, 739–48.

Carlos, T. M. & Harlan, J. M. (1994). Leukocyte-endothelial adhesion molecules. *Blood*, **84**, 2068–101.

Cohen, R. A. (1995). The role of nitric oxide and other endothelium derieved vasoactive substances in vascular disease. (1995). *Progress in Cardiovascular Disease*, **XXXVIII**, 105–28.

Collins, T., Palmer, H. J., Whitley, M. Z., Neish, A. S. & Williams, A. J. (1993). A common theme in endothelial activation – insights from the structural analysis of the genes for E-selectin and VCAM-1. *Trends in Cardiovascular Medicine*, **3**, 92–7.

Cochrane, C. G. & Koffler, D. (1973). Immune complex disease in experimental animals and men. *Advances in Immunology*, **16**, 185.

Cophen, M. V. & Downey, J. M. (1993). Ischaemic preconditioning: can the protection be bottled? *Lancet*, **342**, 6.

Creasey, A. A., Chang, A. C. K., Feigen, L., Wun, T. C., Taylor, F. B. Jr. & Hinshaw, L. B. (1993). Tissue factor pathway inhibitor reduces mortality from E Coli septic shock. *Journal of Clinical Investigation*, **91**, 2850–60.

Csernok, E., Ludemann, J., Gross, W. L. & Bainton, D. F. (1994). Ultrastructural localisation of proteinase 3 the target antigen of ANCA in Wegener's granulomatosis. *American Journal of Pathology*, **137**, 1113–20.

Davies, K. A. A., Mathieson, P., Winearls, C. G., Rees, A. J. & Walport, M. J. (1990). Serum sickness and acute renal failure after streptokinase therapy for myocardial infarction. *Clinical and Experimental Immunology*, **80**, 83–99.

Davies, M. G., Fulton, G. J. & Hagen, P. O. (1995). Clinical biology of nitric oxide. *British Journal of Surgery*, **82**, 1598–610.

Dinarello, C. A., Gelfand, J. A. & Wolff, S. M. (1993). Anticytokine strategies in the treatment of the systemic inflammatory response syndrome. *Journal of the American Medical Association*, **269**, 1829–35.

Drake, T. A., Morissey J. H. & Edgington, T. S. (1989). Selective cellular expression of tissue factor in human tissues. Implications for disorders of haemostasis and thrombosis. *American Journal of Pathology*, **134,** 1087–97.

Emeis, J. J. & Kooistra, T. (1986). IL-1 and lipopolysaccharide induce an inhibitor of tissue type plasminogen activator in vivo and in culturd endothelial cells. (1986). *Journal of Experimental Medicine*, **163**, 1260–6.

Esmon, C. T. & Owen, W. G. (1989). Identification of an endothelial cell cofactor for the factor in human tissues. Implications for disorders of haemostasis and thrombosis. *American Journal of Pathology*, **134**, 1087–97.

Falk, R. J., Terrell, R. S., Charles, L.A. & Jennette, J. C. (1990). Anti-neutrophil cytoplasmic autoantibodies induce neutrophils to degranulate and produce oxygen radicals in vivo. *Proceedings of the National Acadamy of Sciences of the USA*, **87**, 4115–19.

Ferri, C., Zignego, A. L. & Bombardieri, S. (1995). Etiopathogenetic role of hepatitis C virus in mixed cryoglobulinaemia, chronic liver disease and lymphomas. *Clinical and Experimental Rheumatology*, **13**, 3135–40.

Fourier, F., Chopin, F. C., Huart, J. J. et al. (1993). Double-blind placebo controlled trial of antithrombin III concentrates in septic shock with disseminated intravascular coagulation. *Chest*, **104**, 882–8.

Fournie, G. J. (1988). Circulating DNA and lupus nephritis. *Kidney International*, **33**, 487–97.

Gando, S., Nakanishi, Y. & Tedo, I. (1995). Cytokines and plasminogen activator inhibitor-1 in post-trauma disseminated intravascular coagulation: relationship to multiple organ dysfunction syndrome. *Critical Care in Medicine*, **23**, 1835–42.

Gocke, D. J., Hsu, K., Morgan, C. et al. (1970). Association between polyarteritis and Australian antigen *Lancet*, **2**, 1149–53.

Goldschmeding, R., van der Schoot, C. E., ten Bokkel Huinink, D. et al. (1989). Wegener's granulomatosis autoantibodies identify a novel diisopropylfluorpkosphate binding protein with lyosomes of normal human neutrophils. *Journal of Clinical Investigation*, **84**, 1577–87.

Grace, P. A. (1994). Ischaemia-reperfusion injury. *British Journal of Surgery*, **81**, 637–47.

Gross, S. S., Stuehr, D. J., Aisaka, K. et al. (1990). Cell type selective inhibition by N^Gaminoarginine, N^G-nitroarginine, N^Gmethylarginine. *Biochemistry and Biophysics Research Commununication*,**170**, 96–103.

Hamblin, T. J. (1990). Endothelins. *British Medical Journal*, **301**, 568.

Henkel, T., Machleidt, T., Alkalay, I., Kronke, M., Benneriah, Y. & Baeuerle, P. A. (1993). Rapid proteolysis of IκBα is necessary for activation of transcription factor NF-κB. *Nature*, **365**, 182.

Ihrcke, N. S., Wrenshall, L. E., Lindman, B. J., Platt, J. L. (1996). Role of heparan sulphate in immune system-blood vessel interactions. *Immunology Today*, **14**, 500–5.

Jeanette, J. C., Falk, R. J., Andrassy, K., Bacon, P. A., Churg, J., Gross, W. L., et al. (1994). Nomenclature of systemic vasculitides: the proposal of an international consensus conference. *Arthritis and Rheumatism*, **37**, 187–92.

Karmazyn, M., Mailer, K. & Curie, R. W. (1990). Acquisition and decay of heat-shock enhanced postischaemic ventricular recovery. *American Journal of Physiology*, **259**, 424–31.

Keaney, J. F., Puyana, J.-C., Francis, S. et al. (1994). Methylene blue reverses endotoxin-induced hypotension. *Circulation Research*, **74**, 1121–5.

Kekow, J., Szymkowiak, C. & Gross, W. L. (1992). Involvement of cytokines in granuloma formation within primary systemic vasculitis. In *Cytokines: Basic Principles and Clinical Application*, ed. S. Romagni, pp. 341–8. New York: Raven Press.

Kniker, W. & Cochrane, C. G. (1965). Pathogenic factors in vascular lesions of experimental serum sickness. *Journal of Experimental Medicine*, **122**, 83–98.

Kopp, E. & Ghosh, S. (1994). Inhibition of NF-κB by sodium salicylate and aspirin. *Science*, **265**, 956–9.

Levi, M., ten Cate, H., Bauer, K., Van der Poll, T., Edington, T. S., Buller, H. R., van Deventer, S. J. & Rosenberg, R. D. (1994). Inhibition of endotoxin-induced activation of coagulation and fibrinolysis by pentoxifylline or by monoclonal anti-tissue factor antibody in chimpanzees. *Journal of Clinical Investigation*, **93**, 114–20.

Lindquist, S. (1986). The heat-shock response. *Annual Review of Biochemistry*, **55**, 1151–91.

Lorente, J. A., Garcia-Frade, L. J., Landin, L., de Pablo, R., Torrado, C., Renes, E. & Garcia-Avello, A. (1993). Time course of haemostatic abnormalities in sepsis and its relation to outcome. *Chest*, **103**, 1536–42.

Mantovani, A. & Dejana, E. (1989). Cytokines as communication signals between leucocytes and endothelial cells. *Immunology today*, **10**, 370–5.

Marber, M. S., Latchman, D. S., Walker, J. M. & Yellon, D. M. (1993). Cardiac stress protein elevation 24 hours after brief ischaemia or heat stress is associated with resistance to myocardial infarction. *Circulation*, **88**, 1264–72.

Marcus, A. J. (1994). Thrombosis and inflammation as multicellular processes: significance of cell-cell interaction. *Seminars in Haematology*, **31**, 261–9.

Marcus, A. J., Safier, L. B., Hajjar, K. A., Ullman, H. L., Islan, N., Brockman, M. J. & Eiroa, A. M. (1991). Inhibition of platelet function by an aspirin-insensitive endothelial cell membrane ADPase. Thromboregulation by endothelial cells. *Journal of Clinical Investigation*, **88**, 1690.

Marx, J. (1995). How the glucocorticoids suppress immunity. *Science*, **270**, 232–3.

Mayet, W. J. & Meyer, K. H. (1993). Antibodies to PR increase adhesion of neutrophils to human endothelial cells. *Blood*, **22**, 1221–9.

Meroni, P., Khamashta, M. A., Youinou, P. & Shoenfeld, Y. (1995). Mosaic of anti-endothelial cell antibodies. Review of the first International Workshop on antiendothelial cell antibodies, clinical and pathological significance. *Lupus*, **4**, 95–9.

Moore, K. L., Esmon, C. T. & Esmon, C. L. (1989). TNF leads to the internalization and degradation of thrombomodulin from the surface of bovine endothelial cells in culture. *Blood*, **73**, 159–65.

Nava, E., Palmer, R. M. J. & Moncada S. (1992). The role of nitric oxide in endotoxic shock. *Journal of Cardiovascular Pharmacology*, **20**, 5132–4.

Nawroth, P. P. & Stern, D. M. (1986). Modulation of endothelial cell haemostatic properties by TNF. *Journal of Experimental Medicine*, **163**, 740–5.

Nusinow, S. R., Federeci, A. D., Zimmerman, T. S. & Curd, J. G. (1984). Increased von Willebrand factor antigen in the plasma of patients with vasculitis. *Arthritis and Rheumatism*, **27**, 1405–10.

Pall, A. A., Adu, D., Richard, N. T. & Michael, J. (1994). Circulating soluble adhesion molecules in systemic vasculitis. *Nephrology Dialysis and Transplantation*, **9**, 770–4.

Petro, A., Bennet, D. & Vallance, P. (1991). Effect of nitric oxide synthase inhibitors on hypotension in patients with septic shock. *Lancet*, **338**, 1557–8.

Pober, J. S. (1988). Cytokine-mediated activation of vascular endothelium. *American Journal of Pathology*, **133**, 426–33.

Pober, J. S. & Cotrans, R. S. (1991). The role of endothelial cells in inflammation. *Transplantation*, **50**, 536–44.

Pober, J. S., Orosz, C. G., Rose, M. L. & Savage, C. O. (1996). Can graft endothelial cells initiate a host antigraft immune response? *Transplantation*, **61**, 343–9.

Rangel-Frauso, M. S., Pittet, D., Costigan, M., Hirang, T., Davis, C. S. & Wenzel, R. P. (1995). The natural history of the systemic inflammatory response syndrome. *Journal of the American Medical Association*, **273**, 117–23.

Rao, J. K., Allen, N. B., Feussner, J. R. & Weinberger, M. (1995). A prospective study of antineutrophil cytoplasmic antibody (c-ANCA) and clinical criteria in diagnosing Wegener's granulomatosis. *Lancet*, **346**, 926–31.

Rapaport, S. I. (1991). The extrinsic pathway inhibitor: a regulator of tissue factor-dependent blood coagulation. *Thrombosis and Haemostasis*, **66**, 6–15.

Sandset, P. M., Abildgaard, U. & Larsen, M. L. (1988). Heparin induces release of extrinsic pathway inhibitor (EPI). *British Journal of Haematology*, **72**, 391–6.

Savage, C. O. S., Pottinger, B. E., Gaskin, G., Pusey, C. D. & Pearson, J. D. (1992). Autoantibodies developing to myeloperoxidase and proteinase 3 in systemic vasculitis stimulate neutrophil cytotoxicity towards cultured endothelial cells. *American Journal of Pathology*, **141**, 335–42.

Schleef, R. R., Bevilacqua, M. P., Sawdey, M., Gimbone, M. A. Jr & Loskntoff, D. J. (1988). Cytokine activation of vascular endothelium: effects on tissue type plasminogen activator and type one plasminogen activator inhibitor. *Biology and Chemistry*, **263**, 5797–803.

Schur, P. H. & Sandson, J. (1968). Immunological factors and clinical activity in systemic lupus erythematosus. *New England Journal of Medicine*, **278**, 533–8.

Shultz, P. H. & Raij, L. (1992). Endogenously synthesised nitric oxide prevents endotoxin – induced glomerular thrombosis. *Journal of Clinical Investigation*, **90**, 1718–25.

Shusterman, M. & London, W. T. (1984). Hepatitis B and immune complex disease. *New England Journal of Medicine*, **310**, 43–5.

Suffredini, A. F., Harpel, P. C. & Parillo, J. E. (1989). Promotion and subsequent inhibition of plasminogen activation after administration of intravenous endotoxin to normal subjects. *New England Journal of Medicine*, **320**, 1165–72.

Tann, E. M. & Kunkel, H. G. (1966). An immunofluorescent study of skin lesions in systemic lupus erythematosus. *Arthritis and Rheumatism*, **9**, 37–46.

Tannenbaum, S. H., Finsko, R. & Cines, D. B. (1986). Antibody and immune complexes induce tissue factor production by human endothelial cells. *Journal of Immunology*, **137**, 1532–7.

Taylor, F. B., Chang, A., Esmon, C. T., D'Angelo, A., Vigano D'Angelo, S. & Blick, K. E. (1987). Protein C prevents the coagulopathic and lethal effects of *E. coli* infusion in the baboon. *Journal of Clinical Investigation*, **79**, 918–25.

Van Deventer, S. J.H., Buller, H. R. & ten Cate, J. W. (1990). Experimental endotoxaemia in humans: analysis of cytokine release and coagulation , fibrinolytic and complement pathways. *Blood*, **76**, 2520–6.

Van Zee, K. J., DeForge, L. E., Fischer, E., Marano, M. A., Kennys, J. S., Remick, D. G., Lowry, S. F. & Moldawer, L. L. (1991). IL-8 in septic shock, endotoxaemia and after Il-8 administration. *Journal of Immunology*, **146**, 3478–82.

Wagner, D. D. (1990). Cell biology of von Willebrand factor. *Annual Review of Cell Biology*, **6**, 217–46.

Watanabe, T., Suzuki, N., Shimamoto, N. *et al.* (1991). Contribution of endogenous endothelin to the extension of myocardial infarct size in rats. *Circulation Research*, **69**, 370–7.

Weiss, M. A. & Crissman, J. D. (1984). Renal biopsy findings in Wegner's granulomatosis: segmental necrotising glomerulonephritis with glomerular thrombosis. *Human Pathology*, **15**, 943–56.

Weiss, S. J. (1986). Oxygen, ischaemia and revascularization injury. *Acta Physiology Scan (Suppl.)*, **548**, 9–37.

Willms-Kretschmer, K., Flax, M. H. & Cotran, R. S. (1967). The fine structure of the vascular response in hapten-specific delayed hypersensitivty and contact dermatitis. *Laboratory Investigation*, **17**, 334–49.

15

Role of endothelial cells in transplant rejection

M. L. ROSE

Introduction

Approximately 36 000 transplants are performed throughout the world each year, of which the majority are kidney transplants. About 5000 hearts, 6500 livers and 1200 lung transplant are performed. Rejection remains the most common complication following transplantation and is the major cause of morbidity and mortality. Endothelial cells form the interface between donor tissue and recipient blood and so are the first donor cells to be recognized by the host's immune system. This fact, and the observation that they express numerous molecules able to stimulate lymphocytes, has led to much research into their precise role in transplant rejection. It is our view that endothelial cells are pivotal both in controlling the egress of inflammatory cells into the allografted organ but also as specific antigen presenting cells, by presenting foreign molecules to the immune system (Fig. 15.1).

Rejection is mediated by both cell-mediated and humoral mechanisms but the relative importance of these pathways differs in acute and chronic rejection. This chapter briefly describes the features of acute and chronic rejection and then outlines the role of endothelial cells in this process.

Basic mechanism of rejection

The major stimulus for rejection of allografted organs is recognition that the donor cells are foreign, by recognition of antigens that are coded by the major histocompatibilty complex (MHC). There are two classes of MHC: class I (HLA-ABC) and class II (HLA-DR, DP, DQ). Both sets of antigens are highly polymorphic glycoproteins encoded by the MHC locus found on chromosome 6 in humans. The number of T cells which are able to recognize foreign MHC molecules is very large (estimated at an astounding 0.1–1% of circulating T cells) – a fact which almost certainly accounts for the vigour of the rejection response.

Rejection is initiated by the CD4 + T cell subset recognizing MHC class II antigens on antigen presenting cells (APC) within the graft (Fig. 15.2). This recognition results in activation of recipient CD4 + T cells and the release of cytokines (IL-2, IL-4, IL-5, IL-6,

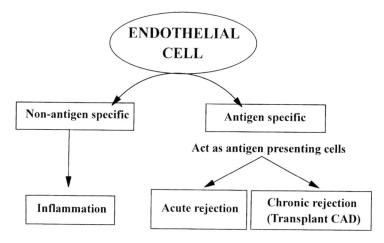

Fig. 15.1. Diagram to illustrate role of endothelial cells in transplant rejection.

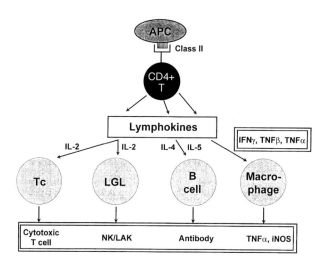

Fig. 15.2. Diagrammatic representation of T cell activation, illustrating the pivotal role of MHC class II antigens (presented by antigen presenting cells within the graft) in initiating rejection. Activation of CD4$^+$ T cells results in a cascade of lymphokines causing the maturation of a number of possible effector mechanisms (in double lined boxes). Note that the cytokines IFN-γ, TNF-β and TNFα may be directly damaging to tissues.

IFNγ, TNF-α, TNF-β) by these cells. This produces the effector mechanisms of rejection, namely maturation of CD8⁺ cytotoxic T cells, infiltration of macrophages, maturation of natural killer (NK) cells and lymphokine activated killer cells (LAK) and antibody formation (Fig. 15.2). These effector mechanisms have been listed for the sake of completeness, but there is little evidence that NK or LAK cells are important in allograft rejection. Indeed, the precise mediators which cause graft dysfunction are unknown; for although CD8⁺ cytotoxic T cells can cause graft destruction they are not essential for rejection, it is quite possible that a direct effect of cytokines, in particular TNF-α and IFNγ are toxic to the allografted cells. For example, TNF-α has a negative inotropic effect on cardiac myocytes. Similarly, induction of inducible nitric oxide synthase (NOS) by activated macrophages and endothelial cells may be an important effector mechanism (Chapter 3).

Activation of CD4⁺ T cells is thus a pivotal event in initiating acute rejection (Fig. 15.2). Foreign MHC class II molecules initiate activation of CD4⁺ T cells and so understanding the distribution and density of these molecules on the allografted organ is important. Advances in immunocytochemical techniques, including the use of monoclonal antibodies and frozen sections, have revolutionized knowledge about the normal distribution of MHC molecules in different tissues. Class II (HLA-DR and DP) antigens were originally thought to be restricted to macrophages, dendritic cells, monocytes and activated T cells, have now been described on human endothelial cells and epithelial cells (for a review see Rose, 1992). The expression of class II antigens on human endothelial cells has been described in every organ (Rose, 1992) and it is particular striking on the microvessels, i.e. capillaries, arterioles and venules. The large vessel endothelium (such as aorta, pulmonary artery, saphenous vein), however, do not express MHC class II.

The expression of MHC antigens is not a constant feature of a cell, they can be upregulated or induced by cytokines (Halloran et al, 1986). Thus, the distribution of MHC class I and class II antigens changes during acute rejection of the graft. After cardiac transplantation there is massive upregulation of MHC class I antigens (normally only on the interstitial cells) so that cardiac myocytes become MHC class I positive (Rose, 1992). Upregulation of MHC class I antigens has also been described after renal, liver and pancreatic transplantation. There is upregulation of MHC class II antigens on renal tubular epithelial cells (Fuggle et al, 1986) after renal transplantation. There is also upregulation of adhesion molecules on endothelial cells during acute rejection (Briscoe et al, 1991: Taylor et al, 1992 and see below). The upregulation of these molecules is almost certainly mediated by local production of cytokines by infiltrating cells; thus some cytokines (such as TNF-α and IFNγ) have been directly visualized in graft biopsies using immunocytochemical methods (Arbustini et al, 1991), others (IL-2, IL-1, IL-4, IL-6, IL-10) have been detected using polymerase chain reaction to amplify cytokine mRNA (Cunningham et al, 1994).

The consequences of T cell activation described above leads to infiltration of the graft with inflammatory cells (T cells and monocytes) – this process is termed acute rejection. The majority of heart transplant recipients have one or two acute rejection episodes in the first 6 months following transplantation. Acute rejection may be suspected clinically but it is always confirmed by histological assessment of endomyocardial biopsy tissue; this is an essential part of the management of patients following cardiac transplantation.

Chronic rejection

Chronic rejection in heart transplant recipients produces a rapidly progressing obliterative vascular disease in the transplanted heart. It is the major cause of late death and repeat transplantation after cardiac transplantation. This disease is variously termed cardiac allograft vasculopathy or transplant associated coronary artery disease. This same phenomenon is also present in renal, lung and liver allografts and has been designated chronic rejection, obliterative bronchiolitis and vanishing bile duct syndrome, respectively. The reported incidence of transplant coronary artery disease, as detected by routine coronary artery angiography, varies greatly between cardiac transplant centres. Incidences of 18% at 1 year progressing to 44% at 3 years have been reported (Gao et al, 1989). There are a number of reviews which describe the histological differences between transplant associated coronary artery disease and naturally occurring coronary artery disease and the various risk factors, both immunological and non-immunological have been described (Hosenpud et al, 1992) . Transplant coronary artery disease is a more diffuse disease, affecting the entire length of all coronary vessels, compared with spontaneous coronary artery disease. There is concentric intimal proliferation down the length of the coronary arteries in transplant coronary artery disease as opposed to the eccentric plaques found in spontaneous coronary artery disease. These differences suggest the whole endothelium is the target of damage in transplant coronary artery disease. As the epicardial branches, including the intramyocardial branches, are affected by transplant associated coronary artery disease, coronary artery bypass surgery for revascularization is usually precluded.

This vasculopathy of allografted organs is almost certainly of multifactorial aetiology. It is highly likely that the obstructive vascular lesions progress through repetitive endothelial injury followed by repair, smooth muscle cell (SMC) proliferation and hypertrophy, all of which gradually produce luminal obliteration. It is useful to think of the disease in term of the Ross hypothesis (Ross, 1993) – namely an initial damage to the endothelium resulting in release of growth factors and intimal proliferation. The latter process will be assisted by risk factors (circulating cholesterol, insulin resistance) common to both spontaneous and transplant-asssociated coronary artery disease. Most investigators would acknowledge that the initial damage to the endothelium is mediated by the allo-immune response, although it can also be argued that non-immunological damage such as ischaemia, surgical manipulation, and perfusion/reperfusion injury could also initially damage the endothelial cells (Tullius & Tilney, 1995). Precisely which pathways of antigen presentation are involved , which endothelial antigens are recognized and the relative importance of cell-mediated and humoral immunity in this process are unknown (see below for discussion of these topics).

Properties of endothelial cells

The phenotypic properties of endothelial cells and their response to cytokines gives them pivotal role in controlling rejection in three distinct ways:

1. They allow extravasation of inflammatory cells into the graft
2. They act as antigen presenting cells
3. They are the target of the alloimmune response.

Adhesion molecules and lymphocyte migration

There is currently extensive research on the role of endothelial adhesion molecules in controlling lymphocyte recirculation and extravasation of inflammatory cells. These processes are controlled by sequential interactions between different families of molecules on the endothelial cells (the selectins, $\beta1$ and $\beta2$ integrins and members of the immunoglobulin family) and their respective ligands on leukocytes. There are excellent reviews of this subject (Springer, 1994) and they are also discussed in Chapter XX. Our own studies have investigated the expression of Platelett adhesion molecules (PECAM-1), intercellular (ICAM-1), vascular cell (VCAM-1) and E-selectin and other markers of endothelial cells (such as von Willebrand factor) on endothelial cells within the cardiovascular system and have explored how these change during rejection (Taylor et al, 1992; Page et al, 1992). Immunocytochemistry of frozen sections of human heart, coronary artery, aorta, pulmonary artery and endocardium have revealed differences with regard to basal expression of these molecules (Table 15.1). PECAM or CD31, generally acknowledged to be a marker of endothelial cells, was strongly expressed on all endothelium. In contrast, von Willebrand factor, also used as a marker of endothelial cells, was strongly expressed on the larger vessels but was very weakly expressed on capillaries. ICAM -1 was constitutively expressed on endothelial cells from all vessels but was particularly strong on capillaries and endothelial cells (EC) lining the coronary artery. The coronary arteries were rather surprising, as they were found to basally express VCAM-1 as well as ICAM-1. VCAM-1 was not found to be expressed on any of the other large vessels. All coronary arteries investigated at this centre have expressed an 'activated phenotype', possible explanations are discussed below. Immunocytochemistry of frozen sections of normal endomyocardial biopsies show weak expression of E-selectin and VCAM-1: the capillaries being negative for these markers and venules showing patchy expression of E-selectin and VCAM-1. During acute (cell mediated) rejection, there is upregulation of VCAM-1 on capillary endothelial cells in close apposition to infiltrating T cells. This is not surprising as interaction between endothelial VCAM-1 with the T cell $\beta1$ integrins ($\alpha4\beta1$) is a requirement for T cell migration across endothelial cells.

Endothelial expression of MHC molecules

As MHC antigens initiate allograft rejection, it is of interest to describe the distribution of these molecules on endothelial cells of different origins (Table 15.1). All endothelial cells constitutively express MHC class I molecules and many endothelial cells constitut-

Table 15.1. *Distribution of adhesion molecules, MHC molecules and von Willebrand factor in endothelial cells derived from microvessels and large vessels of the human cardiovascular system*

	Myocardial biopsies			Large vessels		
	Capillaries	Arterioles	Venules	Coronary	PA	Aorta
CD31	+ +	+ +	+ +	+ +	+ +	+ +
ICAM-1	+ +	+	+	+ +	+	+
VCAM-1	−	±	±	+	−	−
E-selectin	−	−	±	+	±	±
von Willebrand factor	±	+ +	+ +	+ +	+ +	+ +
Class I	+ +	+	+	+ +	+	+
Class II	+ +	±	±	+ +	−	−

Note: + +: strong, even expression; +: strong but patchy expression; ±: weak and patchy expression; −: negative.
Source: summarized from Page et al (1992); Rose (1992); Taylor et al (1992)

ively express MHC class II molecules (for a review see Fuggle 1989); however, there is an interesting heterogeneity with regard to constitutive expression of class II antigens; the large vessels (aorta, pulmonary artery, endocardium, umbilical vein, umbilical artery) are negative but the capillaries within all organs examined are strongly positive (Table 15.1) (Pober & Cotran, 1990; Page et al, 1992). Arterioles and venules within the heart show weak or patchy basal expression of MHC class II antigens. It was surprising to find that all pieces of coronary artery we examined expressed MHC class II molecules, as well as VCAM-1. The coronaries were either obtained from heart donors deemed unsuitable for transplantation , or they were removed from the explanted heart of patients requiring transplantation (for diseases not involving the coronary artery). These molecules may therefore have been upregulated during procedures prior to harvest. The most common endothelial cells used in cell culture are those derived from umbilical vein endothelial cells. These cells do not express MHC class II antigens in situ and it is therefore not surprising that they are also negative in vitro. Interestingly, cardiac microvascular endothelial cells , which are positive in situ, lose their class II after two weeks in culture (McDougall et al, 1996). This observation raises the intriguing possibility that factors in normal serum act to maintain class II expression in vivo. In vitro, cytokines are used extensively to upregulate MHC and adhesion molecules in a variety of cell types, but endothelial cells are unique in the sense that only IFN-γ upregulates MHC class II expression in vitro (Pober & Cotran, 1990).

Pathways of antigen presentation and antigen presenting cells

The term antigen presenting cell (APC) has a specific meaning to immunologists: it means the cell is able to present antigen to resting T cells, i.e. is able to cause activation of resting T cells. Only specialized cells (traditionally recognized as B cells, dendritic cells and monocytes) can perform this task. T cells recognize nominal antigen as processed peptides presented by self MHC molecules . An important step in the understanding of alloreactivity came with the discovery that T cells can engage and respond to allogeneic MHC molecules directly (Fig. 15.3). This form of antigen recognition , termed direct presentation or the direct pathway, is responsible for the strong proliferative response to alloantigens seen in vitro and quite possibly the early acute rejection seen in non-immunosuppressed animals after transplantation of MHC mismatched organs. T cells can also recognize allogeneic peptides that have been processed and presented within self MHC molecules by recipient APC in the same manner that T cells recognize nominal antigen (Fig. 15.3). This pathway is termed the indirect route or indirect pathway of T cell activation (Shoskes & Wood, 1994). Alloantigens shed from the graft are likely to be treated as exogenous antigen by recipient APC and will therefore be presented within MHC class II molecules to activate recipient CD4$^+$ T cells.

Any graft cell expressing class II antigens will be able to activate the indirect pathway – is likely that damaged endothelial cells are an important source of graft-derived MHC class II antigens – as these are the only parenchymal cells expressing class II in the heart. The contribution indirect recognition of endothelial MHC class II makes to cellular rejection is currently not known. The question which has received much attention from a number of groups in recent years is whether endothelial cells can cause direct allostimulation of resting T lymphocytes (for a review see Pober et al, 1996). The reason for this is that direct recognition of allo-MHC molecules results in a 'strong' response, the number of T cells recognizing MHC molecules directly is 10–100 higher than those recognizing nominal antigen, resulting in a strong in vitro proliferative response.

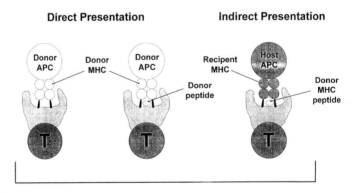

Fig. 15.3. Diagrammatic representation of mechanisms whereby recipient T cells recognize allo-class II determinants. Recipient T cells recognize donor MHC determinants on donor APC (direct presentation) or they recognise donor MHC peptides which have been released from donor cells and processed and presented by host APC within self MHC molecules (indirect presentation). Drawing modified from Shoskes & Wood (1994) with permission.

In order to discover whether endothelial cells directly cause allostimulation of resting T cells, we and others (Page et al, 1994: Savage et al, 1993) have cultured stringently purified CD4$^+$ T cells with pure passaged endothelial cells and looked for T cell proliferation (measured by uptake of [^{3}H]thymidine) at day 6. The endothelial cells are treated with mitomycin C to stop them proliferating; any cell proliferation which is detected is thus due to responding T cells (Fig. 15.4). The results in Fig. 15.5 show the response of CD4$^+$ T cell to human endothelial cells (Eahy.926), porcine aortic endothelial cells (PAEC) and foetal lung fibroblasts. It can be seen that provided IFN-γ is used to upregulate MHC class II, there is a strong proliferative response to human endothelial cells, but not to fibroblasts. There is also a strong response to PAEC, which is independent of IFN-γ treatment. The reason for this is that PAEC class II expression persists in culture. That the response was direct and not indirect was proven by the findings that responder T cells were free of contaminating APC (Page et al, 1994a).

It must be concluded therefore that donor endothelial cells can present alloantigen to recipient T cells. It is interesting to note that there is a species difference between rodents and humans, as rodents do not constitutively express MHC class II antigens on their

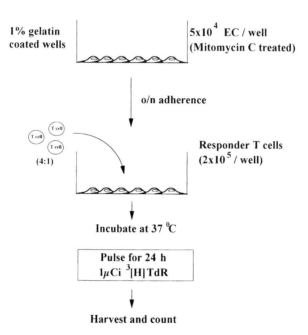

Fig. 15.4. Method of measuring the proliferative response of purified CD4$^+$ T cells to human endothelial cells. Addition of mitomycin C (or irradiated) human endothelial cells to gelatin coated tissue culture wells results in a monolayer of endothelial cells to which can be added appropriate numbers of responder T cells. The endothelial cells and T cells are cocultured for 6 days, in the presence of ^{3}[H]thymidine (^{3}[H]TdR) for the last 24 h. The cultures are harvested and counted on beta counter – the counts (CPM) represent the proliferative response of T cells.

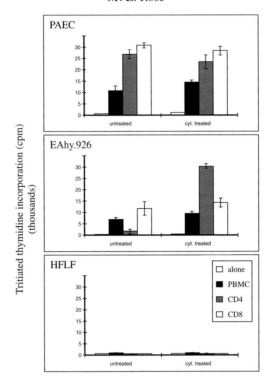

Fig. 15.5. Response at day 6 of purified PBMC (peripheral blood mononuclear cells) CD4[+] and CD8[+] T cells to untreated and IFN-γ treated porcine aortic endothelial cells (PAEC), human endothelial cells (EAhy.926) and human foetal lung fibroblasts (HFLF). CD4[+] and CD8[+] T cells respond strongly to PAEC , regardless of cytokine treatment. CD4[+] T cells respond well to human endothelial cells, providing they have been pretreated with IFN-γ to upregulate MHC class II antigens. CD8[+] T cells respond to human endothelial cells in the absence of cytokine treatment. There is no proliferative response of human lymphocytes to the fibroblasts.

endothelial cells. This difference may explain why it is easier to suppress transplant rejection in rodents than it is in humans. It follows, therefore, that understanding the signals that allow human endothelial cells to stimulate T cells may lead to new strategies of preventing rejection. One of the important concepts to emerge in recent years is the knowledge that T cells require two signals to become activated (Janeway & Bottomly, 1994), one is occupancy of the T cell receptor and the second is activation of one of the many 'accessory molecules' present on T cells (Fig. 15.6). Much attention has focused on the B7 family of receptors, known to be essential as second signals on APC of bone marrow origin (e.g. monocytes, B cells and dendritic cells) ; blockade of this pathway inhibits dendritic cell stimulated mixed lymphocyte responses in vitro and also inhibits allograft and indeed xenograft rejection in rodents (Pearson et al, 1994). We have

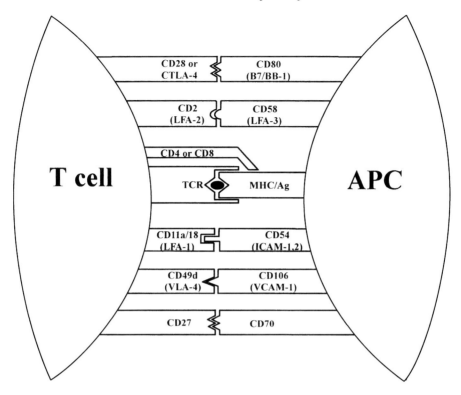

Fig. 15.6. Diagrammatic representation of possible interactions between receptors on T cells and their appropriate ligands on APC.

questioned whether endothelial cells utilize the B7 pathway to stimulate T cells, and our results (Page et al, 1994*b*)) and those of others (Pober et al, 1996) demonstrate that endothelial cells do not express B7 receptors and stimulate T cells via another accessory molecule, LFA-3.

Role of endothelial cells in chronic rejection

It is paradoxical that despite the heavy immunosuppression received by patients after solid organ transplantation, the majority make a vigorous antibody response against the allografted organ (for a review see Rose, 1993). The most common way of detecting these antibodies is a complement-dependent cytotoxicity test against a panel of HLA typed leukocytes (termed panel reactive antibodies or PRA test) or donor cells (termed a donor specific response). Many clinical studies have reported an association between antibody producers and development of chronic rejection (Rose, 1993). Thus SuciuFoca et al reported a 90% 4 year actuarial survival in patients who had not made antibody

following cardiac transplantation versus a 38% 4 year survival in the antibody producers (Suciu-Foca et al, 1991). These authors looked for anti-HLA antibodies, but our
own studies have shown a correlation between anti-endothelial antibodies and chronic
rejection (Dunn et al, 1992). Using gel electrophoreses to separate endothelial peptides
according to molecular weight followed by probing blots with patients'sera, we found
that the majority of patients who had TxCAD had antibodies against endothelial
peptides of 56–58 kDa. We have subsequently confirmed this association in a separate
study of new patients using both western blotting and flow cytometry (unpublished
results). A similar association between anti-endothelial antibodies, detected by flow
cytometry, and chronic rejection has been reported after renal transplantation. As this
test (Dunn et al, 1992) detected antibodies against unrelated (HUVEC), it is clear that
donor specific HLA antigens could not be involved. Use of SDS gel electrophoresis and
amino acid sequencing revealed that the most immunogeneic endothelial peptide (at
56–58 kDa) was the intermediate filament vimentin and other immunoreactive peptides
were identified as triose phosphate isomerase and glucose regulating protein. In all, 40
different proteins were identified which reacted with patients IgM (Wheeler et al, 1995).
Vimentin is the intermediate filament characteristic of but not restricted to endothelial
cells and fibroblasts. Whereas smooth muscle cells (SMCs) predominantly express
desmin as their intermediate filament they coexpress desmin and vimentin when migrating or proliferating. Vimentin is diffusely expressed in the intima and media of normal
and diseased coronary arteries. Our working hypothesis is that antibodies to vimentin
reflect disease activity in the coronary arteries – but the outstanding questions are how
vimentin, a cytosolic protein is exposed to the immune system and whether and how the
antibodies are damaging.

It is highly likely that endothelial cells are damaged early after transplantation
(possibly by non-immunological factors such as ischaemia–reperfusion injury) and
vimentin is released into the circulation. There it binds to host B cells. Our hypothesis to
explain the presence of antivimentin antibodies after transplantation is that host T cells
recognize vimentin fragments, presented indirectly by host B cells. A database of MHC
binding peptides has revealed sequence homology between epitopes of vimentin and
class II presented peptides, these being an HLA-DRα peptide and a heat shock protein
peptide (HSP65), suggesting that the T cells 'see' vimentin as a foreign class II peptide.
Such cross-reactions between DRα and infectious agents/ normal components of tissues
have been suggested as a mechanism for a number of autoimmune diseases (Baum et al,
1996). It is likely that damaged endothelial cells are a source of many other peptides
which will be presented indirectly to recipient T cells.

One of the major drawbacks to ascribing a role for antibodies in the pathogenesis of
rejection is lack of understanding about the way antibodies interact with their cellular
targets. Serum derived from our transplant patients does not exhibit complement
dependent or antibody dependent cellular cytotoxicity against endothelial cells derived
from HUVEC or aorta . Complement mediated lysis is a severe and acute form of
damage, usually associated with hyperacute rejection. Perhaps it is not surprising that
(with the exception of serum from patients with Kawasaki disease , where IgM antibo-

dies are directly cytotoxic to endothelial cells in the presence of complement (Leung et al, 1986), antiendothelial antibodies have not been found to mediate complement-mediated damage to endothelial cells. It may be more important to investigate whether antiendothelial antibodies can cause more subtle forms of change, such as endothelial cell activation (Chapter 3). Recently a number of reports have demonstrated that antibodies from patients with autoimmune disease (Carvalho et al, 1996) or transplant patients (Pidwell et al, 1995) can upregulate adhesion molecules on endothelial cells. We believe the information that antibodies can activate endothelial cells is very promising and should be explored as a mechanism whereby antibodies could damage endothelial cells in both autoimmune disease and chronic rejection after solid organ transplantation.

In conclusion, the immunological properties of endothelial cells suggest they perform a pivotal role in rejection following solid organ transplanation. Expression of MHC class II molecules allows them to activate recipient T cells by the direct and indirect route. Release of non-HLA antigens as a result of immunological or non-immunological damage provides a stimulus for antibody formation which may further damage or activate donor endothelial cells. The costimulatory molecules used by endothelial cells appear to differ to those used by traditional APC such as B cells and dendritic cells. Further understanding of the molecules involved is warranted as development of specific strategies to block endothelial cell recogniton may provide better ways of preventing rejection than methods currently used.

References

Arbustini, E., Grasso, M., Diegoli, M., Bramerio, M., Scott Foglienei, A., Albertario, M., Matinelli, L., Gavazzi, A., Goggi, C., Campana, C. & Vigano, M. (1991). Expression of tumour necrosis factor in human acute cardiac rejection. An immunohistochemical and immunoblotting study. *American Journal of Pathology*, **139**, 709–15.

Baum, H., Davies, H. & Peakman, M. (1996). Molecular mimicry in the MHC: hidden clues to autoimmunity? *Immunology Today*, **17**, 64–70.

Briscoe, D. M., Schoen, F. J., Rice, G. E., Bevilacqua, M. P., Ganz, P. & Pober, J. S. (1991). Induced expression of endothelial-leukocyte adhesion molecules in human cardiac allografts. *Transplantation*, **51**, 537–9.

Carvalho, D., Savage, C. O. S., Black, C. M. & Pearson, J. D. (1996). IgG antiendothelial cell autoantibodies from scleroderma patients induce leukocyte adhesion to human vascular endothelial cells in vitro. *Journal of Clinical Investigation*, **97**, 1–97.

Cunningham, D. A., Dunn, M. J., Yacoub, M. J. & Rose, M. L. (1994). Local production of cytokines in the human cardiac allograft. *Transplantation*, **57**, 1333–7.

Dunn, M. J., Crisp, S. J., Rose, M. L., Taylor, P. M. & Yacoub, M. H. (1992). Antiendothelial antibodies coronary artery disease after cardiac transplantation. *Lancet*, **339**, 1566–70.

Fuggle, S. V., McWhinnie, D. L., Chapman, J. R., Talylor, H. M. & Morris, P. J. (1986). Sequential analysis of HLA-class II antigen expression in human renal allografts. *Transplantation*, **42**, 144–9.

Fuggle, S. V. (1989) MHC antigen expression in vascularized organ allografts: clinical correlations and significance. *Transplantation Reviews* (P. J. Morris, N. L. Tilney, eds) **3**, 81–102.

Gao, S. J., Schroeder, J. S., Alderman, E. L., Hunt, S. A., Valantine, H. A. & Weiederhold, V. (1989). Prevalence of accelerated coronary artery disease in heart transplant survivors. Comparison of cyclosporine and axathiprine regimens. *Circulation*, **8**, 100–5.

Halloran, P. F., Wadgymar, A. & Autenreid, P. (1986). The regulation of the expression of major histocompatibitly complex products. *Transplantation*, **4**, 413–20.

Hosenpud, J. D., Shipley, G. D. & Wagner, C. R. (1992). Cardiac allograft vasculopathy; current concepts, recent developments, and future directions. *Journal of Heart and Lung Transplantation*, **11**, 9–23.

Janeway, C. A. & Bottomly, K. (1994). Signals and signs for lymphocyte responses. *Cell*, **76**, 275–85.

Leung, D. Y., Collins, M. T., Lapierre, L. A., Geha, R., S. & Pober, J. S. (1986). Immunoglobulin M antibodies present in the acute phase of Kawasaki syndrome lyse cultured vascular endothelial cells stimulated by gamma interferon. *Journal of Clinical Investigation*, **77**, 1428–35.

McDougall, R. M., Yacoub, M. H. & Rose, M. L. (1996). Isolation, culture and characterisation of MHC class II positive microvascular endothelial cells from the human heart. *Microvascular Research*, **51**, 137–52.

Page, C. S., Holloway, N., Smith, H., Yacoub, M. H. & Rose, M. L. (1994). Alloproliferative responses of purified CD4$^+$ and CD8$^+$ T cell subsets to human vascular endothelial cells in the absence of contaminating accessory cells. *Transplantation*, **57**, 1628–1637.

Page, C., Rose, M. L., Yacoub, M. H. & Pigott, R. (1992). Antigenic heterogeneity of vascular endothelium. *Amercian Journal of Pathology*, **141**, 673–83.

Page, C. S., Thompson, C., Yacoub, M. H. & Rose, M. L. (1994b). Human endothelial cell stimulation of allogeneic T cells via a CTLA-4 independent pathway. *Transplant Immunology*, **2**, 342–7.

Pearson, T. C., Alexander, D. Z., Winn, K. J., Linsley, P. S., Lowry, R. P. & Larsen, C. P. (1994). Transplantation tolerance induced by CTLA4-Ig. *Transplantation*, **57**, 1701–6.

Pidwell, D. W., Heller, M. J., Gabler, D. & Orosz, C (1995). In vitro stimulation of human endothelial cells by sera from a subpopulation of high percentage panel reactive antibody patients. *Transplantation*, **60**, 563–9.

Pober, J. S. & Cotran, R. S. (1990). The role of endothelial cells in inflammation. *Transplantation*, **50**, 537–44.

Pober, J. S., Orosz, C. G., Rose, M. L. & Savage, C. O. S. (1996). Can graft endothelial cells initiate a host anti-graft immune response ? *Transplantation*, **61**, 343–9.

Rose, M. L. (1992). HLA antigens in tissues. In *Methods in Clinical Histocompatibilty Testing*, ed. P. Dyer & D. Middleton, pp. 192–210. IRL: Oxford University Press.

Rose, M. L. (1993). Antibody mediated rejection following cardiac transplantation. *Transplantation Reviews*, **7**, 140–52.

Ross, R. (1993). The pathogeneis of atherosclerosis: a perspective for the 1990s. *Nature*, **362**, 801–9.

Savage, C. O. S., Hughes, C. C. W., McIntyre, B. W., Picard, J. K. & Pober, J. S. (1993). Human CD4$^+$ T cells proliferate to HLA-DR$^+$ allogeneic vascular endothelium: identification of accessory interactions. *Transplantation*, **56**, 128–134.

Shoskes, D. A. & Wood, K. J. (1994). Indirect presentation of MHC antigens in transplantation. *Immunology Today*, **15**, 32–8.

Springer, T. A. (1994). Traffic signals for lymphocyte recirculation and leukocyte emigration. The multistep paradigm. *Cell*, **76**, 301–14.

Suciu-Foca, N., Reed, E., Marboe, C., Harris, P., Ping-Xi, Y., Yu-Kai, S., Ho, E., Rose, E., Reemsta, K. & King, D. W. (1991). The role of anti-HLA antibodies in heart transplantation. *Transplantation*, **51**, 716–24.

Taylor, P. M., Rose, M. L., Yacoub, M. H. & Piggott, R. (1992). Induction of vascular adhesion molecules during rejection of human cardiac allografts. *Transplantation*, **54**, 451–7.

Tullius, S. G. & Tilney, N. J. (1995). Both alloantigen-dependent and independent factors influence chronic allograft rejection. *Transplantation*, **59**, 313–18.

Wheeler, C. H., Collins, A., Dunn, M. J., Crisp, S. J., Yacoub, M. H. & Rose, M. L. (1995). Characterisation of endothelial antigens associated with transplant associated coronary artery disease. *Journal of Heart and Lung Transplantation*, **14**, S188–S97.

Index